Nature and Health

Experiences in nature are now recognized as being fundamental to human health and well-being. Physical activity in nature has been posited as an important well-being facilitator because the presence of nature augments the benefits of physical activity while also enhancing motivation and adherence. This volume brings together a mix of cutting edge ideas in research, theory and practice from a wide set of disciplines with the purpose of exploring interdisciplinary or trans-disciplinary approaches to understanding the relationship between physical activity in nature and health and well-being.

Nature and Health: Physical Activity in Nature is structured to facilitate ease of use for the researcher, policy maker, practitioner or theorist. Section 1 covers research on physical activity in nature for a number of important health and well-being issues. Each chapter in this section considers how policy and practice might be shaped by current research findings and knowledge. Section 2 considers contemporary theoretical and conceptual understandings that help explain how physical activity in nature enhances health and well-being and also how best to design interventions and research. Section 3 provides examples of current approaches.

This book is an ideal resource for both researchers and advanced students interested in designing future-proofed research, for policy makers interested in improving community well-being and for practitioners interested in best practice applications.

Eric Brymer is a Reader in the School of Sport and Head of Person-Environment Research Lab at Leeds-Beckett University, UK. He is a behavioral scientist who specializes in researching the reciprocal nature of health and wellbeing from nature-based experiences. Eric collaborates with multidisciplined teams across the world and holds research positions in health, exercise and outdoor studies in the UK, Europe and Australia.

Mike Rogerson is a Lecturer in the School of Sport, Rehabilitation and Exercise Sciences at the University of Essex, UK. He is a sport and exercise psychologist with expertise in the role of environments for exercise behaviors, experiences and outcomes.

Jo Barton is a Reader in the School of Sport, Rehabilitation and Exercise Sciences at the University of Essex, UK. She is a Sport and Exercise Scientist and leading expert in 'green exercise', analyzing how exercise settings shape behaviors and health outcomes.

Nature and Health
Physical Activity in Nature

Edited by Eric Brymer, Mike Rogerson, and Jo Barton

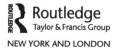
NEW YORK AND LONDON

First published 2021
by Routledge
52 Vanderbilt Avenue, New York, NY 10017

and by Routledge
2 Park Square, Milton Park, Abingdon, Oxon, OX14 4RN

Routledge is an imprint of the Taylor & Francis Group, an informa business

© 2021 Taylor & Francis

The right of Eric Brymer, Mike Rogerson, and Jo Barton to be identified as the authors of the editorial material, and of the authors for their individual chapters, has been asserted in accordance with sections 77 and 78 of the Copyright, Designs and Patents Act 1988.

All rights reserved. No part of this book may be reprinted or reproduced or utilised in any form or by any electronic, mechanical, or other means, now known or hereafter invented, including photocopying and recording, or in any information storage or retrieval system, without permission in writing from the publishers.

Trademark notice: Product or corporate names may be trademarks or registered trademarks, and are used only for identification and explanation without intent to infringe.

Library of Congress Cataloging-in-Publication Data
A catalog record for this title has been requested

ISBN: 978-0-367-72332-3 (hbk)
ISBN: 978-1-032-01903-1 (pbk)
ISBN: 978-1-003-15441-9 (ebk)

DOI: 10.4324/9781003154419

Typeset in ITC New Baskerville Std

Contents

List of Figures		viii
List of Tables		xi
Contributors		xii

1 Nature, Physical Activity, and Health   1
MIKE ROGERSON, ERIC BRYMER, AND JO BARTON

PART I
Research on Physical Activity in Nature   5

**2 Understanding the Affective Benefits of Interacting
with Nature**   7
KATHRYN E. SCHERTZ, KIMBERLY L. MEIDENBAUER, AND MARC G. BERMAN

**3 Green Exercise as a Potential Treatment Strategy for
Type 2 Diabetes**   23
MATT FRASER

4 Green Exercise: Actively Flourishing in Nature   35
OTIS GEDDES AND HOLLI-ANNE PASSMORE

**5 Mind the Gap - On the Necessity of a Situational Taxonomy
for Designing and Evaluating Gait Interventions**   47
STEVEN VAN ANDEL, MICHAEL COLE, AND GERT-JAN PEPPING

PART II
Theoretical Approaches   61

6 Resilience   63
JOHN F. ALLAN

vi *Contents*

7 **Phenomenology and Human Wellbeing in Nature: An Eco-phenomenological Perspective** 83

ROBERT D SCHWEITZER, ERIC BRYMER, AND HARRIET LOUISE GLAB

8 **Developing Integrated Conceptual Green Exercise Models** 95

CLAIRE WICKS, JO BARTON, AND MIKE ROGERSON

9 **Physical Activity in Nature: An Ecological Dynamics Perspective** 112

HSIAO-PU YEH, DUARTE ARAÚJO, ERIC BRYMER, AND KEITH DAVIDS

10 **Physical Activity and Virtual Nature: Perspectives on the Health and Behavioral Benefits of *Virtual* Green Exercise** 127

GIOVANNA CALOGIURI, SIGBJØRN LITLESKARE, AND FRED FRÖHLICH

11 **Emerging Psychological Wellbeing Frameworks for Adventure Recreation, Education, and Tourism** 147

SUSAN HOUGE MACKENZIE

12 ***In Vivo* Nature Exposure as a Positive Psychological Intervention: A Review of the Impact of Nature Interventions on Wellbeing** 160

JILLIAN T. HUNT, ANDREW J. HOWELL, AND HOLLI-ANNE PASSMORE

PART III
Real-World Application 175

13 **Care Farms: A Health-Promoting Context for a Wide Range of Client Groups** 177

SIMONE DE BRUIN, JAN HASSINK, LENNEKE VAANDRAGER, BRAM DE
BOER, HILDE VERBEEK, INGEBORG PEDERSEN, GRETE GRINDAL PATIL,
LINA H. ELLINGSEN-DALSKAU, AND SIREN ERIKSEN

14 **The Next Frontier: Wilderness Therapy and the Treatment of Complex Trauma** 191

GRAHAM PRINGLE, WILL W. DOBUD, AND NEVIN J. HARPER

15 **What Can We Learn About Nature, Physical Activity, and Health from *parkrun*?** 208

GARETH WILTSHIRE AND STEPHANIE MERCHANT

Contents vii

16 Students' Appropriation of Space in Education Outside the Classroom. Some Aspects on Physical Activity and Health from a Pilot Study with 5th-Graders in Germany 223

CHRISTOPH MALL, JAKOB VON AU, AND ULRICH DETTWEILER

17 Outdoor and Adventurous Activities in Supporting Wounded, Injured and Sick Military Personnel and Veterans 233

CHRISTOPHER WILLIAM PHILIP KAY AND REBECCA JENA SUTTON

18 Implications, Impact and Future Directions: Translation into Wider Policy and Practice 249

JO BARTON, MIKE ROGERSON, AND ERIC BRYMER

Index 260

Figures

5.1 Relationship between affordances (the action possibilities offered by the environment) that is informed by calibration (scaling) and exploration. *Note that exploration itself is a possibility for action and thus a cyclical relation exists between these terms.*   49

5.2 Introduction of the continuum between open and closed skills, including labels (top) as introduced by Poulton (1957). *The boxes below illustrate how different modes of gait fit in this continuum. Evidence suggests that to train any skill for benefits in retention and transfer, one should practice in an environment with increased openness.*   50

5.3 Examples of walking environments that present varying degrees of perceptual-motor challenge. *From left to right, presented environments decrease in regularity, that is from more closed environments on the left (A, D) to more open walking challenges on the right (B, C, E, F). Bottom row images present environments without slope (D–F), top row presents more demanding slope conditions (A–C). Key points: in the statement that the use of walking interventions is limited for fall prevention (Sherrington et al., 2019), there is an assumption that the training effect in all environments is equal. We reason that making a distinction between environments could lead to a more refined knowledge from experimental results and better exercise prescription.*   53

5.4 Situational Taxonomy for Environment-Person Pairing In Natural Gait (STEPPING). The horizontal dimension relates to the perceptual demands of closed to less-closed environments, whereas the vertical dimension relates to the physical demands of the environment.   54

5.5 Reanalyzed data from Andel, Cole and Pepping (2019), with falls incidence categorized using the STEPPING classification. The main cause of falls per categories is noted in the table. When categorization was unclear from the

Figures ix

6.   collected reports, the falls were categorized conservatively (closer to 1A). For instance, if a participant reported to have "tripped over a rock" this does not specify any incline of the walk or cluttering of the environment, it only specifies that there was a rock to trip on, resulting in a conservative 2A categorization.   55

6.1 Camp Rating Scale (CRS), Mean (SD) responses.   72

6.2 Perceived Competencies Scale (PCS), Mean (SD) responses.   73

7.1 Sculpture by Dylan Lewis representing a shamanic figure.   87

7.2 The sculptures of Dylan Lewis give expression to the self in relation to the rest of nature. In this image, he reflects the link between self and nature, highlighting both form and disintegration in a natural setting.   92

8.1 The hierarchical model proposed by Bedimo-Rung et al. (Bedimo-Rung et al., 2005) as redrawn by Lawrence, Forbat and Zufferey (2019).   97

8.2 On the left, the more typical approach of nature and health research, and on the right, the proposed integrative approach (Lawrence, Forbat & Zufferey, 2019).   98

8.3 Lachowycz and Jones' socioecological framework for the relationship between greenspace access and health.   98

8.4 Hartig et al.'s model.   99

8.5 Kuo's model.   100

8.6 Merkevych et al.'s model.   101

8.7 Lawrence, Forbat & Zufferey (2019).   102

8.8 The theoretical model of principles for green physical activity research from an Ecological Dynamics perspective (Yeh et al., 2015).   104

8.9 Two intertwining pathways showing how environments influence exercise and health-related outcomes (Rogerson et al., 2019).   105

9.1 A public seat used by children for playing rather than sitting.   114

10.1 A snapshot of two different IVNs reproducing the same environment, which were created using different techniques: 3-dimensional modeling (top image) and commercial 360° camera (bottom image). Images developed by the research team of the project "Green VR: Nature experiences in IVE 2.0: developing virtual settings for green-exercise and health promotion research." Credits to Fred Fröhlich, Ole Einar Flaten, Sigbjørn Litleskare, and Giovanna Calogiuri.   136

10.2 A participant in the study Calogiuri et al. (2018) walking on a manually driven treadmill while viewing a first-person 360° video showing a walk by a river. Picture by Tore L. Rydgren.   137

x *Figures*

11.1 Proposed conceptual framework of adventure and psychological wellbeing (adapted from Houge Mackenzie & Hodge, 2020). 153
13.1 Photo by Arjo Buijs, the Netherlands. 180
13.2 Photo by Anita Janssen, the Netherlands. 181
13.3 Photo by Martin Lundsvoll, Norway. 181
16.1 Ternary plots of the compositions of students' mean time spent in sedentary behavior (SB), light physical activity (LPA), and moderate-to-vigorous physical activity PA (MVPA). Panel A shows the regular classroom students; panel B shows the EOtC students; both panels are segregated by season (fall; spring; summer). A) Regular classroom students B) EOtC students 227
17.1 Sustainable improvements in participant's positive mental well-being 12 months after a multi activity course. 243

Tables

12.1	Summary of well-being measures used in articles reviewed	163
12.2	Summary of randomized controlled trials of in vivo nature interventions: Effects on well-being	164

Contributors

John F. Allan Leeds Beckett University, UK

Duarte Araújo University of Lisbon, PT

Jakob von Au Heidelberg University of Education, USA

Jo Barton University of Essex, UK

Marc G. Berman University of Chicago, US

Eric Brymer Australian College of Applied Psychology, AU

Giovanna Calogiuri University of South-Eastern Norway, NO

Michael Cole Australian Catholic University, AU

Keith Davids Sheffield Hallam University, UK

Bram de Boer Maastricht University, NL

Ulrich Dettweiler University of Stavanger, NO

Simone de Bruin Dutch National Institute for Public Health and the Environment, NL; Wageningen University & Research, NL

Will W. Dobud Charles Sturt University, AU

Lina H. Ellingsen-Dalskau Norwegian University of Life Sciences, NO

Siren Eriksen Lovisenberg Diaconal University College, NO

Matt Fraser University of the Highlands and Islands, UK

Fred Fröhlich Inland Norway University of Applied Sciences, Norway

Otis Geddes University of British Columbia, CA

Harriet L. Glab Queensland University of Technology, AU

Nevin J. Harper University of Victoria, CA

Jan Hassink Wageningen University & Research, NL

Andrew J. Howell MacEwan University, Canada

Contributors xiii

Jillian T. Hunt MacEwan University, CA

Christopher W.P. Kay Leeds Beckett University, UK

Sigbjørn Litleskare Inland Norway University of Applied Sciences, NO

Susan, H. Mackenzie University of Otago, NZ

Christoph Mall Technical University of Munich, DE

Kimberly L. Meidenbauer University of Chicago, US

Stephanie Merchant University of Bath, UK

Holli-Anne Passmore University of Derby, UK

Grete Grindal Patil Norwegian University of Life Sciences, NO

Ingeborg Pedersen Norwegian University of Life Sciences, NO

Gert-Jan Pepping Australian Catholic University, Brisbane, Australia

Graham Pringle Griffith University

Mike Rogerson University of Essex, UK

Kathryn E. Schertz University of Chicago, US

Robert D. Schweitzer Queensland University of Technology, AU

Rebecca J. Sutton Leeds Beckett University, UK

Steven van Andel Australian Catholic University, AU; University of Innsbruck, AT

Lenneke Vaandrager Wageningen University & Research, NL

Hilde Verbeek Maastricht University, NL

Claire Wicks University of Essex, UK

Gareth Wiltshire Loughborough University, UK

Hsiao-Pu Yeh Sheffield Hallam University, UK

1 Nature, Physical Activity, and Health

Mike Rogerson, Eric Brymer, and Jo Barton

Modern living, especially in westernized societies, is associated with a range of public health challenges, such as increasing levels of noncommunicable physical and mental health disorders, and significant health consequences from stressful living conditions. These are often attributable to physical inactivity, daily stresses, and other behavioral opportunities and choices (or lack thereof). Engagement with and physical activity in nature are increasingly being recognized as fundamental to human health and wellbeing and offer powerful mechanisms to counteract many of these challenges (Brymer et al., 2020). Evidence points to benefits for physical health (e.g. lower prevalence of high blood pressure and allergies), mental health (e.g. lower prevalence of depression, anxiety and stress) and social wellbeing outcomes. Further, in contrast to less formal leisure and recreational activities, opportunity for physical activity in nature is sometimes via purposefully designed strategies, structured interventions, and programmes with the specific goal of achieving improved health and wellbeing outcomes (Shanahan et al., 2019). Despite this, there is significant concern that in addition to the health antecedents at the population level, urbanization and the challenges of modern life are leading to reduced engagement with the natural environment.

Since the turn of the century, there has been a renewal of research effort elucidating relationships between physical activity, nature, and health. Research shows that physical activity in nature is an important health and wellbeing facilitator because the presence of nature augments the benefits of physical activity, while also enhancing motivation and adherence to healthy and proenvironmental behaviors. Access to local greenspaces increases the probability that individuals will achieve the recommended physical activity guidelines by over four times (Flowers et al., 2016). However, as residential distance from green space increases, the likelihood of being sufficiently active to prevent ill health gradually diminishes. There is a growing body of evidence demonstrating that being active in nature reduces stress, increases heart rate variability and parasympathetic cardiac contribution during sleep, improves cognitive functioning, and restores mental fatigue (Gidlow et al., 2016; Gladwell et al., 2016). In addition, it

DOI: 10.4324/9781003154419-1

facilitates social interaction and can instill a sense of community (Francis et al., 2012). Nature-based experiences can promote universal positive physiological and psychological stress responses (Kondo et al., 2018). This reduction in stress may occur via multiple mechanisms such as restored directed attention, increased opportunity for social contact, and engaging in physical activity. The recognition that physical activity in nature provides benefits for people, beyond the risk approach (e.g. where nature is seen as solely as a risk-factor for insect-borne diseases or the impacts of disasters), represents a major shift in public health thinking for both the prevention and treatment of health issues.

In recent years, this growing body of research has started to inform governments, nongovernmental organizations, and public and private stakeholders in their development of policy and planning support for the implementation of real-world actions. Examples of actions across the globe include minimum area targets for public green space, provision of inclusive and equitable access to public green space, improving the quality of green infrastructure in public spaces; promoting more opportunities for active travel, and "nature prescriptions," where doctors or other health practitioners prescribe nature-based experiences for patients living with specific health conditions; the 25-year plan for the environment in the UK; and the United Nations sustainable development goals.

Despite this growing evidence base and interest from policymakers, there is a relative dearth of guidance for designing and implementing nature-based physical activity interventions and programs for health. Equally, there seems to be a shortage of such programs designed on evidence-based principles or evaluations that can determine specific health outcomes. This can only limit the potential leveraging of nature to improve health and wellbeing outcomes for individuals and communities, potentially leading to inefficient and ill-targeted investment decisions. Without a coherent picture of the evidence, ability to influence wider policy and practice will remain low.

This book draws together a unique mix of cutting-edge ideas from internationally recognized research, theory, and practice from a wide set of disciplines. It explores the interdisciplinary or trans-disciplinary approaches to understanding the relationship between physical activity in nature, health, and wellbeing. It is split into three sections: (i) overview of the research evidence that nature-based physical activity improves health and wellbeing; (ii) informative frameworks to support designers and researchers; and (iii) examples of good practice. Importantly, many of the chapters include crosscutting key themes that explicitly consider how policy and practice might be informed by the findings and knowledge presented.

The first section of this book outlines research evidence across selected topics within the physical activity, nature, and health context. Chapters in this section outline research that shows benefits for mental health, mood, affect and flourishing, physical conditions such as diabetes, and how the unique properties of nature can support interventions for falls and individuals experiencing post-traumatic stress disorder (PTSD) and depression. Key themes from this section point to nature as beneficial for promotion of wellbeing, prevention of illness and disease as well as reducing ill health. The unique determinants of physical activity in nature can support attempts to reduce obesity, manage diabetes, and support interventions designed to prevent falls in older adults. Nature-based physical activity is also promoted for alleviating immediate psychological ill health as well as promoting high-level wellness.

The middle section, Chapters 6–12, discuss theoretical approaches, models, conceptualizations, and understanding of the dynamic, functional relationships between physical activity, nature, and health. They intentionally explore alternative theoretical approaches, advancing beyond previous narrow theories, such as the Stress Reduction Theory (Ulrich et al., 1991) and the Attention Restoration Theory (Kaplan & Kaplan, 1989). They also cover a range of contexts, such as the virtual world, adventure recreation, education and tourism, *in vivo* nature exposure, and ecophenomenological perspectives. These are deliberately broad in order to capture the variety of possible interventions and provide guidance for a broad range of policy and practice possibilities.

The final section reports on real-world applications, often including not only description of the practice, but also of the evidence or theory that informed its design, and the evaluated efficacy of that practice. These chapters adopt an international lens and cover a wide spectrum of contexts across the life-course – from wilderness therapy for youth at risk in the US and Australia to care farming for adults with dementia in the Netherlands. They provide evidence for real-world applications in German educational settings, for UK-based sick, wounded, and injured military personnel, and from the globally delivered parkrun. It is evident that nature-based interventions offer applicability for a diverse range of cohorts and contexts. Collectively, they demonstrate how evidence can inform practice, public health funding, government health, and social care policies and should therefore be valued by decision makers.

Nature-based activities can be an effective vehicle to drive behavioral change and promote a cost-effective, all-inclusive approach to physical, psychological, and social health and wellbeing. This edited volume offers a coherent picture of current academic understanding on the topic of nature, physical activity, and health, alongside illustrative evidence-based international practice, resonating loudly toward policymaking that links nature and health.

References

Brymer, E., Freeman, E., & Richardson, M. (2019). One Health: The wellbeing impacts of human-nature relationships, Frontiers.

Brymer E., Araújo D., Davids K., & Pepping G-J. (2020). Conceptualizing the Human Health Outcomes of Acting in Natural Environments: An Ecological Perspective. Front. Psychol. 11:1362. doi: 10.3389/fpsyg.2020.01362

Flowers E. P., Freeman P., & Gladwell V. F. (2016). A cross-sectional study examining predictors of visit frequency to local green space and the impact this has on physical activity levels. *BMC Public Health*, 16:420. doi: 10.1186/s12889-016-3050-9. PMID: 27207300; PMCID: PMC4875629.

Francis, J., Giles-Corti, B., Wood, L., & Knuiman M. (2012). Creating sense of community: The role of public space, *Journal of Environmental Psychology*, *32*(4), 401–409.

Gidlow, C. J., Jones, M. V., Hurst, G., Masterson, C., Clark-Carter, D., Tarvainen, M. P., Smith, G., & Nieuwenhuijsen, M. (2016). Where to put your best foot forward: Psycho-physiological responses to walking in natural and urban environments, *Journal of Environmental Psychology*, *45*, 22–29.

Gladwell, V. F., Kuoppa, P., Tarvainen, M. P., & Rogerson, M. (2016). A Lunchtime Walk in Nature Enhances Restoration of Autonomic Control during Night-Time Sleep: Results from a Preliminary Study. *International Journal of Environmental Research and Public Health*, *13*(3), 280. https://doi.org/10.3390/ijerph13030280

Kaplan, R. & Kaplan, S. (1989). *The Experience of Nature: A Psychological Perspective*. New York: Cambridge University Press.

Kondo, M. C., Jacoby, S. F., & South, E. C. (2018). Does spending time outdoors reduce stress? A review of real-time stress response to outdoor environments. *Health & Place*, *51*, 136–150. https://doi.org/10.1016/j.healthplace.2018.03.001

Shanahan, D. F., et al. (2019). Nature-based interventions for improving health and wellbeing: The purpose, the people and the outcomes. *Sports (Basel)*. 7(6):141. doi: 10.3390/sports7060141.

Ulrich, R. S., Simons, R. F., Losito, B. D., Fiorito, E., Miles, M. A., & Zelson, M. (1991). Stress recovery during exposure to natural and urban environments. *Journal of Environmental Psychology*, *11*(3), 201–230. https://doi.org/10.1016/S0272-4944(05)80184-7.

Part I

Research on Physical Activity in Nature

2 Understanding the Affective Benefits of Interacting with Nature

Kathryn E. Schertz, Kimberly L. Meidenbauer, and Marc G. Berman

2.1 Introduction

The documented benefits from interacting with natural environments (such as parks) are vast and include improvements in physical health (Hartig, Mitchell & de Vries, 2014; Kardan et al., 2015), mental health (Bratman et al., 2019; Hartig, Mitchell & de Vries, 2014; Kardan et al., 2015), cognitive functioning (Berman, Jonides & Kaplan, 2008; Bratman, Hamilton & Daily, 2012; Schertz & Berman, 2019), and prosocial behavior (Guéguen & Stefan, 2016; Kuo & Sullivan, 2001b; Zhang et al., 2014). One of the most reliable outcomes of nature interactions is that of improved affect and greater emotional wellbeing (McMahan & Estes, 2015).

One major reason for studying nature interventions as a source of mood improvement is that state affect influences several significant behavioral and health outcomes. The link between emotional state and improved mental health is relatively clear, as day-to-day affective responses are linked to resilience against psychopathology (Gloria & Steinhardt, 2016; Wichers et al., 2010). In addition, researchers have demonstrated the vital influence of emotional state on physical health outcomes such as longevity, lower morbidity, and lessened pain (Pressman & Cohen, 2005; Salovey et al., 2000). Positive affect is also implicated in increasing prosocial tendencies (Aknin, Van de Vondervoort & Hamlin, 2018), and this is particularly true of "self-transcendent" emotions like awe and gratitude (Stellar et al., 2017). It's worth noting here that the terms affect and mood will be used interchangeably in this chapter, as most of the research cited does not distinguish between them. Though the two are sometimes differentiated by their duration (i.e. a mood is longer than an affective state), there lacks a broad consensus regarding the functional difference between mood and affect (Serby 2003).

Another reason to study how nature improves mood is to generate mechanistic accounts of the variety of domains in which nature-elicited gains are documented. For example, greater positive affect may be one potential mechanism for the stress-buffering effects of nature interventions (Tsunetsugu et al., 2013; van den Berg & Custers, 2011). This is not the

DOI: 10.4324/9781003154419-3

only potential mechanism at play, however. Nature exposure has also been shown to improve cognitive functioning, particularly on tasks requiring attention and working memory (Berman, Jonides & Kaplan, 2008; Berman et al., 2012; Stenfors et al., 2019; Stevenson, Schilhab & Bentsen, 2018). As there is evidence that these cognitive benefits are independent of the affective ones (Stenfors et al., 2019), this distinction is necessary to understand why nature is beneficial. In the context of social behavior, nature-associated reductions in aggression appear to be mediated by improvements in attention (Kuo & Sullivan, 2001a). However, increased prosociality after nature exposure has primarily been observed as a consequence of improved affective state (Guéguen & Stefan, 2016; Joye & Bolderdijk, 2014). As such, elucidating the affective benefits of exposure to nature, though important in its own right, also has clear consequences for benefits gained in other domains of research.

Increasingly, humans are spending a disproportionate amount of time indoors and away from nature (Kahn et al., 2010) and research has demonstrated that people may underestimate the affective benefits of nature exposure (Nisbet & Zelenski, 2011). Given these behaviors and overall increasing urbanization (Turner, Nakamura & Dinetti, 2004), it is important to distinguish between what the optimal dose/form of nature exposure is for improved mood and what is realistic and achievable for a typical individual who may or may not have easy access to nearby nature. Though much of the extant research on nature's affective benefits looks at nature walks, it is far from the only domain in which the benefits of nature exposure on mood have been observed. As such, we will review the evidence of affective benefits across several domains of nature exposure and across multiple forms of measurement.

2.2 The Benefits of Natural Environments on Self-Reported Affect and Physiology

In most studies, affect change is measured using either self-reported emotional state or changes in psychophysiological responses. Experimental studies examining self-reported affect in response to the environment have primarily used the Positive and Negative Affect Schedule (PANAS) (Watson, Clark & Tellegen, 1988) or the Zuckerman Inventory of Personal Reactions (ZIPERS) (Zuckerman, 1977). Other measures less frequently used to assess affect in this field include the Subjective Vitality Scale (Ryan & Frederick, 1997), the Profile of Mood States (POMS) (McNair et al., 1971), and the Stress-Refresh Scale (Mackay et al., 1978). Studies using physiological measures have examined changes in heart rate variability (HRV), salivary cortisol levels, blood pressure (BP), and skin conductance during and after exposure to the environment of interest (Alvarsson, Wiens & Nilsson, 2010; Brown, Barton & Gladwell, 2013; Lee et al., 2011; Olafsdottir et al., 2020; Ulrich et al., 1991).

Understanding the Affective Benefits 9

In general, the types of nature exposures which have been shown to affect mood can be placed into a few categories: virtual or simulated nature studies (e.g. images, videos, virtual reality (VR), sounds, etc.), passively viewing real nature (e.g. through a window or sitting in a park), nature walk studies, green exercise studies (green exercise: physical activity whilst experiencing nature), and larger-scale survey-based or observational studies of nature exposure on mood. Though consistent benefits have been observed across these domains, the magnitude and type of such benefits (e.g. self-reported emotion, physiological markers, etc.) can vary. Perhaps unsurprisingly, simulated nature generally produces less robust mood effects than does actual nature (Mayer et al., 2009; McMahan & Estes, 2015). However, dose, as measured by either duration or immersiveness, and activity level (passive viewing vs. exercising in vs. walking in) also has an effect on mood (Barton, Griffin & Pretty, 2012; Barton & Pretty, 2010).

Perhaps the most passive and least immersive type of nature exposure is that of viewing images of natural environments. Studies utilizing a pre-/post-design (i.e. designs that gather affect measures before and after image viewing) typically use reasonably short durations of exposure. Beute and de Kort (2014) utilized a 3-minute image viewing procedure and found significantly greater changes in positive affect after nature exposure versus an urban exposure. Other studies with brief exposures (less than 10 minutes) have also documented improvements in positive feelings, and reductions in negative feelings (Lohr & Pearson-Mims, 2006), as well as increased vitality (Ryan et al., 2010). Hartig and colleagues (Hartig et al., 1996) found similar effects with a slightly longer image viewing duration (12–14 minutes), where participants who viewed nature scenes reported greater positive affect after viewing the scenes, but those who viewed urban images showed no change in emotional state. There is also some evidence that viewing images of nature before experiencing a stressor may have a buffering effect on the processing of that stress, as indexed by changes in HRV (Brown, Barton & Gladwell, 2013). Several other studies, which did not use a nature image "intervention," but rather had participants evaluate varied images (natural scenes, built scenes, tree-lined streets, etc.) found that the nature images elicited the most favorable emotional responses on a per image basis (Sheets & Manzer, 1991; Valtchanov & Ellard, 2015; White et al., 2010). Though some studies using image interventions have not found a significant change in self-reported mood (Berman, Jonides & Kaplan, 2008; Brown, Barton & Gladwell, 2013), it is notable that there is considerable evidence that even brief and passive exposures to nature can have a demonstrable effect on mood.

Another passive, but slightly more immersive, approach involving simulated nature is to use videos or VR. Brief videos (7–10 minutes) of natural environments have been shown to improve a variety of self-reported emotions, including depression, tension, anger, happiness, stress, positive affect, reflection, and feelings of connectedness to nature (Mayer et al., 2009; van den Berg, Koole & van der Wulp, 2003). These effects can be particularly pronounced when an individual begins in an unpleasant affective state. After experiencing a stress induction, participants who viewed a 10-minute video of a natural environment showed significantly greater affective recovery on measures of fear, anger/aggression, and positive emotions in comparison to those who saw a pedestrian mall or heavy traffic video (Ulrich et al., 1991). The participants in Ulrich's (1991) study also experienced lower skin conductance and BP during the nature video. Though less commonly employed, researchers using VR to create a more immersive simulation have also demonstrated the mood-enhancing properties of virtual natural environments (Valtchanov, Barton & Ellard, 2010) (also see Chapter 10).

Research on passive viewing of actual natural environments, sometimes referred to as forest-bathing, typically involves participants sitting in an environment for 10–15 minutes. This approach has yielded significant changes in self-reported affect and physiological measures. A number of studies conducted in Japan demonstrated that forest bathing in nature elicited changes in HRV and cortisol consistent with increased parasympathetic nervous system activity, which is often associated with less stress, as well as large decreases in negative affect and increases in positive emotion (Lee et al., 2011; Lee et al., 2009; Park et al., 2007). Though these initial studies had relatively small sample sizes, subsequent research with larger sample sizes replicated these effects, finding improvements in self-reported affective state and several psychophysiological measurements (Tsunetsugu et al., 2013). However, one important limitation of these forest-bathing studies is that they were exclusively conducted on Japanese male participants. A similar study conducted by Hartig et al. (Hartig et al., 1999) had both male and female participants, but found very small effects on mood for individuals seated for 10 minutes in a botanical garden versus at a heavily trafficked intersection. Whether these differences were due to the study sample demographics or in the type of natural environment (i.e. forest vs. garden) is an open question. Therefore, more research is required to fully examine the salubrious effects of simply sitting in a natural environment across a more diverse group of participants and across more types of natural environments.

Some of the most compelling work on this topic comes from studies which assess changes in affect after actual nature walks. Many studies have shown that a relatively short, 40–50-minute walk in a natural environment versus an urban walk reliably improves positive affect (Berman, Jonides & Kaplan, 2008, 2012; Hartig et al., 2003; Hartig, Mang & Evans, 1991; Johansson, Hartig & Staats, 2011) and may reduce negative emotions such as anger, aggression, rumination, and anxiety (Bratman et al., 2015; Hartig et al., 2003; Hartig, Mang & Evans, 1991). Changes in positive affect, as measured by the PANAS, Subjective Vitality Scale, and reports of fascination and relaxation, have been elicited by even shorter nature walks, in the order of 10 to 20 minutes (Mayer et al., 2009; Nisbet & Zelenski, 2011; Ryan et al., 2010). As reviewed by McMahan and Estes (2015), effect sizes for

Understanding the Affective Benefits 11

exposure to real nature (including passive viewing and walk studies) are generally larger than those for lab-based nature interventions. Effect size, quantified by Pearson's product-moment correlation, was $r = 0.37$ (a moderate effect) for real nature and $r = 0.26$ (a small effect) for lab-based nature. However, it is unclear whether these results are due to the "real vs. simulated" distinction or due to the limited sensory experience of lab-based exposures, which are typically limited to the visual modality. Thus, while the patterns of improvement in mood may be consistent across virtual and real nature, there appears to be an additional benefit in terms of the magnitude of the mood boost when experiencing actual nature.

Experience sampling studies have been effectively used to investigate how incidental contact with nature is also associated with changes in affect. These types of studies notify participants several times throughout the day to take surveys which ask about their mood, surroundings, and activities, which allows for the study of everyday experiences (Hektner, Schmidt & Csikszentmihalyi, 2007). One experience sampling study found that different types of nature had different magnitudes of association with happiness. For example, being in a marine/coastal environment was associated with a happiness score that was 6 points higher than being in an urban environment, on a 100-point scale, while being in woodlands and grasslands was associated with a 2-point higher happiness score compared to urban environments (MacKerron & Mourato, 2013). These effects can be compared to those of companionship – being with a partner or spouse was 4.5 points higher than being alone, while being with one's children was only associated with 0.27 more points (MacKerron & Mourato, 2013).

As experience sampling studies assess measures at multiple time points, they can also be used to investigate how long-lasting the mood benefits of nature are. One such study measured contact with four different types of nature stimuli – hearing birds, seeing water, seeing the sky, and being outdoors. They found that being outdoors and hearing birds were associated with an immediate mood boost, but that the mood boost was not observed at the next assessment 2.5 hours later (Bakolis et al., 2018). In comparison, the mood boost associated with seeing trees or sky had a delayed effect, where the increases in mood were present at the next assessment, but not at the immediate assessment. More studies are required to determine how long-lasting the mood benefits are after intentional vs. incidental nature contact, and how the type of nature (e.g. beach vs. forest) impacts mood benefits. In all, empirical and observational studies have shown that interactions with nature improve mood and that these interactions can also come from simulated natural environments.

2.3 Theories for Nature's Mood Effects

The observation of nature's positive effect on mood has spawned a great number of theoretical accounts for why nature exposure can improve our moods. Many of these theories use an evolutionary framework. They propose that because humans evolved in natural environments, and only a small portion of our history has occurred in more urbanized societies, this evolution in nature has left a trace on our collective psyche, and results in a positive response toward natural environments (Ulrich, 1993). This idea is central to the Biophilia Hypothesis, which focuses on the idea of a human evolved affinity for natural environments, but this theory does not specify how nature impacts emotional functioning (Kellert & Wilson, 1995). Ulrich's stress reduction theory (SRT) builds on the Biophilia Hypothesis, proposing that the emotional benefits of nature exposure are due to our evolved preference for these environments (Ulrich, 1983). Specifically, SRT proposes that unthreatening natural environments increase positive affect and reduce negative affect, which allows a person to return to baseline after a stress response.

Another evolutionary theory is that of Prospect-Refuge Theory (Appleton, 1975), which does not focus on differences between natural and urban environments, but rather on the characteristics that make a natural landscape aesthetically preferred. The theory posits that people prefer landscapes that offer prospect (clear field of view), but also some level of refuge (places to hide). The characteristics of prospect and refuge may then influence how people experience an environment and any affective changes that are observed.

The perceptual fluency account (PFA) suggests that positive affective responses to natural environments are due to the ease with which we process natural stimuli (Joye & van den Berg, 2011). For example, features such as fractalness (amount of recursive patterns) and coherence (how well the features of a scene go together) are found more common in natural than urban environments, and are associated with greater ease of scene processing (Joye et al., 2016). In this framework, stress reduction is simply a byproduct of the positive affect that effortless processing induces.

Kaplan's (1987) theory on environmental preference shares ideas with both SRT and PFA. Kaplan suggested that our positive affective response to natural environments is because they are highly preferred. This preference comes from a combination of nature placing fewer demands on information processing and nature's evolutionary significance (Kaplan, 1987). Preference and positive affect have been found to load together in several studies looking at characteristics of preference and environment (Calvin, Dearinger & Curtin, 1972; Ibarra et al., 2017). Additionally, natural environments are typically so much more preferred than urban environments that it is hard to find overlapping distributions of preference for these types of environments (Kaplan, Kaplan & Wendt, 1972).

Another explanation proposed that feelings of connectedness to nature mediate the link between nature exposure and its beneficial effects on emotion and wellbeing (Mayer et al., 2009). This account suggests that exposure to natural environments leads to a short-term (state) increase in connectedness to nature, which at a trait level is associated with life satisfaction and happiness, and can also provide a sense of belonging (Mayer & Frantz, 2004; Mayer et al., 2009). Thus, this theory proposes that this temporary increase in connectedness to nature is a mechanism for the overall positive affective response occurring after nature exposure.

It is noteworthy that some, though not all, of these theoretical accounts mention nature's status as a highly preferred environment in their explanations. Though the theories do not fully agree on why nature is preferred (e.g. evolutionary mechanisms vs. the ease of stimulus/information processing from natural stimuli), aesthetic preferences for nature are a necessary component of SRT, Prospect-Refuge, and Kaplan's Environmental Preferences theory. In contrast, PFA proposes that preference and affect are both a result of the ease of processing natural stimulation, rather than a mechanism. Connectedness to nature is, in a way, a type of preferential response, but proposes that this connectedness fulfills a fundamental need to belong to the natural world, which appears qualitatively different from an aesthetic preference.

Thus, there appears to be a distinction between mechanistic accounts which propose that nature's affective benefits arise because humans have a strong aesthetic response to nature (e.g. SRT, Kaplan's Theory of Environmental Preference, and Prospect-Refuge) and those which suggest there is something special about nature above and beyond this preference (e.g. Biophilia, PFA, and nature connectedness). The theory regarding connectedness to nature, for example, would fall into the latter category of treating nature as special (Mayer et al., 2009). PFA also places nature in a special place, as it proposes that both preference and mood change arise from nature having stimuli that are easily processed, i.e. that there is something special/unique to nature stimulation (Joye & van den Berg, 2011). A related idea to PFA is that the visual spatial frequencies common in natural scenes are endogenously visually rewarding, and this, in turn, causes a positive affective response (Valtchanov & Ellard, 2015). This account also suggests unique properties of natural stimuli that are not simply due to aesthetics.

In contrast, evidence for a primary role of aesthetics comes from work showing that positive affect change in response to viewing a nature slideshow compared to an urban one was fully mediated by participants' preferences for the slideshows (Beute & de Kort, 2014). Additionally, White et al. (2010) found that images which were rated most highly on preference also evoked the largest positive emotional responses, and that by incorporating bodies of water in images of built environments, these environments were also rated very highly on both preference and affect. Recent work by Meidenbauer et al. (2019) found that individuals who saw preference-equated nature and urban images did not show any differences in affect change. This study also demonstrated that individuals' aesthetic preference ratings for the images that they saw were highly predictive of mood change, but image category (i.e. nature vs. urban) itself did not have significant predictive value beyond absolute preference (i.e. once preference was accounted for, environment did not matter in terms of affect change). All of these studies were performed with simulated nature (i.e. images), therefore, it is possible that these effects would be different in real environments. However, the convergence of effects for real vs. simulated nature suggests that mood changes after interactions with natural environments may be completely driven by preference just as the simulated nature stimuli are.

Understanding the mechanism for nature's emotional benefits is of scientific interest and is relevant for the purposes of optimizing the efficacy of nature interventions. However, it is important to clarify that even if aesthetics are the primary driver of nature's mood effects, this does not mean we should not invest in urban green infrastructure (UGI) or encourage walks in natural environments. Indeed, nature exposure (irrespective of preference) is associated with a variety of other benefits, such as increased contemplative thought (Schertz et al., 2018), greater neighborhood social cohesion (de Vries et al., 2013), and restoration of attentional resources (Berman, Jonides & Kaplan, 2008; Schertz & Berman, 2019). Further, UGI is a relatively low-cost intervention for the emotional wellbeing of residents, lending it practical significance.

2.4 Studies in Populations with Mood Disorders

When considering environmental impacts on affect, it is important to consider how these effects might be different for individuals with affective disorders. Individuals with these conditions may be more or less susceptible to nature exposure compared to the general population. While solitary walks in natural settings have been shown to have mood benefits for healthy adults, these walks could exacerbate certain symptoms for individuals with depressive or anxiety conditions. For example, going on a walk alone provides the potential for rumination, a maladaptive pattern of self-referential thought, which characterizes depression, and can maintain negative affect (Nolen-Hoeksema, Wisco & Lyubomirsky, 2008). Although few studies have been performed that examine the affective influence of the natural environment in individuals with mood disorders, two populations have been studied more extensively in this area: adults with depression and military veterans with post-traumatic stress disorder (PTSD).

Most studies looking at depressive symptoms in relation to natural environments have been observational. Several epidemiological studies have found that neighborhood greenspace is negatively associated with rates for depression in adults (Beyer et al., 2014; Engemann et al., 2019; Gascon et al., 2015; Kardan et al., 2015; Nutsford, Pearson & Kingham, 2013). To date, two experimental studies, using very different paradigms, have been conducted which exposed participants diagnosed with depression to natural

Understanding the Affective Benefits 15

environments. In the first, participants took a 50-minute walk in both a natural or urban environment, separated by a week (i.e. nature the first week and urban the second week or vice versa) (Berman et al., 2012). In this study, mood was assessed using the PANAS before and after the walk. Positive affect increased in both conditions, but there was a condition by time interaction, such that positive mood improved more after the nature walk compared to after the urban walk. Negative affect decreased in both conditions, with no significant differences between conditions. This study can be directly compared to an earlier study, which employed the same interventions, but with a nonclinical sample (Berman, Jonides & Kaplan, 2008). The effect size (as defined by Pearson's product-moment correlation, r) for positive affect was much larger in the depression patient sample (r = 0.47) than in the nonclinical sample (r = 0.29) (Berman, Jonides & Kaplan, 2008, Berman et al., 2012; McMahan & Estes, 2015).

In a different paradigm, a natural environment was used as the setting for cognitive-behavioral therapy (CBT), in comparison to a hospital environment, and a control outpatient group that was not receiving CBT (Kim et al., 2009). The intervention lasted 4 weeks, with participants attending therapy once a week for 3 hours, and participants were tested for remission at a 3-month follow-up. The forest-CBT group showed greater improvement in their depressive symptoms, with over 60% of participants in remission at the 3-month follow-up, compared to 21% in the hospital-CBT group, and 5% in the control group. The forest-CBT group also showed lower cortisol levels at the end of the program, as well as higher high-frequency heart rate variability, which is related to healthy parasympathetic nervous system activity (Kim et al., 2009). Taken together, the evidence is promising that passive exposure to natural elements (through local greenspace) can offer protective benefits against depressive symptoms, while active exposure (through walks and therapy in natural environments) can improve affect for those already diagnosed with depression, which is characterized by low levels of positive affect (Watson & Naragon-Gainey, 2010).

Another population of participants that have demonstrated affective benefits from exposure to nature are military veterans with PTSD. Nature-assisted therapies (NAT) have been the most commonly tested way to assess the effects of nature in veterans (Poulsen, Stigsdotter & Refshage, 2015). For example, a large randomized clinical trial (n = 219; treatment n = 108; control n = 111) found qualitative effects on affect for a group of veterans who completed a 1-week fully immersive Outward Bound experience as part of a 14-week therapy intervention, compared to a group that just completed the standard therapy (Hyer et al., 1996). In interviews with the participants several weeks after the Outward Bound trip, they reported less anhedonia, more control over negative emotions, and more positive emotions. Hyer and colleagues did not find any statistical differences in PTSD symptoms between the two groups. In a smaller study that used a 1-year treatment time with weekly 3-hour sessions in nature (thus longer but less immersive than Outward Bound), participants saw statistically significant improvements in their PTSD symptoms, depressive symptoms, social and emotional quality of life, and sense of hope, compared to a wait-list control group (n = 42; treatment n = 22; control n = 20) (Gelkopf et al., 2013). Thus, while a 1-year nature-related intervention may be more successful in reducing PTSD symptomology, both short and long programs seem to provide some improvements in affect.

2.5 Policy and Practice

Overall, there is a large body of evidence that interacting with natural environments and stimuli can have mood benefits, for both the general population and for those suffering from mood disorders. There is evidence that natural stimuli are highly preferred, which leads to the following question: are nature's mood benefits solely due to nature being a preferred stimulus, or is nature special in some way? A speculation for one difference between nature stimuli and other well-liked stimuli is that the mood effects of nature do not seem to saturate. Thus, while people may tire of their favorite movie or favorite food, rarely do people tire of watching sunsets or seeing waterfalls. This allows nature to be a source for greater well-being over time.

Governments at different levels (e.g. local, state and federal), as well as private institutions, can take steps to help citizens experience the mood benefits of nature by providing equitable access to urban greenspace. Different groups may prefer to engage with nature in different ways, whether grouped by age, mobility, gender, or ethnicity (Ho et al., 2005). By providing spaces with facilities attuned to the needs of different groups, cities can help improve the overall wellbeing of their citizens. Although longer, more immersive natural engagements with environments seem to have the largest effects on mood, it might not be feasible for everyone to engage with nature in that same immersive manner. Cities can provide different types of nature experiences that allow individuals to experience nature in many ways. Larger natural areas can be supplemented with small urban "pocket parks," and, importantly, parks like this have been shown to provide a location for positive, contemplative thought (Schertz et al., 2018). Tree-lined streets can increase the pleasantness and likelihood of walking trips within one's neighborhood (Tilt, 2010), as well as improve the perceived health of residents (Kardan et al., 2015). Institutions such as schools, hospitals, and prisons should consider how adding or allowing the utilization of pre-existing natural areas in and around their buildings may increase affect and wellbeing amongst students (Holt et al., 2019), patients (Ulrich, 2002), prisoners (Moran & Turner, 2019), and employees at all of those locations. In doing so, these institutions not only help individuals, but also demonstrate that access to nature should not be viewed as a luxury, but rather a societal value.

Understanding the Affective Benefits 17

One study found that people systematically underestimate the mood benefit they'll experience by engaging with nearby nature (Nisbet & Zelenski, 2011). This may mean that people do not choose to interact with nature as often as they should, given how much happier they will feel afterward. Thus, education campaigns may play a critical role in which individuals are reminded of the affective benefits that even short periods of time in nature can provide. This can be paired with resources that make it easier to find sites for outdoor activities. One example of this comes from the Chicago-based nonprofit, Openlands, which created the "Get Outside" interactive map. This map of locations for engaging with nature, both in and around Chicago, can be filtered by access (such as served by public transit), facilities, or available activities. Additionally, public service announcements, such as those sponsored by the U.S. Forest Service with the tagline "every neighborhood has a naturehood," as part of their *Discover the Forest* campaign, may encourage more people to explore their local natural environments. It would be important for researchers and practitioners to evaluate the efficacy of these campaigns via experimental means.

In conclusion, there is a large body of work supporting the idea that natural stimuli and environments have affective benefits. While the effects of different exposure types, such as image-based vs. real-world, incidental vs. intentional exposure, active vs. passive interactions, may be different in terms of duration and magnitude, each of these exposures has empirical support for positively influencing affect. Work remains to be done on determining the mechanism of these benefits, and, in turn, accepting or modifying one or more of the proposed theories for why nature interactions produce these affective benefits. However, practitioners, private institutions, and governments are already in a position to encourage people to choose to engage more with natural environments as an inexpensive and effective way to enhance their emotional wellbeing.

References

Aknin, L. B., Van de Vondervoort, J. W., & Hamlin, J. K. (2018). Positive feelings reward and promote prosocial behavior. *Current Opinion in Psychology, 20*, 55–59.

Alvarsson, J. J., Wiens, S., & Nilsson, M. E. (2010). Stress recovery during exposure to nature sound and environmental noise. *International journal of environmental research and public health, 7*(3), 1036–1046.

Appleton, J. (1975). Landscape evaluation: the theoretical vacuum. *Transactions of the Institute of British Geographers*, 120–123.

Bakolis, I., Hammoud, R., Smythe, M., Gibbons, J., Davidson, N., Tognin, S., & Mechelli, A. (2018). Urban mind: Using smartphone technologies to investigate the impact of nature on mental well-being in real time. *Bioscience, 68*(2), 134–145.

Barton, J., Griffin, M., & Pretty, J. (2012). Exercise-, nature- and socially interactive-based initiatives improve mood and self-esteem in the clinical population. *Perspectives in Public Health, 132*(2), 89–96.

18   K.E. Schertz, K.L. Meidenbauer, and M.G. Berman

Barton, J., & Pretty, J. (2010). What is the best dose of nature and green exercise for improving mental health? A multi-study analysis. *Environmental Science & Technology, 44*(10), 3947–3955.

Berman, M. G., Jonides, J., & Kaplan, S. (2008). The cognitive benefits of interacting with nature. *Psychological Science, 19*(12), 1207–1212.

Berman, M. G., Kross, E., Krpan, K. M., Askren, M. K., Burson, A., Deldin, P. J., ... Jonides, J. (2012). Interacting with nature improves cognition and affect for individuals with depression. *Journal of Affective Disorders, 140*(3), 300–305.

Beute, F., & de Kort, Y. A. W. (2014). Natural resistance: Exposure to nature and self-regulation, mood, and physiology after ego-depletion. *Journal of Environmental Psychology, 40*, 167–178.

Beyer, K. M. M., Kaltenbach, A., Szabo, A., Bogar, S., Nieto, F. J., & Malecki, K. M. (2014). Exposure to neighborhood green space and mental health: Evidence from the survey of the health of Wisconsin. *International Journal of Environmental Research and Public Health, 11*(3), 3453–3472.

Bratman, G. N., Anderson, C. B., Berman, M. G., Cochran, B., de Vries, S., Flanders, J., ... Daily, G. C. (2019). Nature and mental health: An ecosystem service perspective. *Science Advances, 5*(7), eaax0903.

Bratman, G. N., Daily, G. C., Levy, B. J., & Gross, J. J. (2015). The benefits of nature experience: Improved affect and cognition. *Landscape and Urban Planning, 138*, 41–50.

Bratman, G. N., Hamilton, J. P., & Daily, G. C. (2012). The impacts of nature experience on human cognitive function and mental health. *Annals of the New York Academy of Sciences, 1249*, 118–136.

Brown, D. K., Barton, J. L., & Gladwell, V. F. (2013). Viewing nature scenes positively affects recovery of autonomic function following acute-mental stress. *Environmental Science & Technology, 47*(11), 5562–5569.

Calvin, J. S., Dearinger, J. A., & Curtin, M. E. (1972). An attempt at assessing preferences for natural landscape. *Environment and Behavior, 4*(4), 447.

de Vries, S., van Dillen, S. M. E., Groenewegen, P. P., & Spreeuwenberg, P. (2013). Streetscape greenery and health: Stress, social cohesion and physical activity as mediators. *Social Science & Medicine, 94*, 26–33.

Engemann, K., Pedersen, C. B., Arge, L., Tsirogiannis, C., Mortensen, P. B., & Svenning, J.-C. (2019). Residential green space in childhood is associated with lower risk of psychiatric disorders from adolescence into adulthood. *Proceedings of the National Academy of Sciences of the United States of America, 116*(11), 5188–5193.

Gascon, M., Triguero-Mas, M., Martínez, D., Dadvand, P., Forns, J., Plasència, A., & Nieuwenhuijsen, M. J. (2015). Mental health benefits of long-term exposure to residential green and blue spaces: A systematic review. *International Journal of Environmental Research and Public Health, 12*(4), 4354–4379.

Gelkopf, M., Hasson-Ohayon, I., Bikman, M., & Kravetz, S. (2013). Nature adventure rehabilitation for combat-related posttraumatic chronic stress disorder: A randomized control trial. *Psychiatry Research, 209*(3), 485–493.

Gloria, C. T., & Steinhardt, M. A. (2016). Relationships among positive emotions, coping, resilience and mental health. *Stress and Health: Journal of the International Society for the Investigation of Stress, 32*(2), 145–156.

Guéguen, N., & Stefan, J. (2016). "Green altruism": Short immersion in natural green environments and helping behavior. *Environment and Behavior, 48*(2), 324–342.

Hartig, T., Böök, A., Garvill, J., Olsson, T., & Gärling, T. (1996). Environmental influences on psychological restoration. *Scandinavian Journal of Psychology*, *37*(4), 378–393.

Hartig, T., Evans, G. W., Jamner, L. D., Davis, D. S., & Garling, T. (2003). Tracking restoration in natural and urban field settings. *Journal of Environmental Psychology*, *23*, 109–123.

Hartig, T., Mang, M., & Evans, G. W. (1991). Restorative effects of natural environment experiences. *Environment and Behavior*, 23(1), 3–26.

Hartig, T., Mitchell, R., & de Vries, S. (2014). Nature and health. *Annual Review of Public Health*, 35, 207–228.

Hartig, T., Nyberg, L., Nilsson, L.-G., & Gärling, T. (1999). Testing for mood congruent recall with environmentally induced mood. *Journal of Environmental Psychology*, *19*(4), 353–367.

Hektner, J. M., Schmidt, J. A., & Csikszentmihalyi, M. (2007). *Experience Sampling Method: Measuring the Quality of Everyday Life*. SAGE. Thousand Oaks, CA, USA

Ho, C.-H., Sasidharan, V., Elmendorf, W., Willits, F. K., Graefe, A., & Godbey, G. (2005). Gender and ethnic variations in urban park preferences, visitation, and perceived benefits. *Journal of Leisure Research*, *37*, 281–306. https://doi.org/10.1080/00222216.2005.11950054

Holt, E. W., Lombard, Q. K., Best, N., Smiley-Smith, S., & Quinn, J. E. (2019). Active and passive use of green space, health, and well-being amongst university students. *International journal of environmental research and public health*, *16*(3), 424.

Hyer, L., Boyd, S., Scurfield, R., Smith, D., & Burke, J. (1996). Effects of outward bound experience as an adjunct to inpatient PTSD treatment of war veterans. *Journal of clinical psychology*, *52*(3), 263–278.

Ibarra, F. F., Kardan, O., Hunter, M. R., Kotabe, H. P., Meyer, F. A. C., & Berman, M. G. (2017). Image feature types and their predictions of aesthetic preference and naturalness. *Frontiers in Psychology*, *8*, 632.

Johansson, M., Hartig, T., & Staats, H. (2011). Psychological benefits of walking: Moderation by company and outdoor environment: Environmental moderation of walking benefits. *Applied Psychology: Health and Well-Being*, *3*(3), 261–280.

Joye, Y., & Bolderdijk, J. W. (2014). An exploratory study into the effects of extraordinary nature on emotions, mood, and prosociality. *Frontiers in Psychology*, *5*, 1577.

Joye, Y., Steg, L., Ünal, A. B., & Pals, R. (2016). When complex is easy on the mind: Internal repetition of visual information in complex objects is a source of perceptual fluency. *Journal of Experimental Psychology: Human Perception and Performance*, *42*(1), 103–114.

Joye, Y., & van den Berg, A. (2011). Is love for green in our genes? A critical analysis of evolutionary assumptions in restorative environments research. *Urban Forestry & Urban Greening*, *10*(4), 261–268.

Kahn, P. H., Ruckert, J. H., Severson, R. L., Reichert, A. L., & Fowler, E. (2010). A nature language: An agenda to catalog, save, and recover patterns of human–nature interaction. *Ecopsychology*, *2*, 59–66. https://doi.org/10.1089/eco.2009.0047

Kaplan, S. (1987). Aesthetics, affect, and cognition: Environmental preference from an evolutionary perspective. *Environment and Behavior*, *19*(1), 3–32.

Kaplan, S., Kaplan, R., & Wendt, J. S. (1972). Rated preference and complexity for natural and urban visual material. *Perception & Psychophysics*, *12*(4), 354–356.

20 *K.E. Schertz, K.L. Meidenbauer, and M.G. Berman*

Kardan, O., Gozdyra, P., Misic, B., Moola, F., Palmer, L. J., Paus, T., & Berman, M. G. (2015). Neighborhood greenspace and health in a large urban center. *Scientific Reports, 5*, 11610.

Kellert, S. R., & Wilson, E. O. (1995). *The Biophilia Hypothesis.* Island Press. Washington, DC.

Kim, W., Lim, S.-K., Chung, E.-J., & Woo, J.-M. (2009). The effect of cognitive behavior therapy-based psychotherapy applied in a forest environment on physiological changes and remission of major depressive disorder. *Psychiatry Investigation, 6*, 245. https://doi.org/10.4306/pi.2009.6.4.245

Kuo, F. E., & Sullivan, W. C. (2001a). Aggression and violence in the inner city: Effects of environment via mental fatigue. *Environment and Behavior, 33*(4), 543–571.

Kuo, F. E., & Sullivan, W. C. (2001b). Environment and crime in the inner city: Does vegetation reduce crime? *Environment and Behavior, 33*(3), 343–367.

Lee, J., Park, B.-J., Tsunetsugu, Y., Kagawa, T., & Miyazaki, Y. (2009). Restorative effects of viewing real forest landscapes, based on a comparison with urban landscapes. *Scandinavian Journal of Forest Research, 24*(3), 227–234.

Lee, J., Park, B.-J., Tsunetsugu, Y., Ohira, T., Kagawa, T., & Miyazaki, Y. (2011). Effect of forest bathing on physiological and psychological responses in young Japanese male subjects. *Public Health, 125*(2), 93–100.

Lohr, V. I., & Pearson-Mims, C. H. (2006). Responses to scenes with spreading, rounded, and conical tree forms. *Environment and Behavior, 38*(5), 667–688.

Mackay, C., Cox, T., Burrows, G., & Lazzerini, T. (1978). An inventory for the measurement of self-reported stress and arousal. *British journal of social and clinical psychology, 17*(3), 283–284.

MacKerron, G., & Mourato, S. (2013). Happiness is greater in natural environments. Global Environmental Change: Human and Policy Dimensions, *23(5), 992-1000.*

Mayer, F. S., & Frantz, C. M. (2004). The connectedness to nature scale: A measure of individuals' feeling in community with nature. *Journal of Environmental Psychology, 24*(4), 503–515.

Mayer, F. S., Frantz, C. M., Bruehlman-Senecal, E., & Dolliver, K. (2009). Why is nature beneficial?: The role of connectedness to nature. *Environment and Behavior, 41*(5), 607–643.

McMahan, E. A., & Estes, D. (2015). The effect of contact with natural environments on positive and negative affect: A meta-analysis. *The Journal of Positive Psychology, 10*(6), 507–519.

McNair, D. M., Lorr, M., & Droppleman, L. F. (1971). Manual for the profile of mood states (POMS). *San Diego: Educational and Industrial Testing Service.*

Meidenbauer, K. L., Stenfors, C. U. D., Bratman, G. N., Gross, J. J., Schertz, K. E., Choe, K. W., & Berman, M. G. (2020). The affective benefits of nature exposure: What's nature got to do with it?. *Journal of environmental psychology, 72*, 101498.

Moran, D., & Turner, J. (2019). Turning over a new leaf: The health-enabling capacities of nature contact in prison. *Social Science & Medicine, 231*, 62–69.

Nisbet, E. K., & Zelenski, J. M. (2011). Underestimating nearby nature: Affective forecasting errors obscure the happy path to sustainability. *Psychological Science, 22*(9), 1101–1106.

Nolen-Hoeksema, S., Wisco, B. E., & Lyubomirsky, S. (2008). Rethinking rumination. *Perspectives on Psychological Science: A Journal of the Association for Psychological Science, 3*(5), 400–424.

Nutsford, D., Pearson, A. L., & Kingham, S. (2013). An ecological study investigating the association between access to urban green space and mental health. *Public Health, 127*(11), 1005–1011.

Olafsdottir, G., Cloke, P., Schulz, A., Van Dyck, Z., Eysteinsson, T., Thorleifsdottir, B., & Vögele, C. (2020). Health benefits of walking in nature: A randomized controlled study under conditions of real-life stress. *Environment and Behavior, 52*(3), 248–274.

Park, B.-J., Tsunetsugu, Y., Kasetani, T., Hirano, H., Kagawa, T., Sato, M., & Miyazaki, Y. (2007). Physiological effects of Shinrin-yoku (taking in the atmosphere of the forest): Using salivary cortisol and cerebral activity as indicators. *Journal of Physiological Anthropology, 26*(2), 123–128.

Poulsen, D. V., Stigsdotter, U. K., & Refshage, A. D. (2015). Whatever happened to the soldiers? Nature-assisted therapies for veterans diagnosed with post-traumatic stress disorder: A literature review. *Urban Forestry & Urban Greening, 14*(2), 438–445.

Pressman, S. D., & Cohen, S. (2005). Does positive affect influence health? *Psychological Bulletin, 131*(6), 925–971.

Ryan, R. M., & Frederick, C. (1997). On energy, personality, and health: Subjective vitality as a dynamic reflection of well-being. *Journal of personality, 65*(3), 529–565.

Ryan, R. M., Weinstein, N., Bernstein, J., Brown, K. W., Mistretta, L., & Gagné, M. (2010). Vitalizing effects of being outdoors and in nature. *Journal of Environmental Psychology, 30*(2), 159–168.

Salovey, P., Rothman, A. J., Detweiler, J. B., & Steward, W. T. (2000). Emotional states and physical health. *The American Psychologist, 55*(1), 110.

Schertz, K. E., & Berman, M. G. (2019). Understanding nature and its cognitive benefits. *Current Directions in Psychological Science*, https://doi. org/10.1177/0963721419854100.

Schertz, K. E., Sachdeva, S., Kardan, O., Kotabe, H. P., Wolf, K. L., & Berman, M. G. (2018). A thought in the park: The influence of naturalness and low-level visual features on expressed thoughts. *Cognition, 174*, 82–93. https://doi.org/10.1016/j. cognition.2018.01.011

Serby, M. (2003). Psychiatric resident conceptualizations of mood and affect within the mental status examination. *American Journal of Psychiatry, 160*(8), 1527–1529.

Sheets, V. L., & Manzer, C. D. (1991). Affect, cognition, and urban vegetation: Some effects of adding trees along city streets. *Environment and Behavior, 23*(3), 285–304.

Stellar, J. E., Gordon, A. M., Piff, P. K., Cordaro, D., Anderson, C. L., Bai, Y., … Keltner, D. (2017). Self-transcendent emotions and their social functions: Compassion, gratitude, and awe bind us to others through prosociality. *Emotion Review: Journal of the International Society for Research on Emotion*, https://doi. org/10.1177/1754073916684557.

Stenfors, C. U. D., Van Hedger, S. C., Schertz, K. E., Meyer, F. A. C., Smith, K. E. L., Norman, G. J., … Berman, M. G. (2019). Positive effects of nature on cognitive performance across multiple experiments: Test order but not affect modulates the cognitive effects. *Frontiers in Psychology, 10*, 1413.

Stevenson, M. P., Schilhab, T., & Bentsen, P. (2018). Attention restoration theory II: A systematic review to clarify attention processes affected by exposure to natural environments. *Journal of Toxicology and Environmental Health, Part B*, 21, 227–268. doi:10.1080/10937404.2018.1505571

22   K.E. Schertz, K.L. Meidenbauer, and M.G. Berman

Tilt, J. H. (2010). Walking trips to parks: Exploring demographic, environmental factors, and preferences for adults with children in the household. *Preventive Medicine, 50*(Suppl 1), S69–S73.

Tsunetsugu, Y., Lee, J., Park, B.-J., Tyrväinen, L., Kagawa, T., & Miyazaki, Y. (2013). Physiological and psychological effects of viewing urban forest landscapes assessed by multiple measurements. *Landscape and Urban Planning, 113*, 90–93.

Turner, W. R., Nakamura, T., & Dinetti, M. (2004). Global urbanization and the separation of humans from nature. *Bioscience, 54*(6), 585–590.

Ulrich, R. S. (1983). Aesthetic and affective response to natural environment. In I. Altman & J. F. Wohlwill (Eds.), *Behavior and the Natural Environment* (pp. 85–125). Boston, MA: Springer US.

Ulrich, R. S. (1993). Biophilia, biophobia, and natural landscapes. *The Biophilia Hypothesis, 7*, 73–137.

Ulrich, R. S. (2002, April). Health benefits of gardens in hospitals. In Paper for conference, Plants for People International Exhibition Floriade (Vol. 17, No. 5, p. 2010). TX: College State.

Ulrich, R. S., Simons, R. F., Losito, B. D., Fiorito, E., Miles, M. A., & Zelson, M. (1991). Stress recovery during exposure to natural and urban environments. *Journal of Environmental Psychology, 11*(3), 201–230.

Valtchanov, D., Barton, K. R., & Ellard, C. (2010). Restorative effects of virtual nature settings. *Cyberpsychology, Behavior and Social Networking, 13*(5), 503–512.

Valtchanov, D., & Ellard, C. G. (2015). Cognitive and affective responses to natural scenes: Effects of low level visual properties on preference, cognitive load and eye-movements. *Journal of Environmental Psychology, 43*, 184–195.

van den Berg, A. E., & Custers, M. H. G. (2011). Gardening promotes neuroendo-crine and affective restoration from stress. *Journal of Health Psychology, 16*(1), 3–11.

van den Berg, A. E., Koole, S. L., & van der Wulp, N. Y. (2003). Environmental preference and restoration: (How) are they related? *Journal of Environmental Psychology, 23*(2), 135–146.

Watson, D., Clark, L. A., & Tellegen, A. (1988). Development and validation of brief measures of positive and negative affect: The PANAS scales. *Journal of Personality and Social Psychology, 54*(6), 1063–1070.

Watson, D., & Naragon-Gainey, K. (2010). On the specificity of positive emotional dysfunction in psychopathology: Evidence from the mood and anxiety disorders and schizophrenia/schizotypy. *Clinical Psychology Review, 30*(7), 839–848.

White, M., Smith, A., Humphryes, K., Pahl, S., Snelling, D., & Depledge, M. (2010). Blue space: The importance of water for preference, affect, and restorativeness ratings of natural and built scenes. *Journal of Environmental Psychology, 30*(4), 482–493.

Wichers, M., Peeters, F., Geschwind, N., Jacobs, N., Simons, C. J. P., Derom, C., … van Os, J. (2010). Unveiling patterns of affective responses in daily life may improve outcome prediction in depression: A momentary assessment study. *Journal of Affective Disorders, 124*(1–2), 191–195.

Zhang, J. W., Piff, P. K., Iyer, R., Koleva, S., & Keltner, D. (2014). An occasion for unselfing: Beautiful nature leads to prosociality. *Journal of Environmental Psychology, 37*, 61–72.

Zuckerman, M. (1977). Development of a situation-specific trait-state test for the prediction and measurement of affective responses. *Journal of Consulting and Clinical Psychology, 45*(4), 513–523.

3 Green Exercise as a Potential Treatment Strategy for Type 2 Diabetes

Matt Fraser

Green exercise research has most frequently focused on "healthy" participants. However, there are many specific populations for whom green exercise participation might be particularly useful. This chapter offers an initial discussion of green exercise in relation to type 2 diabetes. This condition, its associated comorbidities, current prevention, and treatment strategies are briefly outlined. Green exercise is then considered in relation to the prevention and management of type 2 diabetes, and some of its comorbidities, and issues that may be barriers to participation for this population are considered. Despite very few studies having yet been published on the effects of green exercise and type 2 diabetes, this chapter draws on a range of highly relevant and applicable literature in its consideration of this topic. In this way, it is intended that this chapter provokes further thoughts in relation to the application of green exercise for other specific health conditions.

3.1 Type 2 Diabetes, Comorbidities, Risk Factors, and Treatments

Type 2 diabetes is a chronic health condition that occurs when either the body does not produce enough insulin to regulate blood glucose or it does not effectively use the insulin produced (World Health Organization, 2020). The disease can occur as a result of nonchangeable factors such as genetics and ethnicity, but also more changeable factors such as poor diet and a sedentary lifestyle (Zheng, Ley & Hu, 2018). Type 2 diabetes accounts for 90–95% of diabetes cases worldwide (American Diabetes Association, 2020). Current figures from the International Diabetes Federation show that in 2019, 9.3% of adults (20–79 years old) were living with diabetes (overwhelmingly type 2 diabetes). If current trends continue by the year 2030, 578 million people will be living with diabetes and by the year 2045, this figure will have increased to 700 million. For further information including prevalence and costs, statistics, epidemiology and pathology of type 2 diabetes, visit the websites of the International Diabetes Federation and the World Health Organization.

DOI: 10.4324/9781003154419-4

24 *M. Fraser*

Comorbidities of type 2 diabetes range from disturbances in metabolism and organ damage to cardiovascular diseases such as atherosclerosis, cardiomyopathy and hypertension. Other issues include retinopathy and foot ulceration, which can make conducting regular physical activity challenging (Colberg, 2017). In addition to the physical complications, type 2 diabetes is often associated with experiencing psychological stress (Madhu et al., 2019), depression (Fisher et al., 2008), reduced quality of life and psychological wellbeing (Hadjiconstantinou et al., 2016; Trikkalinou, Papazafiropoulou & Melidonis, 2017) and anxiety (Chaturvedi et al., 2019). Moreover, Nouwen et al. (2019) highlight that as a result of depressive symptoms, individuals living with type 2 diabetes can exhibit reduced self-care and increases in negative physical health-related outcomes (de Groot et al., 2001), and thus greater mortality rates are evident (Zhang et al., 2005).

The highest risk factor for the development of type 2 diabetes is obesity (Belkina & Denis, 2010). Other risk factors include family history, race, dietary factors, air pollution and lifestyle factors such as smoking, alcohol consumption and physical activity and inactivity levels (Bellou et al., 2018). The most widely-used treatments to minimize negative health impacts of type 2 diabetes are consumption of a balanced diet, calorie restriction, physical activity and medication (American Diabetes Association, 2020). Many treatments target reductions in plasma glucose and body fat, so to delay the onset of diabetes-related comorbidities (American Diabetes Association, 2020).

3.2 Physical Activity and Type 2 Diabetes

Physical activity, which is inversely related to BMI (Schmidt et al., 2015) – the measure by which obesity is most commonly identified, can result in a 30–50% reduction in likelihood of developing type 2 diabetes (Wu et al., 2014). Improved glucose tolerance and weight loss are prominent mechanisms underpinning this (Telford, 2007). However, Nolan, Damm and Prentki (2011) note that adherence to physical activity interventions outside of clinical trials is low. Current global diabetes physical activity guidelines recommend at least 150 minutes a week of moderate (50–70% maximum heart rate) to vigorous (> 70% maximum heart rate) exercise to contribute to ongoing management of the disease (Colberg et al., 2010). Hamasaki (2016) highlights that these recommendations can be a burden to many individuals living with type 2 diabetes because of their lower physical performance threshold compared to healthy individuals, in terms of physical capability and fatigue; which may lead to nonadherence to physical activity.

Physical activity completed as part of diabetes treatment often takes place indoors, with resistance training and gym prescriptions most commonly employed (Williams et al., 2020). The stable indoor exercise environment has been shown to promote individuals' focus on internal cues such as heart rate or breathing (Goode & Roth, 1993), leading to boredom (Calogiuri, Nordtug & Weydahl, 2015) and reduced motivation (Fraser, Munoz & MacRury, 2019). Comparatively, research has shown that individuals can exercise at a greater intensity whilst perceiving the activity as easier, in outdoor, nature-based environments (Brown & Stanforth, 2017; Rogerson et al., 2016). This is an important finding toward increasing exercise behaviors of individuals living with type 2 diabetes, as Korkiakangas, Alahuhta and Laitinen (2009) highlight that individuals living with type 2 diabetes often lack the required motivation to adhere to new physical activity interventions; and research across the past 15 years has hinted toward a pathway linking exercise intensity to intentions for future exercise behaviors, via affective responses (Lee, Emerson & Williams, 2016). Summarizing, these outlined effects of green exercise in promoting adherence to regular physical activity can play a key role in prevention and treatment of type 2 diabetes via obesity reductions.

As one of the prominent treatments for managing type 2 diabetes, findings in relation to the influences of physical activity on psychological comorbidities of type 2 diabetes have been mixed. A systematic review by Van der Heijden et al. (2013) found statistically significant effects on quality of life in only one of sixteen investigated studies. From four depression studies, only one showed an improvement. Two from four studies into general wellbeing found significant positive effects and in the only study to examine anxiety, a significant improvement was found. Another review by Cai et al. (2017) concluded that aerobic activity was a safe and effective way to improve the quality of life of those living with type 2 diabetes. Both reviews failed to identify which elements of exercise contributed most to positive results. Across many reviews of this kind, the factor of the environment where exercise is performed is largely overlooked. In an initial step to address this, Fraser et al. (2019) reviewed the reported effects of exercise interventions specifically performed in outdoor areas, on the mental health of individuals living with type 2 diabetes. Only four studies met the inclusion criteria and there were mixed findings for depression, quality of life, and wellbeing. Two hundred and thirty-one (231) participants were sampled across the four studies and each intervention utilized a form of walking. An issue identified by the review was the limited description of the environments where the exercise took place. Two studies included in the review investigated Nordic walking (Gram et al., 2010; Fritz et al., 2011); however, little to no significant effects were found in either study following a 4-month intervention, and in the study by Gram et al. (2010), a year follow-up found no significant effects. Positive effects were found by Guglani, Shenoy and Sandhu (2014) for 16 of 19 quality of life subscales and general wellbeing, following a 4-month intervention. Finally, in a study by Delevatti et al. (2018), no significant effects were found for depression, however physical and psychological measures of quality of life were significantly improved following a dry land training intervention.

3.3 Green Exercise, Exercise Adherence, and Vitamin D for Type 2 Diabetes

Here, the combination of physical activity conducted in nature should boost prevention and management of type 2 diabetes, as research has reported greater adherence to green exercise than to exercise conducted indoors (Lacharité-Lemieux, Brunelle & Dionne, 2015).

Creating enjoyable experiences is paramount in promoting uptake and adherence to physical activity (Calogiuri & Chroni, 2014). Previous research has shown adherence to long-term physical activity programmes is typically low in type 2 diabetics, although it varies from 10–80% (Praet & van Loon, 2009). Praet and van Loon (2009) state that those living with type 2 diabetes find it challenging to adhere to activities which are not preferred. When considered that regular physical activity is essential to treatment and management of the condition, identifying activities that individuals enjoy will promote uptake and adherence.

To this point, research has shown exercise conducted in natural areas to often be more enjoyable in comparison to indoor and artificial exercise environments (Lahart et al., 2019). For individuals who do not frequently visit natural areas, greater levels of enjoyment occur from factors including escapism from everyday routines, the social aspect provided through such environments and the entertainment value from the unpredictable stimuli from nature (Gladwell et al., 2013). Green exercise has also been found to increase levels of mood and positive affect following a session (Thompson Coon et al., 2011). Activities that increase positive affect can close the intention–behavior gap which is important in undertaking exercise (Ekkekakis, Hall & Petruzzello, 2004). Moreover, positive changes in affect during exercise have been found to be predictive of self-efficacy, enjoyment, long-term motivation for adherence to exercise (Kwan & Bryan, 2010), and is positively linked to future exercise behaviors (Rhodes & Kates, 2015). Another aspect by which green exercise can function well for type 2 diabetes patients is that of the social experience. Work by Rogerson et al. (2016) found that compared to indoor exercise settings, outdoor environments promote greater levels of social interaction during exercise, and that social interaction was a significant predictor of intention to repeat green space exercise behaviors, but this was not the case for indoor exercise. This suggests the importance of the social aspect that green exercise can promote, which should be an important consideration when designing physical activity as a preventative or prescribed treatment to ameliorate diabetes.

Of course, as part of green exercise participation, the exercise functions as a vehicle for attaining other salutogenic benefits of nature environments (Rogerson et al., 2019). Research has demonstrated that vitamin D can improve the body's sensitivity to insulin (Teegarden & Donkin, 2009) and there is moderate evidence that recreational sun exposure is associated with a reduced risk of developing type 2 diabetes (Shore-Lorenti et al.,

2014). Safe exposure to sunlight for those already living with diabetes can be a cost-effective therapy to help manage the condition. Further research is required to confirm the effects of vitamin D in managing diabetes, but the combination of exercise and concurrent exposure to sunlight, as green exercise often offers, is an interesting topic for further investigation.

3.4 Green Exercise and Comorbidities of Type 2 Diabetes

Where evidence from type 2 diabetes samples is still currently lacking, findings from research sampling "healthy" participants suggest green exercise to be an effective modality to manage the previously outlined psychological comorbidities of type 2 diabetes. Green exercise has been shown to reduce stress (Rogerson et al., 2016; Wooller et al., 2018), self-reported depression (Bodin & Hartig, 2003; Glover & Polley, 2019; Townsend, 2006), and anxiety (Lawton et al., 2017; Martyn & Brymer, 2016), whilst improving quality of life and wellbeing (Klaperski et al., 2019; Rogerson et al., 2020).

Green exercise research has begun sampling participants living with other specific health conditions and a review by Wendelboe-Nelson et al. (2019) reported that 70% of the included studies found a positive health-related outcome from green space interventions (many of which could be considered to be green exercise) in a range of participants from healthy individuals *and* those living with mental health conditions and other disabilities. Chun, Chang and Lee (2017) examined individuals living with chronic effects of strokes. Participants assigned to a forest exercise condition experienced significant reductions in anxiety and depression in comparison to the group assigned to an urban condition. Further, Sonntag-Öström et al. (2014) noted that visits to forest environments were perceived as more restorative than urban city environments in females living with exhaustion disorder. However, whilst Askari et al. (2017) demonstrated exercise-associated improvements in affective, cognitive, or somatic measures in individuals living with depression, there were no statistically significant differences in these outcomes, between indoor and green exercise conditions. Similar to research that has focused on "healthy" participants, despite no specific green exercise research yet having sampled individuals living with type 2 diabetes, the initial research into the efficacies of green exercise for individuals living with *other* specific health conditions offers food for thought in relation to some of the aforementioned associated comorbidities.

3.5 Forms of Green Exercise for Type 2 Diabetes and Barriers to Participation

Walking is the most common form of green exercise examined in the literature (Lahart et al., 2019). Epidemiological studies have suggested that walking is associated with a reduced risk of type 2 diabetes (Hamasaki, 2016). However, there are a range of other activities that can be considered to be

28   M. Fraser

green exercise. Interventions cited in the literature include green gyms (Nałęcz, Ostrowska-Tryzno & Pawlikowska-Piechotka, 2018), community gardening (participants plant trees, dig beds, etc.) (Draper & Freedman, 2010), care farms, and horticultural therapy (Murray et al., 2019). These activities can be conducted by a range of capabilities and ages. For some, identifying activities that individuals find enjoyable or remove the thought of "doing" physical activity may prove to be the most effective. Indeed, aside from walking and other typically aerobic, traditional exercise modes, research has also shown that resistance training improves physiological parameters such as glycemic control and muscle substrate metabolism, and mental health parameters, in type 2 diabetics (Pesta et al., 2017; Ramirez & Kravitz, 2012). Traditionally, the majority of resistance training is undertaken indoors; however, it would be interesting to consider the effects of resistance training in the form of "green gym" activities, which are becoming increasingly popular and available in public areas, for both the general public and more specifically, those living with long-term health conditions such as type 2 diabetes. It should also be considered that the increasing number of outdoor green gyms can be engaged with free of charge and thus are more inclusive and accessible to the public, especially as finance has been identified as a barrier to conducting physical activity (Salmon et al., 2003).

Additionally to being associated with obesity, which brings both perceived and real challenges and risks to exercise participation, type 2 diabetes is most common in older adults (Rashedi et al., 2017). This brings additional challenges in finding accessible forms of green exercise to engage in. The Ecological Dynamics Theory (Brymer, Davids & Mallabon, 2014) describes that natural settings help provide affordances for more diverse physical, psychological, and social exercise experiences, compared to indoor or urban environments. However, as functional affordances are the result of characteristics of both the environment and the individual, these affordances can be altered by complications associated with the disease such as pain, fear of hypoglycaemia, or a coexisting disease (Colberg, 2017). There are a number of possible reasons why to date, green exercise interventions have been largely underutilized in the treatment of type 2 diabetes. Exercise can induce hypoglycaemia, which can make exercise in relatively more remote rural areas or nature environments, such as a forest, a safety concern. Additionally, as indicated earlier in this chapter, diabetes brings increased likelihood of hypertension, retinopathy, and foot ulceration. As well as making conducting regular physical activity more challenging, it also makes it more risky. More generally, the terrain and topography of the environments can be a barrier for many, as it can lead to complications such as foot ulcerations or musculoskeletal injuries (Riddell & Burr, 2011). This is perhaps where green exercise's other, "less traditional" exercise forms, mentioned earlier in this section, can be particularly useful for this population. These are important considerations when designing new policies to manage type 2 diabetes. Green exercise can be conducted all year round in a vast range of natural areas. Individuals living with or without type 2 diabetes should look to incorporate regular forms of green exercise or activities into their everyday lifestyle. Activities such as nature walks, cycles or jogs in forests, beaches, public parks or trails, are a great way to enhance health, although additional diabetes-related safety issues should be prepared for, for example, packing adequate sources of sugar or medication.

Virtual nature, or bringing nature experiences indoors, is one interesting approach to address such barriers experienced by individuals living with type 2 diabetes. This would be particularly useful for individuals living with type 2 diabetes who have mobility issues, reduced muscular strength or associated disabilities, which are particularly common in older and obese adults living with the disease (Rejeski et al., 2012), as these comorbidities often prevent them regularly visiting natural areas. Many studies have examined virtual green exercise experiences – either showing images or videos of nature on a screen during exercise, or more recently, using virtual reality headsets. Compared to other virtual environments (typically of urban settings), viewing nature during exercise boosts positive affect and reduced levels of stress (Valtchanov, Barton & Ellard, 2010), which can help ameliorate psychological comorbidities of type 2 diabetes. Chapter 10 in this book further discusses virtual nature experiences.

This chapter provides a number of insights into the relevance of green exercise for the prevention and management of a specific health condition – type 2 diabetes and its comorbidities. Examples included better adherence to physical activity through increased enjoyment, mood and affect, and social opportunities, specific psychological comorbidities, and benefits of exposure to vitamin D. Although there is already clear merit for public health bodies to promote green exercise for prevention of type 2 diabetes, it seems likely that more research focusing specifically on this cohort is required before health practitioners and policymakers more widely endorse prescription of green exercise (rather than exercise per se) to directly manage pre-existing type 2 diabetes.

References

American Diabetes Association, 2020. 2. *Classification and diagnosis of diabetes: Standards of medical care in diabetes—2020. Diabetes Care, 43*(Supplement 1), pp. S14–S31. DOI: https://doi.org/10.2337/dc20-S002

Askari, J., Saberi-Kakhki, A., Taheri, H. and Yassini, S. M., 2017. *The effect of aerobic indoor exercise compared with green exercise on different symptoms of depression: An investigation of psychological mediators of stress and coping. Open Journal of Medical Psychology, 6*(3), pp. 197–212. DOI: 10.4236/ojmp.2017.63016

Belkina, A. C. and Denis, G. V., 2010. *Obesity genes and insulin resistance. Current opinion in endocrinology, diabetes, and obesity, 17*(5), p. 472. DOI: 10.1097/MED.0b013e32833c5c48

30   M. Fraser

Bellou, V., Belbasis, L., Tzoulaki, I. and Evangelou, E. (2018). *Risk factors for type 2 diabetes mellitus: An exposure-wide umbrella review of meta-analyses. PLOS ONE, 13*(3), e0194127.

Bodin, M. and Hartig, T., 2003. *Does the outdoor environment matter for psychological restoration gained through running?. Psychology of Sport and Exercise, 4*(2), pp. 141–153. DOI: https://doi.org/10.1016/S1469-0292(01)00038-3

Brown, K. and Stanforth, D., 2017. *Go green with outdoor activity. ACSM's Health & Fitness Journal, 21*(1), pp. 10–15. DOI: 10.1249/FIT.0000000000000264

Brymer, E., Davids, K. and Mallabon, L., 2014. *Understanding the psychological health and well-being benefits of physical activity in nature: An ecological dynamics analysis. Ecopsychology, 6*(3), pp. 189–197. DOI: http://doi.org/10.1089/eco.2013.0110

Cai, H., Li, G., Zhang, P., Xu, D. and Chen, L., 2017. *Effect of exercise on the quality of life in type 2 diabetes mellitus: A systematic review. Quality of Life Research, 26*(3), pp. 515–530. DOI: https://doi.org/10.1007/s11136-016-1481-5

Calogiuri, G. and Chroni, S., 2014. *The impact of the natural environment on the promotion of active living: An integrative systematic review. BMC Public Health, 14*(1), p. 873. DOI: https://doi.org/10.1186/1471-2458-14-873

Calogiuri, G., Nordtug, H. and Weydahl, A., 2015. *The potential of using exercise in nature as an intervention to enhance exercise behavior: Results from a pilot study. Perceptual and Motor Skills, 121*(2), pp. 350–370. DOI: https://doi.org/10.2466/06. PMS.121c17x0

Chaturvedi, S. K., Gowda, S. M., Ahmed, H. U., Alosaimi, F. D., Andreone, N., Bobrov, A., Bulgari, V., Carrà, G., Castelnuovo, G., de Girolamo, G. and Gondek, T., 2019. *More anxious than depressed: Prevalence and correlates in a 15-nation study of anxiety disorders in people with type 2 diabetes mellitus. General Psychiatry, 32*(4). DOI: 10.1136/gpsych-2019-100076

Chun, M. H., Chang, M. C. and Lee, S. J., 2017. *The effects of forest therapy on depression and anxiety in patients with chronic stroke. International Journal of Neuroscience, 127*(3), pp. 199–203. DOI: https://doi.org/10.3109/00207454.2016.1170015

Colberg, S. R., 2017. *Key points from the updated guidelines on exercise and diabetes. Frontiers in Endocrinology, 8*, p. 33. DOI: https://doi.org/10.3389/fendo.2017.00033

Colberg, S. R., Sigal, R. J., Fernhall, B., Regensteiner, J. G., Blissmer, B. J., Rubin, R. R., Chasan-Taber, L., Albright, A. L. and Braun, B., 2010. *Exercise and type 2 diabetes: The American College of Sports Medicine and the American Diabetes Association: Joint position statement. Diabetes Care, 33*(12), pp. e147–e167. DOI: https://doi.org/10.2337/dc10-9990

de Groot, M., Anderson, R., Freedland, K. E., Clouse, R. E. and Lustman, P. J., 2001. *Association of depression and diabetes complications: A meta-analysis. Psychosomatic Medicine, 63*(4), pp. 619–630. DOI: https://www.diabetes.co.uk/cost-of-diabetes.html

Gladwell, V. F., Brown, D. K., Wood, C., Sandercock, G. R., & Barton, J. L., 2013. *The great outdoors: how a green exercise environment can benefit all. Extreme physiology & medicine, 2*(1), pp. 1–7.

Delevatti, R. S., Schuch, F. B., Kanitz, A. C., Alberton, C. L., Marson, E. C., Lisboa, S. C., Pinho, C. D. F., Bregagnol, L. P., Becker, M. T. and Kruel, L. F. M., 2018. *Quality of life and sleep quality are similarly improved after aquatic or dry-land aerobic training in patients with type 2 diabetes: A randomized clinical trial. Journal of Science and Medicine in Sport, 21*(5), pp. 483–488. DOI: https://doi.org/10.1016/j.jsams.2017.08.024

Draper, C. and Freedman, D., 2010. *Review and analysis of the benefits, purposes, and motivations associated with community gardening in the United States. Journal of Community Practice, 18*(4), pp. 458–492. DOI: https://doi.org/10.1080/1070542 2.2010.519682

Ekelund, U., Griffin, S. J. and Wareham, N. J., 2007. *Physical activity and metabolic risk in individuals with a family history of type 2 diabetes. Diabetes Care, 30*(2), pp. 337–342. DOI: https://doi.org/10.2337/dc06-1883

Ekkekakis, P., Hall, E. E. and Petruzzello, S. J., 2004. *Practical markers of the transition from aerobic to anaerobic metabolism during exercise: Rationale and a case for affect-based exercise prescription. Preventive Medicine, 38*(2), pp. 149–159. DOI: https://doi. org/10.1016/j.ypmed.2003.09.038

Fisher, L., Skaff, M. M., Mullan, J. T., Arean, P., Glasgow, R. and Masharani, U., 2008. *A longitudinal study of affective and anxiety disorders, depressive affect and diabetes distress in adults with type 2 diabetes. Diabetic Medicine, 25*(9), pp. 1096–1101. DOI: https://doi.org/10.1111/j.1464-5491.2008.02533.x

Fraser, M., Munoz, S. A. and MacRury, S., 2019. *What motivates participants to adhere to green exercise?. International Journal of Environmental Research and Public Health, 16*(10), p. 1832. DOI: https://doi.org/10.3390/ijerph16101832

Fraser, M., Polson, R., Munoz, S. A. and MacRury, S., 2019. *Psychological effects of outdoor activity in type 2 diabetes: A review. Health Promotion International.* daz064, https://doi.org/10.1093/heapro/daz064

Fritz, T., Caidahl, K., Osler, M., Östenson, C. G., Zierath, J. R. and Wändell, P., 2011. *Effects of Nordic walking on health-related quality of life in overweight individuals with type 2 diabetes mellitus, impaired or normal glucose tolerance. Diabetic Medicine, 28*(11), pp. 1362–1372. DOI: https://doi.org/10.1111/j.1464-5491.2011.03348.x

Glover, N. and Polley, S., 2019. *Going green: The effectiveness of a 40-day green exercise intervention for insufficiently active adults. Sports, 7*(6), p. 142. DOI: https://doi. org/10.3390/sports7060142

Goode, K. T. and Roth, D. L., 1993. *Factor analysis of cognitions during running: Association with mood change. Journal of Sport and Exercise Psychology, 15*(4), pp. 375–389. DOI: https://doi.org/10.1123/jsep.15.4.375

Gram, B., Christensen, R., Christiansen, C. and Gram, J., 2010. *Effects of Nordic walking and exercise in type 2 diabetes mellitus: A randomized controlled trial. Clinical Journal of Sport Medicine, 20*(5), pp. 355–361. DOI: 10.1227/ NEU.0b013e3181e56e0a

Guglani, R., Shenoy, S. and Sandhu, J. S., 2014. *Effect of progressive pedometer based walking intervention on quality of life and general well being among patients with type 2 diabetes. Journal of Diabetes & Metabolic Disorders, 13*(1), p. 110. DOI: https://doi. org/10.1186/s40200-014-0110-5

Hadjiconstantinou, M., Byrne, J., Bodicoat, D. H., Robertson, N., Eborall, H., Khunti, K. and Davies, M. J., 2016. *Do web-based interventions improve well-being in type 2 diabetes? A systematic review and meta-analysis. Journal of Medical Internet Research, 18*(10), p. e270. DOI: 10.2196/jmir.5991

Hamasaki, H., 2016. *Daily physical activity and type 2 diabetes: A review. World Journal of Diabetes, 7*(12), p. 243. DOI: 10.4239/wjd.v7.i12.243

Klaperski, S., Koch, E., Hewel, D., Schempp, A. and Müller, J., 2019. *Optimizing mental health benefits of exercise: The influence of the exercise environment on acute stress levels and wellbeing. Mental Health & Prevention, 15*, p. 200173. DOI: https://doi. org/10.1016/j.mhp.2019.200173

32 M. Fraser

Korkiakangas, E. E., Alahuhta, M. A. and Laitinen, J. H., 2009. *Barriers to regular exercise among adults at high risk or diagnosed with type 2 diabetes: A systematic review.* Health Promotion International, 24(4), pp. 416–427. DOI: https://doi.org/10.1093/heapro/dap031

Kwan, B. M. and Bryan, A. D., 2010. *Affective response to exercise as a component of exercise motivation: Attitudes, norms, self-efficacy, and temporal stability of intentions.* Psychology of Sport and Exercise, 11(1), pp. 71–79. DOI: https://doi.org/10.1016/j.psychsport.2009.05.010

Lacharité-Lemieux, M., Brunelle, J. P. and Dionne, I. J., 2015. *Adherence to exercise and affective responses: Comparison between outdoor and indoor training.* Menopause, 22(7), pp. 731–740. DOI: 10.1097/GME.0000000000000366

Lahart, I., Darcy, P., Gidlow, C. and Calogiuri, G., 2019. *The effects of green exercise on physical and mental wellbeing: A systematic review.* International Journal of Environmental Research and Public Health, 16(8), p. 1352. DOI: https://doi.org/10.3390/ijerph16081352

Lawton, E., Brymer, E., Clough, P. and Denovan, A., 2017. *The relationship between the physical activity environment, nature relatedness, anxiety, and the psychological wellbeing benefits of regular exercisers.* Frontiers in Psychology, 8, p. 1058. DOI: https://doi.org/10.3389/fpsyg.2017.01058

Lee, H. H., Emerson, J. A. and Williams, D. M. (2016). *The exercise–affect–adherence pathway: An evolutionary perspective.* Frontiers in Psychology, 7(1285). DOI: 10.3389/fpsyg.2016.01285

Madhu, S. V., Siddiqui, A., Desai, N. G., Sharma, S. B. and Bansal, A. K., 2019. *Chronic stress, sense of coherence and risk of type 2 diabetes mellitus.* Diabetes & Metabolic Syndrome: Clinical Research & Reviews, 13(1), pp. 18–23. DOI: https://doi.org/10.1016/j.dsx.2018.08.004

Martyn, P. and Brymer, E., 2016. *The relationship between nature relatedness and anxiety.* Journal of Health Psychology, 21(7), pp. 1436–1445. DOI: https://doi.org/10.1177/1359105314555169

Murray, J., Wickramasekera, N., Elings, M., Bragg, R., Brennan, C., Richardson, Z., Wright, J., Llorente, M. G., Cade, J., Shickle, D. and Tubeuf, S., 2019. *The impact of care farms on quality of life, depression and anxiety among different population groups: A systematic review.* Campbell Systematic Reviews, 15(4), p. e1061. DOI: https://doi.org/10.1002/cl2.1061

Nałęcz, H., Ostrowska-Tryzno, A. and Pawlikowska-Piechotka, A., 2018. *Outdoor gyms as an example of outdoor recreation activity in urbanized areas.* Turyzm, 28(1), pp. 65–71. DOI: https://doi.org/10.2478/tour-2018-0008

Nolan, C. J., Damm, P. and Prentki, M., 2011. *Type 2 diabetes across generations: From pathophysiology to prevention and management.* The Lancet, 378(9786), pp. 169–181. DOI: https://doi.org/10.1016/S0140-6736(11)60614-4

Nouwen, A., Adriaanse, M. C., van Dam, K., Iversen, M. M., Viechtbauer, W., Peyrot, M., Caramlau, I., Kokoszka, A., Kanc, K., de Groot, M. and Nefs, G., 2019. *Longitudinal associations between depression and diabetes complications: A systematic review and meta-analysis.* Diabetic Medicine, 36(12), pp. 1562–1572. DOI: https://doi.org/10.1111/dme.14054

Pesta, D. H., Goncalves, R. L., Madiraju, A. K., Strasser, B. and Sparks, L. M., 2017. *Resistance training to improve type 2 diabetes: Working toward a prescription for the future.* Nutrition & Metabolism, 14(1), p. 24. DOI: https://doi.org/10.1186/s12986-017-0173-7

Praet, S. F. and van Loon, L. J., 2009. *Exercise therapy in type 2 diabetes. Acta Diabetologica,* 46(4), pp. 263–278. DOI: 10.1007/s00592-009-0129-0

Ramirez, A. and Kravitz, L., 2012. *Resistance training improves mental health. IDEA Fitness Journal,* 9(1), pp. 20–22.

Rashedi, V., Asadi-Lari, M., Delbari, A., Fadayevatan, R., Borhaninejad, V. and Foroughan, M., 2017. *Prevalence of diabetes type 2 in older adults: Findings from a large population-based survey in Tehran, Iran (Urban HEART-2). Diabetes & Metabolic Syndrome: Clinical Research & Reviews,* 11, pp. S347–S350. DOI: https://doi.org/10.1016/j.dsx.2017.03.014

Rejeski, W. J., Ip, E. H., Bertoni, A. G., Bray, G. A., Evans, G., Gregg, E. W. and Zhang, Q., 2012. *Lifestyle change and mobility in obese adults with type 2 diabetes. New England Journal of Medicine,* 366(13), pp. 1209–1217. DOI: 10.1056/NEJMoa1110294

Rhodes, R. E. and Kates, A., 2015. *Can the affective response to exercise predict future motives and physical activity behavior? A systematic review of published evidence. Annals of Behavioral Medicine,* 49(5), pp. 715–731. DOI: https://doi.org/10.1007/s12160-015-9704-5

Riddell, M. C. and Burr, J., 2011. *Evidence-based risk assessment and recommendations for physical activity clearance: Diabetes mellitus and related comorbidities. Applied Physiology, Nutrition, and Metabolism,* 36(S1), pp. S154–S189. DOI: https://doi.org/10.1139/h11-063

Rogerson, M., Brown, D. K., Sandercock, G., Wooller, J. J. and Barton, J., 2016. *A comparison of four typical green exercise environments and prediction of psychological health outcomes. Perspectives in Public Health,* 136(3), pp. 171–180. DOI: https://doi.org/10.1177/1757913915589845

Rogerson, M., Colbeck, I., Bragg, R., Dosumu, A. and Griffin, M., 2020. *Affective outcomes of group versus lone green exercise participation. International Journal of Environmental Research and Public Health,* 17(2), p. 624. DOI: https://doi.org/10.3390/ijerph17020624

Rogerson, M., Gladwell, V. F., Gallagher, D. J. and Barton, J. L., 2016. *Influences of green outdoors versus indoors environmental settings on psychological and social outcomes of controlled exercise. International Journal of Environmental Research and Public Health,* 13(4), p. 363. DOI: https://doi.org/10.3390/ijerph13040363

Salmon, J., Owen, N., Crawford, D., Bauman, A. and Sallis, J. F., 2003. *Physical activity and sedentary behavior: A population-based study of barriers, enjoyment, and preference. Health Psychology,* 22(2), p. 178. DOI: https://doi.org/10.1037/0278-6133.22.2.178

Schmidt, F. M., Weschenfelder, J., Sander, C., Minkwitz, J., Thormann, J., Chittka, T., … Stumvoll, M. (2015). *Inflammatory cytokines in general and central obesity and modulating effects of physical activity. PLOS ONE,* 10(3), e0121971.

Shore-Lorenti, C., Brennan, S. L., Sanders, K. M., Neale, R. E., Lucas, R. M. and Ebeling, P. R., 2014. *Shining the light on sunshine: A systematic review of the influence of sun exposure on type 2 diabetes mellitus-related outcomes. Clinical endocrinology,* 81(6), pp. 799–811. DOI: https://doi.org/10.1111/cen.12567

Sonntag-Öström, E., Nordin, M., Lundell, Y., Dolling, A., Wiklund, U., Karlsson, M., Carlberg, B. and Järvholm, L. S., 2014. *Restorative effects of visits to urban and forest environments in patients with exhaustion disorder. Urban Forestry & Urban Greening,* 13(2), pp. 344–354. DOI: https://doi.org/10.1016/j.ufug.2013.12.007

Teegarden, D. and Donkin, S. S., 2009. *Vitamin D: Emerging new roles in insulin sensitivity. Nutrition Research Reviews,* 22(1), pp. 82–92. DOI: https://doi.org/10.1017/S0954422409389301

34 M. Fraser

Telford, R. D., 2007. *Low physical activity and obesity: Causes of chronic disease or simply predictors?*. Medicine & Science in Sports & Exercise, 39(8), pp. 1233–1240. DOI: 10.1249/mss.0b013e31806215b7

Thompson Coon, J., Boddy, K., Stein, K., Whear, R., Barton, J., & Depledge, M. H., 2011. *Does participating in physical activity in outdoor natural environments have a greater effect on physical and mental wellbeing than physical activity indoors? A systematic review.* Environmental science & technology, 45(5), 1761–1772.

Townsend, M., 2006. *Feel blue? Touch green! Participation in forest/woodland management as a treatment for depression.* Urban Forestry & Urban Greening, 5(3), pp. 111–120. DOI: https://doi.org/10.1016/j.ufug.2006.02.001

Trikkalinou, A., Papazafiropoulou, A. K. and Melidonis, A. (2017). *Type 2 diabetes and quality of life.* World Journal of Diabetes, 8(4), 120. DOI: 10.4239/wjd.v8.i4.120

Valtchanov, D., Barton, K. R. and Ellard, C., 2010. *Restorative effects of virtual nature settings.* Cyberpsychology, Behavior, and Social Networking, 13(5), pp. 503–512. DOI: https://doi.org/10.1089/cyber.2009.0308

Van der Heijden, M. M. P., van Dooren, F. E., Pop, V. J. M. and Pouwer, F., 2013. *Effects of exercise training on quality of life, symptoms of depression, symptoms of anxiety and emotional well-being in type 2 diabetes mellitus: a systematic review.* Diabetologia, 56(6), pp. 1210–1225. DOI: https://doi.org/10.1007/s00125-013-2871-7

Wendelboe-Nelson, C., Kelly, S., Kennedy, M. and Cherrie, J. W., 2019. *A scoping review mapping research on green space and associated mental health benefits.* International Journal of Environmental Research and Public Health, 16(12), p. 2081. DOI: https://doi.org/10.3390/ijerph16122081

Williams, A., Radford, J., O'Brien, J. and Davison, K., 2020. *Type 2 diabetes and the medicine of exercise: The role of general practice in ensuring exercise is part of every patient's plan.* Australian Journal of General Practice, 49(4), p. 189.

Wooller, J. J., Rogerson, M., Barton, J., Micklewright, D. and Gladwell, V., 2018. *Can simulated green exercise improve recovery from acute mental stress?*. Frontiers in Psychology, 9, p. 2167. DOI: https://doi.org/10.3389/fpsyg.2018.02167

World Health Organization, 2020. *Diabetes.* [Viewed 1 June 2020]. Available from: https://www.who.int/news-room/fact-sheets/detail/diabetes

Wu, Y., Ding, Y., Tanaka, Y. and Zhang, W., 2014. *Risk factors contributing to type 2 diabetes and recent advances in the treatment and prevention.* International Journal of Medical Sciences, 11(11), p. 1185. DOI: 10.7150/ijms.10001

Zhang, X., Norris, S. L., Gregg, E. W., Cheng, Y. J., Beckles, G. and Kahn, H. S., 2005. *Depressive symptoms and mortality among persons with and without diabetes.* American Journal of Epidemiology, 161(7), pp. 652–660. DOI: https://doi.org/10.1093/aje/kwi089

Zheng, Y., Ley, S. H. and Hu, F. B., 2018. *Global aetiology and epidemiology of type 2 diabetes mellitus and its complications.* Nature Reviews Endocrinology, 14(2), p. 88. DOI: https://doi.org/10.1038/nrendo.2017.151

4 Green Exercise: Actively Flourishing in Nature

Otis Geddes and Holli-Anne Passmore

4.1 Green Exercise: Actively Flourishing in Nature

For the majority of human existence, physical activity was a necessity. Physical activity was simply embedded within our daily lives; moreover, this activity largely occurred outdoors. The landscape of physical activity has changed. Nowadays, if people do build physical exercise into their day, this exercise generally occurs indoors – running on treadmills, "spinning" on stationary exercise bikes (Schriever, 2018). For the bulk of urbanite humans, a sedentary lifestyle, largely spent indoors, is the norm. The number of people who are physically active today is smaller than ever: less than 5% of American adults participate in 30 minutes of physical activity every day (U.S. Department of Health & Human Services, 2017). This decline in physical activity is one aspect of larger cultural shifts in how we live.

In a breakdown of what they call "Anthropocene syndrome," Prescott and Logan (2017) discuss how the modern age has brought about rapid urbanization, gross disturbance of the environment, and a transformation of the places we live in. Their work addresses the phenomenon of "grey space," areas filled to the brim with mass advertising, fast-food, and convenience and liquor stores. The implications of Anthropocene syndrome are many, encompassing rises in obesity (Hurt et al., 2010), heart disease (Benjamin et al., 2019), and depression (Curtin et al., 2016). Equally worrying are rises in feelings of meaninglessness (Softas-Nall & Woody, 2017) and self-reported anxiety (Pitchforth et al., 2019). To address these issues, it has been suggested that our future necessitates movement into the "Symbiocene" – an epoch of reintegration into nature – psychologically and technologically (Prescott & Logan, 2017). In line with this, an urgent call has been made for innovative strategies to improve public health and both physical and mental well-being, close the health inequality gap, and alleviate the financial burden currently facing health services (Robinson & Breed, 2019). We present Green Exercise – being active in "green" or natural places – as one such innovative strategy with the potential to effectively answer this call. Indeed, a host of synergistic health benefits arise from green exercise; together, physical activity and nature are more than the sum of their parts (Barton et al., 2016; Shanahan et al., 2016).

DOI: 10.4324/9781003154419-5

36   O. Geddes and H.-A. Passmore

At its core, this chapter is about the relationship between humans and nature, which has implications for how we view and conduct green exercise.[1] As Antal and Drews (2015) describe, we need to shift the way we talk about nature, away from instrumental and mechanistic terms (which emphasize separateness between humans and nature), and toward talking about nature in terms of interpersonal relationships. Such framing avoids rationalizing and shunning responsibility when it comes to our relationship to nature. Such a shift may also be instrumental in the promotion of green exercise; reframing our view of nature in terms of an interpersonal relationship may make us more interested in interacting actively with our "partner."

For example, Brooks and colleagues (2006) used the relationship/partner metaphor to analyze how visitors to Rocky Mountain National Park formed long-term relationships to the park. They concluded that such long-term relationships become inseparable from a person's relationship with, or sense of value of, the concept of wilderness. It appears there is a bidirectional influence of our attitudes toward nature and our interaction with nature, including green exercise – wherein our attitudes toward nature influence our participation in green exercise and our participation in green exercise influences our attitudes. This idea has roots in philosophy, specifically the deep ecology of Arne Naess who suggested that deep-nature experiences could strengthen one's commitment to nature (1973; see also Gelter, 2000). Naess' thinking starts to get at the root of the idea of Symbiocene: symbiosis. We *are* nature, its health is our health, and the extent to which we value it is the extent, really, to which we value ourselves.

Ecopsychology is a field that focuses on human relationships with the natural world through ecological and psychological perspectives. One concept within ecopsychology is that nature can instill in a person a sense of belongingness, purpose, and meaning (Softas-Nall & Woody, 2017). Existential psychologist Rollo May (1953) echoed this sentiment, emphasizing that humankind and nature are inseparable, interconnected entities, and that connection to nature is an essential value of humans. Green exercise intertwines with our relationship with nature in that it represents active participation in strengthening that relationship. We propose that because of this, green exercise is relevant not only to human flourishing but also to strengthening our relationship with nature.

4.2 Benefits

Flourishing, a state of complete mental health (Keyes & Annas, 2009), goes beyond merely feeling good and experiencing positive emotions (i.e. hedonia); it also requires that an individual be functioning well (i.e. eudaimonia). As incorporated into Seligman's (2011) PERMA model, flourishing comprises positive emotion (P), engagement (E), positive relationships (R), meaning (M), and accomplishment (A) (see also Scorsolini-Comin et al., 2013). Flourishing also relates to resilience, vitality, self-esteem, and self-determination (Crespo & Mesurado, 2015). One route to flourishing is green exercise.

Much evidence has supported physical activity as conducive to boosting both physical and mental health (e.g. Caddick & Smith, 2014; Holley et al., 2011; Penedo & Dahn, 2005; Windle et al., 2010). A growing number of studies also demonstrate the mental and physical benefits of green exercise; even distinguishing those benefits from benefits gained from other forms of exercise, particularly with respect to the hedonic (feeling good) aspect of wellbeing. For example, Pasanen and colleagues (2014) found a significant association between physical activity conducted in natural environments and wellbeing, but not between physical activity conducted in built environments (whether outdoors or indoors). A meta-analysis of 25 studies revealed that walking or running outdoors (vs. indoors) was more beneficial, resulting in significantly lower levels of negative emotions such as sadness and anger (Bowler et al., 2010). Physical activity experiences in environments that are visibly more (vs. less) green have been found to result in significantly lower levels of nervousness and fatigue (Han & Wang, 2018). Green exercise has been found to produce moderate short-term reductions in anxiety, especially for participants who perceived themselves to be exercising in more natural environments (Mackay & Neil, 2010). Even in regular exercisers, individuals who engage in outdoor physical activity report significantly lower somatic anxiety levels, whereas indoor physical activity is predictive of higher somatic anxiety (Lawton et al., 2017). These findings suggest that green exercise contributes to the positive emotion (or hedonic) aspect of PERMA.

Although not as extensive, evidence also supports an association between green exercise and eudaimonic aspects of wellbeing. For example, Rogerson and colleagues (2016) reported that those who exercised in nature had significantly increased social-interaction time compared to indoor exercisers. Green exercise has been found to produce feelings of mindfulness (Wolsko & Lindberg, 2013); evidence has consistently demonstrated the strong relationship between mindfulness and wellbeing (see review Keng et al., 2011). Glackin and Beale (2018) interviewed a group of road cyclists about how the sport contributed to their well-being. They found that, collectively, responses referred to intrinsic motivation, personal achievement, vitality, and the simple joys of riding in the countryside, thus lending support to the role that green exercise plays in the engagement and accomplishment aspects of PERMA.

On the whole, green exercise research is an area of largely untapped potential for positive psychologists. The full contribution that engaging in physical activity in natural settings provides to a holistic and eudaimonic conception of human health remains underappreciated.

4.3 Green Prescriptions

The green prescription movement is attempting to get doctors to prescribe time in nature and green exercise to their patients; its overarching aim is to ensure that such practices are routinely integrated into everyday health care practice (van den Berg, 2017). Barton and Pretty (2010) assessed the optimal "dose" of green exercise via a review of ten studies in various populations; these studies measured self-esteem and mood before and after a variety of green exercise activities. Results evidenced that substantial changes came from only 5 minutes of green activity, with benefits continuing to rise afterward.

Despite such evidence, medical practitioners have been slow to prescribe green exercise. For example, Dutch doctors, while routinely advising patients to be physically active, do not usually mention the benefits of doing so in nature (Maas & Verheji, 2007). It is unclear whether this predicament is caused by a lack of awareness on the part of the medical community or a lack of certainty in the evidence supporting green exercise. Interestingly though, Meyer and Botsch (2017) found that German health professionals generally seem to believe that forests offer health benefits. This suggests that there may be other factors involved in suppressing the number of green prescriptions that are written. What is clear is that more needs to be done with respect to disseminating the mounting evidence for the beneficial effects of green exercise. This information needs to be put into the hands (and prescription pads) of medical professionals. Additional research assessing doctors' beliefs and prescription practices regarding green exercise is vital.

4.4 Mechanisms

Going beyond the benefits of green exercise, the question arises of how it all works. How does the act of engaging in physical activity differ in nature? How does this activity connect to concepts of flourishing?

Attention Restoration Theory (ART; Kaplan & Kaplan, 1989) draws from William James' (1899) concept of "voluntary attention," the attention that we must apply in effortful concentration and that goes "against the grain" of distraction. Kaplan (1995) deemed this "directed attention" and suggested that directed attention can be fatigued and depleted with use. ART proposes that the opposite form of attention, that is, James' involuntary attention, is the form that is manifested when a person is in nature. Specifically, natural environments are restorative because they produce "captivated fascination," distracting us from whatever held our voluntary attention and promoting effortless attention in all directions (Olafsdottir et al., 2017). A distinction is made between "soft fascination" and "hard fascination." Soft fascination is associated with time in nature and with leftover space for mental reflection; whereas hard fascination has been found to be associated with watching television, with no space for contemplation (Basu et al., 2019). From this perspective, green exercise would entail benefits arising through restoring one's resources, and from directing attention away from stressful aspects of one's life.

Brymer and colleagues (Brymer et al., 2014; Araújo et al., 2019) point to an "organismic asymmetry" of evolutionary and restorative theories in which a distinction is made between human behavior and environment, and between subjective experience and objective natural features. Instead, they proposed and discussed an ecological dynamics framework, an interdependent relationship wherein nature and organism continuously redefine each other. Three tenets for this framework are outlined wherein: (1) the person is seen as an inherently active agent, scanning and reacting to the environment; (2) the experience resides in the person–environment relationship; and (3) the environment inhabited by humans contains "affordances," properties which are functionally relevant. Affordances are to be actively engaged with based on momentary decisions to do so by the individual. Objects provide numerous affordances. The main difference between natural and urban environments is that urban objects are limited in their affordances by social convention and design, like a treadmill, which has just one socially prescribed use. A tree trunk, on the other hand, has no prescribed or conventional use. The conclusion is that the natural environment and its variability request holistic, emotional, cognitive, and physical involvement of the person. From an ecological dynamics view, it is the heterogeneity of a natural environment, how unique that is and what it affords us in our actions, that is fundamental in producing the benefits evidence by green exercise.

4.5 Future Research

Given that the groundwork has been laid in establishing green exercise as indeed producing additional important benefits (relative to exercise indoors), refinement is now needed to push these findings into practical use. One such area involves broadening our area of focus beyond physical activity done in groomed, urban neighborhood parks. Bamberg and colleagues (2018) highlighted that much green exercise research focuses on visual green, on the uniformity of activities, and lack of variation in environments. They argued that green exercise includes or even necessitates variable weather, challenging environments, and variation in surfaces. More attention needs to be given toward how we are defining nature with respect to green exercise, whether these definitions are adequately broad, and whether they are practical.

Other researchers suggest that to glean the full effects of green exercise, it may not be enough to merely engage in physical activity in natural settings; rather one must also turn their attention to engagement with the environment (e.g. C. Egger, personal communication, October 4, 2019). In line with this are recent findings that mindfulness in nature enhances not only nature connectedness (a feeling that one is part of, and not separate from nature), but also mood (Nisbet et al., 2019), and previous findings of Lawton and colleagues (2017) evidencing that individuals who regularly exercise outdoors report high levels of nature connectedness. Going forward, research in green exercise should consider where exercisers' attention is allocated to, levels of mindfulness, and exercisers' levels of nature connectedness.

Partially addressing this point of attention is a subset of green research not to be overlooked. Nettleton (2013) provided an ethnography of fell running in the English Lake district – a long-distance running sport which challenges participants to navigate "fells" or hills. The qualitative interviews show a substantial overlap with quantitative results of green exercise literature. One consistent theme which emerged in Nettleton's research is the process of leaving everyday worries behind due to the attention that is needed to navigate and avoid falling. Moreover, when given a moment's respite from the activity itself, attention fell to the environment or on moments described as "magical." Nettleton refers to an existential experience reported by these fell runners, an "embodied reassurance rooted in the connection between the corporeal self and the landscape" and to a further connection between runners who have a common passion. Attention is forefront here – being captivated necessarily by what's underfoot and what's above. Further research in this vein is provided by Glackin and Beale (2018), who interviewed a group of road cyclists. They noted how these cyclists' responses lined up with the ecological dynamics framework (Araújo et al., 2019), emphasizing the unique affordances of the natural environment. It is clear that for these green exercisers (i.e. road cyclists) in Glackin and Beale's study, the green countryside played an active role in affording participants the opportunity and freedom to constantly challenge themselves. As with the fell runners (Nettleton), when the opportunity arose, such as when cyclists paused at the top of a hill, attention was guided toward the environment. The benefits arising from such pauses of attentional allocation lend qualitative support to Egger'supposition. In general, these qualitative studies not only add weight to the substantial quantitative literature in green exercise, these studies also add their own value, providing richer, more personal, and perhaps even more tangible support for the benefits of exercising in natural environments.

As pertains to measurement methods, a case has been made for using neurophysiological measures in order to measure brain activity during green exercise (Flowers et al., 2018; Han & Wang, 2018). Additionally, it has been suggested standardized methods to examine the effects of greenness/naturalness and related environmental variables are what is required to move this field forward (Klaperski et al., 2019). Araújo and colleagues (2019) proposed that eco-variables (e.g. stride length, steps per minute, duration of foot contact with ground) be utilized in studies involving running in nature.

Longitudinal studies are required which observe green exercise participation for periods longer than 24 hours (Wood & Smyth, 2019), and/or for repeated measurements be taken after multiple bouts of green exercise (Pasanen et al., 2018). Recommendations from Wooller and colleagues (2018) include that future research explore the importance and mechanisms of each physical sense pertaining to stress recovery. This recommendation aims to address the somewhat narrow focus that green exercise research has had to this point, wherein vision has been studied almost exclusively (Bamberg et al., 2018). From the smell of pines to the feeling of one's feet interacting with the ground, a wider perspective is important.

Future research is needed that addresses how green exercise contributes to adherence to physical activity in general (Glover & Polley, 2019). That is, does practicing green exercise keep people motivated to exercise more so than does classic physical activity. Further, it has been suggested that research be conducted exploring how role-models, age, and gender influence green exercise behavior (Colley et al., 2019). In the same vein, research is needed to address cultural patterns of green exercise and how country-specific infrastructure can influence green exercise (Pasanen et al., 2019). There is much to be learned about how people from different cultures view green exercise, at what rates they engage in it, and to what extent green exercise is supported around the globe.

Given the paucity of research addressing green exercise and eudaimonic aspects of flourishing, we propose that consideration be lent to the effects of green exercise on meaning in life, personal growth, environmental mastery, and aspects of self-determination theory (i.e. autonomy, competence, and relatedness; Deci & Ryan, 2000). We also propose that further research is necessary exploring how green exercise relates to one's relationship to nature and perceptions of the human-nature relationship in general. We suggest investigating this relationship within a framework of a bidirectional influence between a person's relationship to nature and their participation in green exercise. Lastly, we suggest that consideration of individuals' personal meaning regarding preferred locations for green exercise might reveal insights into how the activity itself can be beneficial. For example, on a broad level, research has demonstrated that place attachment (i.e. feeling connected to familiar places) enhances psychological wellbeing needs related to meaning, relatedness, and happiness (Scannell & Gifford, 2016). Preliminary evidence suggests that emotional attachment to local green spaces is weakly, but significantly, positively related to mental health (Zhang et al., 2015). Moreover, Passmore and colleagues (2019) found that a noticing nature intervention significantly boosted participants' attachment to their local natural environment. Thus, an enhanced sense of place attachment may be one mechanism by which green exercise manifests its demonstrated wellbeing benefits.

4.6 Conclusion

Green exercise – physical activity in natural surroundings – brings with it a host of benefits. Of course, it is by no means a new idea to suggest that individually, getting outside and getting active are good for human health. However, research suggests that these two activities yield benefits to wellbeing greater than the sum of their individual parts. Nonetheless, access to green space and willingness to participate in physical activity are dwindling resources. Current trends of sedentary, consumer lifestyles combined with rapid urbanization and environmental destruction are putting stress on the human-nature relationship. Green exercise is one way to address both of these issues. Green exercise can serve to facilitate a movement toward a health system which emphasizes flourishing along with physical health, while also functioning as a mediator in our complicated (and currently, distant) relationship with the natural world. Moreover, we believe that research evidence is now strong enough to call for green exercise to be integrated into the field of medicine. For as Hippocrates wrote, "The physician treats, but nature heals."

Note

1. A body of research has investigated, and evidenced, the well-being benefits of intense forms of physical activity in nature, for example, extreme sports, such as big-wave surfing, extreme skiing, waterfall kayaking, rope-free climbing, extended wilderness adventures (e.g. Brymer, 2011; Brymer & Gray, 2010). In this chapter, we focus on more common-place types of exercise and physical activity.

References

Antal, M., & Drews, S. (2015). Nature as relationship partner: An old frame revisited. *Environmental Education Research, 21*, 1056–1078.

Araújo, D., Brymer, E., Brito, H., Withagen, R., & Davids, K. (2019). The empowering variability of affordances of nature: Why do exercisers feel better after performing the same exercise in natural environments than in indoor environments? *Psychology of Sport and Exercise, 42*, 138–145. doi.org: 10.1016/j.psychsport.2018.12.020

Antal, M., & Drews, S. (2015). Nature as relationship partner: An old frame revisited. *Environmental Education Research, 21*, 1056–1078.

Bamberg, J., Hitchings, R., & Latham, A. (2018). Enriching green exercise research. *Landscape and Urban Planning, 178*, 270–275. doi: 10.1016/j.landurbplan.2018.06.005

Barton, J., & Pretty, J. (2010). What is the best dose of nature and green exercise for improving mental health: A multi-study analysis. *Environmental Science and Technology, 44*, 3947–3955. doi: 10.1021/es903183r

Barton, J., Wood, C., Pretty, J., & Rogerson, M. (2016). Green exercise for health: A dose of nature. In J. Barton, R. Bragg, C. Wood, & J. Pretty (Eds.). *Green exercise: Linking nature, health, and well-being* (pp. 26–36). London: Routledge.

Basu, A., Duvall, J., & Kaplan, R. (2019). Attention restoration theory: Exploring the role of soft fascination and mental bandwidth. *Environment and Behavior, 51*, 1055–1081. doi: 10.1177/0013916518774400

Benjamin, E. J., Muntner, P., Alonso, A., Bittencourt, M. S., Callaway, C. W., Carson, A. P., ... Virani, S. S. (2019). Heart disease and stroke statistics-2019 update: A report from the American Heart Association. *Circulation, 13*, e56–e66. doi.org: 10.1161/CIR.0000000000000659

Bowler, D. E., Buyung-Ali, L. M., Knight, T. M., & Pullin, A. S. (2010). A systematic review of evidence for the added benefits to health of exposure to natural environments. *BMC Public Health, 10*, 456. doi: 10.1186/1471-2458-10-456

Brooks, J. J., Wallace, G. N., & Williams, D. R. (2006). Place as relationship partner: An alternative metaphor for understanding the quality of visitor experience in a backcountry setting. *Leisure Sciences, 28*, 331–349. doi: 10.1080/01490400600745852

Brymer, E. (2011). Extreme sports as a facilitator of ecocentricity and positive life changes. *World Leisure Journal, 51*, 47–53. doi: 10.1080/04419057.2009.9674581

Brymer, E., & Gray, T. (2010). Developing an intimate "relationship" with nature through extreme sports participation. *Loisir, 34*, 361–374.

Brymer, E., Davids, K., & Mallabon, L. (2014). Understanding the psychological health and well-being benefits of physical activity in nature: An ecological dynamics analysis. *Ecopsychology, 6*, 189–197. doi: 10.1089/eco.2013.0110

Caddick, N., & Smith, B. (2014). The impact of sport and physical activity on the well-being of combat veterans: A systematic review. *Psychology of Sport and Exercise, 15*, 9–18. doi: 10.1016/j.psychsport.2013.09.11

Colley, K., Currie, M. J. B., & Irvine, K. N. (2019). Then and now: Examining older people's engagement in outdoor recreation across the life course. *Leisure Sciences, 41*, 186–202. doi: 10.1080/01490400.2017.1349696

Crespo, R. F., & Mesurado, B. (2015). Happiness economics, eudaimonia and positive psychology: From happiness economics to flourishing economics. *Journal of Happiness Studies, 16*, 931–946. doi: 10.1007/s10902-014-9541-4

Curtin, S. C., Warner, M., & Hedegaard, H. (2016). Increase in suicide in the United States, 1999–2014. NCHS data brief, no 241. Hyattsville, MD: National Center for Health Statistics.

Deci, E. L., & Ryan, R. M. (2000). The "what" and "why" of goal pursuits: Human needs and the self-determination of behavior. *Psychological Inquiry, 11*, 227–268.

Flowers, E. P., Freeman, P., & Gladwell, V. F. (2018). Enhancing the acute psychological benefits of green exercise: An investigation of expectancy effects. *Psychology of Sport and Exercise, 39*, 213–221. doi: 10.1016/j.psychsport.2018.08.014

Gelter, H. (2000). Friluftsliv: The Scandinavian philosophy of outdoor life. *Canadian Journal of Environmental Education, 5*, 77–92.

Glackin, O. F., & Beale, J. T. (2018). "The world is best experienced at 18 mph." The psychological wellbeing effects of cycling in the countryside: An interpretative phenomenological analysis. *Qualitative Research in Sport, Exercise and Health, 10*, 32–46. doi: 10.1080/2159676X.2017.1360381

Glover, N., & Polley, S. (2019). Going green: The effectiveness of a 40-day green exercise intervention for insufficiently active adults. *Sports, 7*(6), 142. doi: 10.3390/sports7060142

Han, K. T., & Wang, P. C. (2018). Empirical examinations of effects of three-level green exercise on engagement with nature and physical activity. *International Journal of Environmental Research and Public Health, 15*. doi: 10.3390/ijerph15020375

44 O. Geddes and H.-A. Passmore

Holley, J., Crone, D., Tyson, P., & Lovell, G. (2011). The effects of physical activity on psychological well-being for those with schizophrenia: A systematic review. *British Journal of Clinical Psychology, 50*, 84–105. doi: 10.1348/014466510X496220

Hurt, R. T., Kulisek, C., Buchanan, L. A., & McClave, S. A. (2010). The obesity epidemic: Challenges, health initiatives, and implications for gastroenterologists. *Gastroenterology and Hepatology, 6*, 780–792.

James, W. (1899/1983). *Talks to teachers on psychology: And to students on some of life's ideals.* Harvard University Press.

Kaplan, R., & Kaplan, S. (1989). *The experience of nature: A psychological perspective.* Cambridge, UK: Cambridge University Press.

Kaplan, S. (1995). The restorative benefits of nature: Toward an integrative framework. *Journal of Environmental Psychology, 15*, 169–182. doi: 10.1016/0272- 4944(95)90001-2

Keng, S.-L., Smoski, M. J., & Robins, C. J. (2011). Effects of mindfulness on psychological health: A review of empirical studies. *Clinical Psychology Review, 31*, 1041–1056. doi: 10.1016.jcor.2011.04.006

Keyes, C. L. M., & Annas, J. (2009). Feeling good and functioning well: Distinctive concepts in ancient philosophy and contemporary science. *The Journal of Positive Psychology, 4*, 197–201.

Klaperski, S., Koch, E., Hewel, D., Schempp, A., & Müller, J. (2019). Optimizing mental health benefits of exercise: The influence of the exercise environment on acute stress levels and wellbeing. *Mental Health & Prevention, 15*, 200173. doi: 10.1016/j.mhp.2019.200173

Lawton, E., Brymer, E., Clough, P., & Denovan, A. (2017). The relationship between the physical activity environment, nature relatedness, anxiety, and the psychological well-being benefits of regular exercisers. *Frontiers in Psychology: Environmental Psychology, 8*, e1058. doi: 10.3389/fpsyg.2017.01058

Maas, J., & Verheij, R. A. (2007). Are health benefits of physical activity in natural environments used in primary care by general practitioners in The Netherlands? *Urban Forestry and Urban Greening, 6*, 227–233. doi: 10.1016/j.ufug.2007.03.003

Mackay, G. J., & Neill, J. T. (2010). The effect of "green exercise" on state anxiety and the role of exercise duration, intensity, and greenness: A quasi-experimental study. *Psychology of Sport and Exercise, 11*, 238–245. doi: 10.1016/j.psychsport.2010.01.002

May, R. (1953). *Man's search for himself.* New York, NY: Norton.

Meyer, K., & Botsch, K. (2017). Do forest and health professionals presume that forests offer health benefits, and is cross-sectional cooperation conceivable? *Urban Forestry and Urban Greening, 27*, 127–137. doi: 10.1016/j.ufug.2017.07.002

Naess, A. (1973). The shallow and the deep, long-range ecology movement: A summary. *Inquiry, 16*, 95–100. doi: 10.1080/00201747308601682

Nettleton, S. (2013). Cementing relations within a sporting field: Fell running in the English Lake District and the acquisition of existential capital. *Cultural Sociology, 7*, 196–210. doi: 10.1177/1749975512473749

Nisbet, E. K., Zelesnki, J. M., & Grandpierre, Z. (2019). Mindfulness in nature enhances connectedness and mood. *Ecopsychology, 11*, 81–91. doi: 10.1089/eco.2018.0061

Olafsdottir, G., Cloke, P., & Vögele, C. (2017). Place, green exercise and stress: An exploration of lived experience and restorative effects. *Health and Place, 46*, 358–365. doi: 10.1016/j.healthplace.2017.02.006

Pasanen, T. P., Ojala, A., Tyrväinen, L., & Korpela, K. M. (2018). Restoration, well-being, and everyday physical activity in indoor, built outdoor and natural outdoor settings. *Journal of Environmental Psychology, 59*, 85–93. doi: 10.1016/j.jenvp.2018.08.014

Pasanen, T. P., Tyrväinen, L., & Korpela, K. M. (2014). The relationship between perceived health and physical activity indoors, outdoors in built environments, and outdoors in nature. *Applied Psychology: Health and Well-Being, 6*, 324–346. doi: 10.1111/aphw.12031

Pasanen, T. P., White, M. P., Wheeler, B. W., Garrett, J. K., & Elliott, L. R. (2019). Neighbourhood blue space, health and wellbeing: The mediating role of different types of physical activity. *Environment International, 131*, 105016. doi: 10.1016/j.envint.2019.105016

Passmore, H.-A., Yang, Y., & Sabine, S. (2019, in preparation). *Noticing Nature as a well-being intervention: Replication and expansion in a Chinese sample.*

Penedo, F. J., & Dahn, J. R. (2005). Exercise and well-being: A review of mental and physical health benefits associated with physical activity. *Current Opinion in Psychiatry, 18*, 189–193.

Pitchforth, J., Fahy, K., Ford, T., Wolpert, M., Viner, R. M., & Hargreaves, D. S. (2019). Mental health and well-being trends among children and young people in the UK, 1995–2014: Analysis of repeated cross-sectional national health surveys. *Psychological Medicine, 49*, 1275–1285. doi: 10.1017/S0033291718001757

Prescott, S., & Logan, A. (2017). Down to earth: Planetary health and biophilosophy in the Symbiocene ewpoch. *Challenges, 8*, 19. doi: 10.3390/challe8020019

Robinson, J., & Breed, M. (2019). Green prescriptions and their co-benefits: Integrative strategies for public and environmental health. *Challenges, 10*, 9. doi: 10.3390/challe10010009

Rogerson, M., Gladwell, V. F., Gallagher, D. J., & Barton, J. L. (2016). Influences of green outdoors versus indoors environmental settings on psychological and social outcomes of controlled exercise. *International Journal of Environmental Research and Public Health, 13*, 363. doi: 10.3390/ijerph13040363

Scannell, L., & Gifford, R. (2016). Place attachment enhances psychological need satisfaction. *Environment and Behavior, 49*, 359–389. doi: 10.1177/0013916516637648

Schriever, N. (2018, July). 30 facts about the gym and fitness industry that will surprise you! *Bluewater Credit.* Retrieved from https://bluewatercredit.com/30-facts-gym-fitness-industry-will-surprise/

Scorsolini-Comin, F., Fontaine, A. M. G. V., Koller, S. H., & dos Santos, M. A. (2013). From authentic happiness to well-being: The flourishing of positive psychology. *Psicologia: Reflexao e Critica, 26*, 663–670. doi: 10.1590/S0102-79722013000400006

Seligman, M. E. P. (2011). *Flourish: A visionary new understanding of happiness and well-being.* New York, NY: Free Press.

Shanahan, D. F., Franco, L., Lin, B. B., Gaston, K. J., & Fuller, R. A. (2016). The benefits of natural environments for physical activity. *Sports Medicine, 46*, 989–995. doi: 10.1007/s40279-016-0502-4

Softas-Nall, S., & Woody, W. D. (2017). The loss of human connection to nature: Revitalizing selfhood and meaning in life through the ideas of Rollo May. *Ecopsychology, 9*, 241–252. doi: 10.1089/eco.2017.0020

U.S. Department of Health and Human Services. Facts and Statistics (2017). Available at: https://www.hhs.gov/fitness/resource-center/facts-and-statistics/index.html.

van den Berg, A. E. (2017). From green space to green prescriptions: Challenges and opportunities for research and practice. *Frontiers in Psychology, 8.* doi: 10.3389/fpsyg.2017.00268

Windle, G., Hughes, D., Linck, P., Russell, I., & Woods, B. (2010). Is exercise effect in promoting mental well-being in older age? A systematic review. *Aging & Mental Health, 14,* 652–669. doi: 10.1080/13607861003713232

Wolsko, C., & Lindberg, K. (2013). Experiencing connection with nature: The matrix of psychological well-being, mindfulness, and outdoor recreation. *Ecopsychology, 5,* 80–91. doi: 10.1089/eco.2013.0008

Wood, C. J., & Smyth, N. (2019). The health impact of nature exposure and green exercise across the life course: A pilot study. *International Journal of Environmental Health Research.* doi: 10.1080/09603123.2019.1593327

Wooller, J. J., Rogerson, M., Barton, J., Micklewright, D., & Gladwell, V. (2018). Can simulated green exercise improve recovery from acute mental stress? *Frontiers in Psychology, 9,* 1–10. doi: 10.3389/fpsyg.2018.02167

Zhang, Y., van Dijk, T., Tang, J., & van den Berg, A. E. (2015). Green space attachment and health: A comparative study in two urban neighborhoods. *International Journal of Environmental Research and Public Health, 12,* 14342–14363.

5 Mind the Gap - On the Necessity of a Situational Taxonomy for Designing and Evaluating Gait Interventions

Steven van Andel, Michael Cole, and Gert-Jan Pepping

5.1 Falls as a Problem of Perception and Action

The examples are abound: *"Please hold handrail"* and *"Mind the gap"*; messages brought to you through public address systems in, for instance, railway stations or airports, where people need to walk to get about. These messages are an interesting summary of the risk aversive nature of our current society. A message with the best intentions to minimize the risk of tripping and sustaining injury but at the same time a message that might also discourage commuters to use locomotor means to get to their destination. Instead they might opt for other, easier, safer, more convenient means of locomotion, such as the elevator, or in the case of the elderly, using a wheelchair or mobility scooter. Consequently, such choices steer people away from using unaided locomotion, and using for instance stairs and subways, as a training tool for balance and leg strength. We have become experts in creating predictable risk free or risk-managed environments. These artificial environments developed with the principal aims of minimizing risk and maximizing safety have one thing in common – they minimize the strain on the perceptual-motor system. Examples like holding a handrail reduce the demand for balance, messages over the public address system and orange cones on the street reduce the demands of visual search for hazards and building smooth and flat pavements reduce the need for adaptation in one's steps when walking.

In the current chapter, we will consider mobility across the lifespan and will argue that mobility, i.e. gait – walking in an unaided fashion, needs to be considered as an exemplar of an open skill. To consider this, and its relevance, we will focus on one of modern-day society's more costly mobility problems; falling of older adults. Falls are one of the main causes of accidental injuries in older adults, leading to fractures, decreases in quality of life and potentially death for an individual, and significant health care costs for society (Burns et al., 2016; Hendrie et al., 2004; World Health Organization, 2007). Falls are most prevalent during gait, in particular, as a result of trips and slips (Andel, Cole, et al., 2019; Berg et al., 1997). Trips and slips do not happen in a totally closed environment, as in a totally

DOI: 10.4324/9781003154419-6

48   S. v. Andel, M. Cole, and G.-J. Pepping

closed environment, there would be no need for adaptation; after all, there is nothing to trip or slip over. Hence, in order to prepare for fall-free ambulation in a dynamic, open, environment, one needs to practice within environments that provide the right challenge to the perceptual-motor system. That is, an environment that has at least the same dynamics and degree of openness as the complex gait tasks during which falls occur.

Like with any physiological system in our body, the principle of "use it or lose it" also applies to the perceptual-motor system. One needs to use this system, and *challenge* it, to improve and maintain the functioning of this system. Research in the field of "ecological psychology" has produced an extensive knowledge base on the function of this system and the means to improve it. Behavior, simplified as decisions about "what to do" is said to be prospectively guided by the perception of future opportunities for action (Gibson, 1979). The opportunities for action or "affordances" are properties of the person-environment system that specify the different movement opportunities that are available to individuals in specific situations (Chemero, 2003; Chemero, 2009). Imagine, for instance, walking through the railway station: You perceive the option to take the elevator or the stairs, the option to either use the handrail or not, to look straight ahead or to look around you. At any moment in time, you are surrounded by an unlimited number of opportunities for action and thereby an unlimited number of affordances. How we pick one affordance over another can be conceptualized to be mediated by how much an affordance *invites* a certain behavior – and whether it is able to be a stronger invitation than the other available affordances (Withagen et al., 2012). In natural, every day, situations the multitude of affordances available to individuals and the relationships they embody, give rise to the emergence and dissipation of synergies that drive individual and social behavior. From this viewpoint, it becomes understandable that for some people, the affordances that are presented by an elevator (perhaps unfortunately) provide more inviting options to get to one's destination, compared to the affordances that are presented by the stairs. Note that the decisions to act on one invitation/ affordance over another can also be influenced by declarative knowledge, e.g. reading the "please hold handrail" sign (Cisek & Kalaska, 2010).

This decision making is possible because the perceptual-motor system can distinguish possible from impossible future actions. This occurs through a scaling of the perception of the affordances in terms of the individuals' own action capabilities; a process known as *calibration* (Andel, Cole, et al., 2017; Gray, 2014). For instance, when perceiving steps, research has shown that one scales the perception of the step height in terms of one's leg length and walking capabilities (Konczak et al., 1992; Warren, 1984). It is important to realize that in order for this calibration process to be successful, one needs to actively *explore* one's environment to get information about how one's action capabilities compare to the future opportunities for action offered by the environment (Andel, Cole, et al., 2017; Andel,

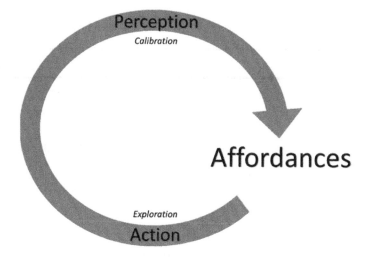

Figure 5.1 Relationship between affordances (the action possibilities offered by the environment) that is informed by calibration (scaling) and exploration. *Note that exploration itself is a possibility for action and thus a cyclical relation exists between these terms.*

McGuckian, et al., 2019). In short, active exploration is the means of the perceptual-motor system to calibrate and successfully perceive affordances and guide behavior (Figure 5.1 – see also Andel, McGuckian, et al., 2019).

Using these processes efficiently is imperative for skills in which a person needs to interact with their environment. From Physical Education (PE) and skill acquisition research, such skills have become known as *open skills* (following Poulton, 1957) as opposed to closed skills in which a person can act without much disturbance from the environment. It is important to emphasize that the distinction between open and closed skills is continuous. The different influences of the environment, as introduced by Poulton (1957), are presented in Figure 5.2. For more open skills like walking, there is a general consensus that the optimal method for training is through diversification and variable practice (following Gentile, 1972). However, some research suggests that, regardless of the skill's classification, training in open environments (using variable or random practice designs) could be beneficial for creating more adaptable movement patterns and maximizing retention and transfer of learning. Summarizing, skills seem to be optimally trained in an environment that is at least as open as the performance environment. This is an important consideration for mobility across the lifespan. All everyday tasks have a different place on the open-to-close continuum and if we should take one message from physical education, sport training, and skill acquisition research, it should be that we need to practice these skills with at least an equal amount of openness.

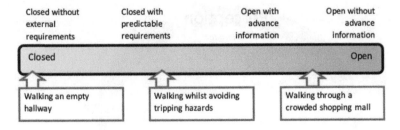

Figure 5.2 Introduction of the continuum between open and closed skills, including labels (top) as introduced by Poulton (1957). *The boxes below illustrate how different modes of gait fit in this continuum. Evidence suggests that to train any skill for benefits in retention and transfer, one should practice in an environment with increased openness.*

So far in this chapter, we have introduced a theoretical model of the processes involved in fall-free ambulation and have come to recommendations for training this skill. It should be apparent that the aims of our built environment (creating predictable, risk-free environments) are in direct contrast with these recommendations gained from the physical education, sport training and skill acquisition/motor learning literature. In fact, our tendencies to place exercise in gyms and rehabilitation in clinics are both powerful movements that result in a more closed motor learning environment. But how does this prepare us for those occasions that we do need to perform in an open environment? In the remainder of this chapter, we will further explore the problem of falls for older adults as an exemplar to introduce the benefits of *green exercise*. Furthermore, we will introduce a taxonomy that helps classify the environmental demands on gait, as a tool for practitioners, to better understand the challenges offered by the natural world and to prescribe green exercise in environments with the right degree of openness.

5.2 The Need for a Situational Taxonomy to Guide Green Exercise Research and Practice

To better understand the problem of fall prevention and the potential scope of green exercise as a part of the solution, it is important to understand the current best practice. Based on a systematic analysis of falls prevention intervention studies, Sherrington and colleagues concluded that successful interventions should include a combination of balance and functional exercises (Sherrington et al., 2019). No mention was made in this systematic review of the opportunities offered by green exercise specifically. Walking interventions were discussed, but based on their statistics, Sherrington and colleagues (2019) could not reach certainty in their conclusions. Only two studies were included that assessed the effects of walking in isolation from other interventions. These studies either reported an increase of falls rate due to the increased exposure in the intervention (Ebrahim et al., 1997) or neither an increase nor a decrease of falls rate (Voukelatos et al., 2015). Based on this, Sherrington and colleagues (2019) concluded that the use of walking interventions is limited for the purposes of falls prevention.

It seems counter-intuitive that most falls occur during gait or gait-related activities (Andel, Cole, et al., 2019; Berg et al., 1997), yet practice-specific training in this activity does not seem to have been particularly effective or helpful in improving walking skills and preventing falls (Sherrington et al., 2017). To better understand why this might be, we can learn from developments in other fields of the movement sciences.

Research within the PE and motor learning domains has accumulated evidence on the importance of transfer of the training task to the performance setting and the need for representative task design; a method that optimizes training effects by keeping the training close to the performance environment (Dicks et al., 2009; Orth et al., 2019; Pinder et al., 2011). The theories underpinning the notion of representative task design are developed through application of general theories of perception and movement (Davids et al., 2008; Gibson, 1979; Newell, 1986) and a similar call for a representative approach is present in allied health disciplines of the movement sciences (Vaz et al., 2017). Furthermore, processes that rely on our motor learning capabilities, such as in a visuomotor rotation task seem to work similarly (albeit slower) in older compared to younger adults (Fernández-Ruiz et al., 2000). As such, it seems likely that these motor learning principles could be generalized to any field of human movement science.

Consider two inter-related explanations for the seeming contradiction that current walking intervention designs do not effectively prevent falls. Firstly, it is possible that within the walking interventions, "fall-free-walking-skill" did improve; however, through the increased exposure to risky environments, falls rates went up. Second, it is possible that the interventions were not truly representative and did not provide the right challenge to improve walking skill. Applying the right degree of openness to a training environment is crucial for the effectiveness of an intervention. However, with increasing openness comes increasing unpredictability, increasing the difficulty level of the task. As such, successful interventions for falls prevention would need to have the right balance in challenge and risk management. Using this interpretation, an intervention, which involved self-paced walking that gradually increased in terms of frequency and duration (Voukelatos et al., 2015), might not have been representative of the walking tasks in which falls occur. Participants were free to only engage in low demand walking. With the emphasis on increasing the time spent walking, it is likely that participants would not go out of their way to look for challenging walks. More likely, one looks for easier walks or perhaps opts for walking on a treadmill. Unfortunately, in the

52   S. v. Andel, M. Cole, and G.-J. Pepping

above intervention, people were not instructed on where to walk – in what kind of environment or with what kind of challenges. In another intervention, participants were asked to briskly walk three times a week for 40 minutes (Ebrahim et al., 1997), which might have been too strenuous. Fatigue changes the dynamics in the perceptual-motor system, creating an increased need for perceptual-motor calibration. These quickly changing dynamics could potentially help explain the increased fall incidence in this study. What is missing within these previous studies is a tool that could aid exercise prescription and could be used to categorize and evaluate the quality of the gait interventions.

5.3 A Situational Taxonomy for Environment-Person Pairing In Natural Gait (STEPPING)

Natural gait can take place in environments that can widely vary in terms of the challenge they present to the perceptual-motor system (see Figure 5.3). To assist practitioners in finding the right degree of challenge in a gait task and to help researchers design interventions in which they can assess the degree of challenge brought on by the environment, we here introduce the *Situational Taxonomy for Environment-Person Pairing In Natural Gait* or *STEPPING* (Figure 5.4). For example, an older person at risk of falls might aim to increase their walking activity, but without further instruction, would do this in a completely closed environment (1A) because this feels safe. However, this might limit the training effect to situations where the person might need to cope with more open environments. The classification system can be used by researchers to understand the exposure within an intervention. Similarly, a health practitioner could use the STEPPING to progressively introduce activities beyond category 1A; to slowly start taking people outside and off the tracks. Naturally, a person at risk for falls should not "jump into the deep end" and start with activities like rock climbing (4C), but a practitioner could use the STEPPING to gradually increase the difficulty level, *one step at the time*. Built environment practitioners (designers, architects, planners, and policymakers) can use the STEPPING to benchmark the challenges that they are creating or aim to implement and can use it as a much-needed counterargument for risk-mitigation policy. To conclude that "walking interventions do not work well for falls prevention" would mean that the effect of all these categories would be the same (and would be zero). Future studies are required to find out what the effects are of practice in higher-level categories of the STEPPING and of progressive increases in difficulty level tailored to the abilities of the participant.

The STEPPING classification system refers, in part, to the continuum from closed to open skills (Poulton, 1957; Figure 5.2). However, it should be noted that the classification system currently only covers the left half of this continuum, describing the degree of openness in what would generally be considered relatively closed environments. To be further

Mind the Gap - On the Necessity 53

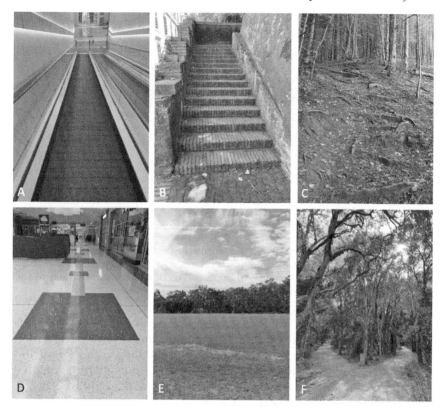

Figure 5.3 Examples of walking environments that present varying degrees of perceptual-motor challenge. *From left to right, presented environments decrease in regularity, that is from more closed environments on the left (A, D) to more open walking challenges on the right (B, C, E, F). Bottom row images present environments without slope (D–F), top row presents more demanding slope conditions (A–C). Key points: in the statement that the use of walking interventions is limited for fall prevention (Sherrington et al., 2019), there is an assumption that the training effect in all environments is equal. We reason that making a distinction between environments could lead to a more refined knowledge from experimental results and better exercise prescription.*

completed, additional columns could be added to Figure 5.4 which refer to increased levels of openness of the environment. In making the decision not to add these further columns at this stage, two reasons were considered. First, the initial aim of this classification was for a clinician to understand the demands of a given walking intervention and see the natural progression in these environments. The further (fifth, sixth, etc.) columns would be dependent upon unpredictable elements of the environment, such as wind, rain, iciness, other humans or animals, etc., which would potentially limit the usefulness of this tool for clinical practice to describe natural environments and prescribe green exercise. Second, even though

	1. Regular	2. Irregular	3. Irregular/Cluttered	4. Visually challenging
	No step-to-step adjustments needed	*Adjustments needed to maintain gait*	*Adjustments needed in cluttered environment*	*Demands of adjustments not visually specified*
C. Steep Incline or Decline (>5 degrees or longer stairs)	*Steep pavement*	*Stairs walking*	*Hill climbing*	*Climbing a hill with loose rocks*
B. Slight Incline or Decline (0-5 degrees or 1-2 steps)	*Wheelchair ramp*	*Stepping onto a kerb*	*Rock hopping*	*Stepping onto a kerb in the dark*
A. Level Walking	*Treadmill walking Indoor walking*	*Walking on grass*	*Bushwalking*	*Slippery sidewalk*

Figure 5.4 Situational Taxonomy for Environment-Person Pairing In Natural Gait (STEPPING). The horizontal dimension relates to the perceptual demands of closed to less-closed environments, whereas the vertical dimension relates to the physical demands of the environment.

the "open environment" would be a natural progression in terms of skills classification, it would not be a progression in terms of risk-taking. Risk is usually measured in terms of the chance of something going wrong and the severity of the potential consequences (Aven et al., 2011). It could be hypothesized that in this aspect, the slippery sidewalk would have bigger odds of leading to a fall than a busy shopping mall.

To better understand the usefulness of the STEPPING, we refer to the results of a recent prospective falls screening collected in our lab (Andel, Cole, et al., 2019). A reanalysis of the used falls questionnaires provides an insight into the circumstances of the falls that occurred during locomotion (Figure 5.5). Most of the falls in this cohort occurred in a complex environment (mainly STEPPING category 2A) and only 6% of the falls in the simplest environment (1A). Also note that many of the higher order categories recorded a low falls incidence. This is probably related to exposure to these categories being limited. To refer to one of the earlier conclusions of this chapter, a successful intervention for falls prevention will need to be set in *an environment that has at least the same openness as the complex gait tasks during which falls occur*. Following this recommendation, successful walking interventions for falls prevention should include demands similar to, but preferably harder than, the STEPPING category 2A.

5.4 Recommendations...

... for research. This chapter introduced a situational taxonomy as a means to assess the demands of different environments on gait. The data presented in Figure 5.4 provides some indication that making this delineation

	1. Regular	2. Irregular	3. Irregular/Cluttered	4. Visually challenging
N = 104 participants 96 total falls reported 53 falls during locomotion	*No step-to-step adjustments needed*	*Adjustments needed to maintain gait*	*Adjustments needed in cluttered environment*	*Demands of adjustments not visually specified*
C. Steep Incline or Decline (>5 degrees or longer stairs)		**11%** *Mainly going up or down stairs*	**4%** *Bushwalking activities*	**4%** *Bushwalking activities*
B. Slight Incline or Decline (0-5 degrees or 1-2 steps)		**2%** *Missed a step*	**7%** *Bushwalking activities*	**4%** *Bushwalking activities*
A. Level Walking	**6%** *Various activities*	**48%** *Mainly trips while walking*	**4%** *Bushwalking activities*	**11%** *Mainly slips while walking*

Figure 5.5 Reanalyzed data from Andel, Cole and Pepping (2019), with falls incidence categorized using the STEPPING classification. The main cause of falls per categories is noted in the table. When categorization was unclear from the collected reports, the falls were categorized conservatively (closer to 1A). For instance, if a participant reported to have "tripped over a rock" this does not specify any incline of the walk or cluttering of the environment, it only specifies that there was a rock to trip on, resulting in a conservative 2A categorization.

between different environments could lead to new insights; however, further study is required to assess how gait and falls risk really change in the different categories. With the STEPPING classification system, the current chapter comes with new hypotheses that can be tested. Future studies within this direction should assess: i, whether walking interventions within particular classifications or with STEPPING-based progressions can be useful for falls prevention. ii, whether studies that show results in one category of the classification system can be generalized to natural gait with greater demands (and vice versa). And iii, whether different environments afford different means of exploration for the successful interaction with the world around us.

... for clinicians. Considering the lack of evidence-based protocols for using the STEPPING for exercise prescription, the clinical impact of this chapter is currently limited, and this chapter should be seen as a starting point to build this evidence base. However, the theoretical principles the taxonomy is founded upon are readily available and we recommend health practitioners to start with getting people more active in more open environments for the benefit of exploration, calibration, and overall functioning.

... for built environment practitioners (designers, architects, and planners). It is necessary to appreciate that creating new environments results in the creation of manifolds of opportunity for action for the individuals that will inhabit and use these environments. In doing so, built environment practitioners shape perception and action in relation to the

56   *S. v. Andel, M. Cole, and G.-J. Pepping*

created available affordances – the field of relevant affordances (Rietveld & Kiverstein, 2014; see also Withagen et al., 2012). How environments are built will invite and encourage certain behaviors and prevent other behaviors from being meaningful. In the context of mobility, healthy aging and falls prevention, as argued in this chapter, it is important to design environments that allow for affordances and gait-related activities that provoke gait-adaptability, such as those that are available in the natural environment (Andel, Cole, et al., 2018; Andel, Cole, et al., 2019; see also Brymer et al., 2020). Related, in the context of green exercise, to invite a broader range of health and wellbeing behaviors, built environment practitioners need to appreciate and provide for key nature affordances, beyond playing fields and picnic areas (van Heezik & Brymer, 2018). The STEPPING can be used as a tool in the design of these environments, for instance, to benchmark designed affordances against developed health standards for activity, mobility, and other relevant topics.

... for policy. Finally, it is important to consider how these insights could help shape policy, as mainly through policy could they have a greater impact on our aging society. Firstly, policymakers could do more to engage people in green exercise. That is, exercise in which people engage with the world around them. It is great development that policymakers understand the function of exercise (World Health Organization, 2018) and there are certainly benefits of getting more people active in gyms. However, for the purposes of gait adaptability and mobility over the lifespan, these benefits are limited. Green exercise would be an alternative that policymakers could focus on, which has potential benefits not only to gait adaptability and falls prevention, but also for mental wellbeing and quality of life (Barton & Pretty, 2010; Pretty et al., 2005).

In describing the function of prescribing green exercise for a healthy society, it is important to consider who will be prescribing this new mode of exercise. In the ruling medical model, we go to a doctor (general practitioner or otherwise) when something is wrong with us and this doctor might refer on to a specialist. However, prescribing exercise does not fit the traditional scope of practice of a doctor. Furthermore, if we wait until a person visits a medical doctor, many opportunities to improve quality of life with exercise have already been missed. Policymakers should bring people closer to those professionals that prescribe exercise (ideally these are Accredited Exercise Physiologists if available, though, in some countries, exercise prescription is done by Physiotherapists). It would be feasible in the prevention of long-term medical costs to make a visit to an exercise professional affordable and universally available as only these professionals can be expected to understand the optimal way to deliver exercise as preventative medicine. These professionals are the ones that should be aware of motor learning principles and could, for instance, use the STEPPING to improve health and wellbeing and use it as a much-needed counterargument for risk-mitigation.

In conclusion, let us return to our introduction, and the sign that reads *"please hold handrail."* We do not mean to say that all of the built environment should give up their risk mitigation strategies and, arguably, a train station would not be the place to embrace risk. Public transport needs to be available and accessible for everyone, also with limited mobility. However, embracing risk should remain an option for people and architects should facilitate this. As discussed above, any training of skill in, for instance, falls risk needs to be done in a situation with increased openness and thus increased risk. Mitigating all risk in our environment results in people not being trained anymore to function in open environments. The option to engage with an open environment should therefore always be readily available for people. One should not have to travel out of cities and into forests or bushland to encounter an open environment; the built environment can be designed to give people the option to train their gait.

References

Andel, S. van, Cole, M. H., & Pepping, G.-J. (2017). A systematic review on perceptual-motor calibration to changes in action capabilities. *Human Movement Science, 51*, 59–71. https://doi.org/10.1016/j.humov.2016.11.004

Andel, S. van, Cole, M. H., & Pepping, G.-J. (2018). Regulation of locomotor pointing across the lifespan: Investigating age-related influences on perceptual-motor coupling. *PLOS ONE, 13*(7), e0200244. https://doi.org/10.1371/journal.pone.0200244

Andel, S. van, Cole, M. H., & Pepping, G.-J. (2019). Associations between gait-related falls and gait adaptations when stepping onto a curb: A prospective falls study. *Journal of Aging and Physical Activity, 27*(3), 309–315. https://doi.org/doi:10.1123/japa.2018-0124

Andel, S. van, McGuckian, T. B., Chalkley, D., Cole, M. H., & Pepping, G.-J. (2019). Principles of the guidance of exploration for orientation and specification of action. *Frontiers in Behavioral Neuroscience, 13*(231), 1–11. https://doi.org/10.3389/FNBEH.2019.00231

Aven, T., Renn, O., & Rosa, E. A. (2011). On the ontological status of the concept of risk. *Safety Science, 49*(8–9), 1074–1079. https://doi.org/10.1016/j.ssci.2011.04.015

Barton, J., & Pretty, J. (2010). What is the best dose of nature and green exercise for improving mental health: A multi-study analysis. *Environmental Science and Technology, 44*(10), 3947–3955. https://doi.org/10.1021/es903183r

Berg, W. P., Alessio, H. M., Mills, E. M. E. M., & Tong, C. (1997). Circumstances and consequences of falls in independent community-dwelling older adults. *Age and Ageing, 26*(4), 261–268. https://doi.org/10.1093/ageing/26.4.261

Brymer, E., Araújo, D., Davids, K., Pepping, G.-J. (2020). *Conceptualizing the Human Health Outcomes of Acting in Natural Environments : An Ecological Perspective. 11*(July), 1–6. https://doi.org/10.3389/fpsyg.2020.01362

Burns, E. R., Stevens, J. A., & Lee, R. (2016). The direct costs of fatal and non-fatal falls among older adults — United States. *Journal of Safety Research, 58*, 99–103. https://doi.org/10.1016/j.jsr.2016.05.001

58　*S. v. Andel, M. Cole, and G.-J. Pepping*

Chemero, A. (2003). An outline of a theory of affordances. *Ecological Psychology*, 15(2), 181–195.

Chemero, A. (2009). *Radical Embodied Cognitive Science*. MIT Press.

Cisek, P., & Kalaska, J. F. (2010). Neural mechanisms for interacting with a world full of action choices. *Annual Review of Neuroscience*, 33, 269–298. https://doi. org/10.1146/annurev.neuro.051508.135409

Davids, K. W., Button, C., & Bennett, S. J. (2008). *Dynamics of Skill Acquisition: A Constraints-led Approach*. Human Kinetics.

Dicks, M., Davids, K., & Button, C. (2009). Representative task designs for the study of perception and action in sport. *International Journal of Sport Psychology*, 40(4), 506–524.

Ebrahim, S., Thompson, P. W., Baskaran, V., & Evans, K. (1997). Randomized placebo-controlled trial of brisk walking in the prevention of postmenopausal osteoporosis. *Age and Ageing*, 26(4), 253–260. https://doi.org/10.1093/ ageing/26.4.253

Fernández-Ruiz, J., Hall, C., Vergara, P., & Díaz, R. (2000). Prism adaptation in normal aging: Slower adaptation rate and larger aftereffect. *Cognitive Brain Research*, 9(3), 223–226. https://doi.org/10.1016/S0926-6410(99)00057-9

Gentile, A. M. (1972). A working model of skill acquisition with application to teaching. *Quest*, 17(1), 3–23. https://doi.org/10.1080/00336297.1972.10519717

Gibson, J. J. (1979). *The Ecological Approach to Visual Perception*. Psychology Press.

Gray, R. (2014). Embodied perception in sport. *International Review of Sport and Exercise Psychology*, 7(1). https://doi.org/10.1080/1750984X.2013.871572

Hendrie, D., Hall, S. E., Arena, G., & Legge, M. (2004). Health system costs of falls of older adults in Western Australia. *Australian Health Review : A Publication of the Australian Hospital Association*, 28(3), 363–373.

Konczak, J., Meeuwsen, H. J., & Cress, M. E. (1992). Changing affordances in stair climbing: The perception of maximum climbability in young and older adults. *Journal of Experimental Psychology. Human Perception and Performance*, 18(3), 691–697.

Newell, K. M. (1986). Constraints on the Development of Coordination. In M. G. Wade & H. T. A. Whiting (Ed.), *Motor development in children: Aspects of coordination and control* (pp. 341–360). Martinus Nijhoff Publishers.

Orth, D., van der Kamp, J., & Button, C. (2019). Learning to be adaptive as a distributed process across the coach–athlete system: Situating the coach in the constraints-led approach. *Physical Education and Sport Pedagogy*, 24(2), 146–161. https://doi.org/10.1080/17408989.2018.1557132

Pinder, R. A., Davids, K., Renshaw, I., & Araújo, D. (2011). Representative learning design and functionality of research and practice in sport. *Journal of Sport and Exercise Psychology*, 33(1), 146–155. https://doi.org/10.1123/jsep.33.1.146

Poulton, E. E. (1957). On prediction in skilled movements. *Psychological Bulletin*, 54(6), 467–478. https://doi.org/10.1037/h0045515

Pretty, J., Peacock, J., Sellens, M., & Griffin, M. (2005). The mental and physical health outcomes of green exercise. *International Journal of Environmental Health Research*, 15(5), 319–337. https://doi.org/10.1080/09603120500155963

Rietveld, E., & Kiverstein, J. (2014). A rich landscape of affordances. *Ecological Psychology*, 26(4), 325–352. https://doi.org/10.1080/10407413.2014.958035

Sherrington, C., Fairhall, N. J., Wallbank, G. K., Tiedemann, A., Michaleff, Z. A., Howard, K., Clemson, L., Hopewell, S., & Lamb, S. E. (2019). Exercise for preventing falls in older people living in the community. *Cohrane Database of Systematic Reviews*, 1. https://doi.org/10.1002/14651858.CD012424.pub2

Sherrington, C., Michaleff, Z. A., Fairhall, N., Paul, S. S., Tiedemann, A., Whitney, J., Cumming, R. G., Herbert, R. D., Close, J. C. T., & Lord, S. R. (2017). Exercise to prevent falls in older adults: An updated systematic review and meta-analysis. *British Journal of Sports Medicine*, *51*(24), 1749–1757. https://doi.org/10.1136/bjsports-2016-096547

van Heezik, Y., & Brymer, E. (2018). Nature as a commodity: What's good for human health might not be good for ecosystem health. *Frontiers in Psychology*, *9*(SEP), 1–5. https://doi.org/10.3389/fpsyg.2018.01673

Vaz, D. V., Silva, P. L., Mancini, M. C., Carello, C., & Kinsella-Shaw, J. (2017). Towards an ecologically grounded functional practice in rehabilitation. *Human Movement Science*, *52*, 117–132. https://doi.org/10.1016/j.humov.2017.01.010

Voukelatos, A., Merom, D., Sherrington, C., Rissel, C., Cumming, R. G., & Lord, S. R. (2015). The impact of a home-based walking programme on falls in older people: The easy steps randomised controlled trial. *Age and Ageing*, *44*(3), 377–383. https://doi.org/10.1093/ageing/afu186

Warren, W. H. (1984). Perceiving affordances: Visual guidance of stair climbing. *Journal of Experimental Psychology. Human Perception and Performance*, *10*(5), 683–703. https://doi.org/10.1037/0096-1523.10.5.683

Withagen, R., de Poel, H. J., Araújo, D., & Pepping, G.-J. (2012). Affordances can invite behavior: Reconsidering the relationship between affordances and agency. *New Ideas in Psychology*, *30*(2), 250–258. https://doi.org/10.1016/j.newideapsych.2011.12.003

World Health Organization (2007). *WHO global report on falls prevention in older age*. World Health Organization. https://doi.org/978 92 4 156353 6

World Health Organization (2018). *Global action plan on physical activity 2018–2030: More active people for a healthier world*. World Health Organization.

Part II

Theoretical Approaches

6 Resilience

John F. Allan

6.1 Introduction

Young people across western society are facing a multitude of risk factors which challenge their capacity to cope with stress and fulfil their potential as adults. This inability to adapt to changing circumstances will result in a marked deterioration of their mental health, which, without help, could lead them to face a lifetime of psychological problems. Highly resourceful individuals with wide functional repertoires for handling stress are considered resilient. Resilient individuals adapt and recover quickly from prevailing stressors (denoting bounce-back ability) and see problems as opportunities for dynamic self-renewal (bounce-beyond ability). Although resilience does not provide immunity from stress or emotional distress, it comprises a healthy, stable trajectory of functionality which can be learned (Bonanno, 2004; Norris, Tracey & Galea, 2009). Given this understanding, the purposeful development of resilience of young people is high on the agenda for education and health care strategists and practitioners.

Resilience enables young people to deal with stress throughout periods of uncertainty in their lives, such as transitions between primary and secondary school, or when starting university (McIntosh & Shaw, 2017). A dearth of research evidence suggests engagement with nature-based and Adventurous Physical Activities (APA) help young people build a range of psychosocial strengths, consistent with resilience, to support their healthy development (e.g. Ewert & Tessneer, 2019; Fuller, Powell & Fox, 2017; Kelly, 2019). Few of these studies, however, contain robust empirical designs which examine the impact and processes of APA experiences upon young people's resilience. This chapter appraises psychological resilience as a viable working construct for the positive development of young people. Firstly, a rationale for the adoption of resilience to build adaptive capacity in young people is critiqued. Following this, a synopsis of our research evaluates the value of nature-based and APA for building resilience in young people in education. This includes evaluating their learned capability to bounce back from setbacks and to constructively harness the stress response to support their happy, well-adjusted growth.

DOI: 10.4324/9781003154419-8

64   *J.F. Allan*

6.2 A Question of Healthy Adaptability

On the journey into adulthood, young people need to be resilient to ever-present threats to their healthy development. Political, social, and economic instabilities present adolescents with wide-ranging challenges at a period in their life of significant adjustments in physical, cognitive, and social-emotional capabilities. Such environmental and personal upheavals leave young people vulnerable to mental ill-health if they cannot adapt to changing circumstances. The prevention of healthy development of adolescents has been attributed to the increased prevalence of mental disorders which represent the major cause of disability worldwide in youth aged 10 to 24 years of age (World Health Organization, 2015, 2020).

Adolescent mental health is increasingly impacted from societal practices which may directly inhibit the resilience of young people. Many young people have been reported as fearful of bullying, stressed by exam workloads, worried about family relationships, experiencing peer pressure, or physical, emotional, or sexual abuse (Holloway, Green & Livingstone, 2013; The Good Childhood Report, 2015). In *The Coddling of the American Mind,* Jonathon Haidt suggests these modern-day maladies are linked with over-reductive education, paranoid parenting, and overzealous bureaucracy which cocoon young people from failure; limiting their capacity to overcome even small problems. Pathological labeling of normal adolescent responses to everyday experiences such as loss of romantic attachments may intensify negative feelings, providing a sense of victimhood and create an even more diminished sense of responsibility (Craig, 2009).

Psychological resilience reflects the adaptive capabilities of individuals to withstand stressors and develop under difficult circumstances (Rutter et al., 2013). Although resilience is not synonymous with mental health (Provencher & Keyes, 2011), such incapacity is likely to lead to permanently sick or disabled middle-aged adults (Kessler et al., 2012). Given over half of all lifetime mental disorders have been diagnosed by mid-teens, adolescence is a prime time for building the resilience of youngsters to make healthy, effective transitions into adulthood (Allan, Slee & Bell, 2017; Allan & McKenna, 2019; Allan & McKenna, 2021; Layhard & Hagell, 2015).

The worldwide prevalence of adolescent mental ill-health suggests educational institutions need to play a more significant role in detecting problems, supporting young people, and providing preventative programmes. In the World Health Organization report, *Health for the World's Adolescents* (2014), authors specifically call upon educational institutions to respond to the needs of adolescents' physical and mental health more urgently. Resilience has long been understood to be significant in learning contexts within school-age education (Bryan, 2005; Cassidy, 2015; Esquivel, Doll & Oades-Sese, 2011) where an ability to build adaptive resources to recover or "bounce back" from unusual situations is linked to success. However, the pressure of school inspections and performance league tables has led to schools delivering overly reductive exam-based education (Hutchings, 2015). There are too few opportunities for young people to take part in authentic "nonformal learning" activities that enable them to build vital character attributes.

Despite the acknowledged mental health benefits of outdoor physical activity for young people (Tillmann et al., 2018; van den Berg et al., 2015), many youngsters are being denied access to nature or authentic risky forms of play to build their resilience. A survey by The Children's Society (2014) found that one-third of children never play outside mainly due to fears surrounding abduction and injury. Those children that do engage in physical activities outside spend more time under adult supervision which tends to stifle their creativity and drive to experiment. Evidence suggests that outdoor skills not only reinforce academic learning but also have a significant positive influence on various later life outcomes, including those relating to health, wellbeing, and careers (Paterson, Tyler & Lexmond, 2014). Coupled with overindulgent parenting and increasing risk-aversive practices, youngsters may be ill-prepared for present and future bumps in the road.

Young people are certainly vulnerable to stress when making transitions in education. Movement between primary and secondary school and starting life at university seems to impact negatively upon an increasing number of students' psychological health and academic achievement (Royal College of Psychiatrists, 2011). For example, UK school children, particularly those from poorer households and ethnic minorities, are finding it increasingly difficult to assimilate into new educational settings (Deieso & Fraser, 2019). Mental ill-health and dropouts from studies within new university student populations have also been reported to be problematically high (Johnson & Crenna-Jennings, 2018; Thorley, 2017) and evidenced from multiple countries (Aljohani, 2016; Glass, 2010; Hussain et al, 2013; Pidgeon et al., 2014; Storrie, Ahern & Tuckett, 2010) making this an important contemporary Public Health issue.

As the case with schoolchildren, resilience has helped university students to perform successfully in educational settings (Ayala & Manzano, 2018; Challen, Machin & Gillham, 2014; Pidgeon et al., 2014). Resilient behaviors have improved their mental health during stressful exam periods (DeBerard, et al., 2004; Elizondo-Omana et al., 2007; Galante et al., 2018) and more strongly influence retention and achievement in higher education (HE) than qualifying grades (Bell & Chang, 2017). Nonetheless, inadequate pedagogy and support strategies for students' assimilation into HE are widely reported, leading to calls for universities to build resilience in learners to enable them to complete their studies (Higher Education Policy Institute, 2019; Hubble & Bolton, 2019; Pereira et al., 2019). To understand positive trajectories by which students can create fulfilling learning experiences, more research is required into the concept of psychological resilience across educational settings. This includes the underlying motivations

66   J.F. Allan

and protective factors which can inform strategies to help young people achieve their potential and influence various later life outcomes, including those relating to health, wellbeing, and careers.

6.3 Understanding Resilience, Concepts, and Origins

Psychological resilience is widely used to refer to a range of phenomena including the prevention of psychopathology, positive adaptive functioning, rapid recovery from adverse circumstances, and post-traumatic psychological growth (Allan & Charura, 2018; Calhoun & Tedeschi, 2004; Fletcher & Sarkar, 2013). The numerous definitions of resilience typically incorporate two facets: (i) the experience of stress or risk, and (ii) positive achievement despite adversity (Gartland et al., 2011; Murphey, Barry & Vaughn, 2013). Young people confronted by adverse circumstances are considered resilient if they continue to function within acceptable bounds on measures of behavioral, social, or intellectual functioning (Harvey & Delfabbro, 2004; Masten, 2014). Four waves of resilience research continue to yield a consistent body of findings, concepts, and theories for understanding the prevention, resistance to, and recovery from, adversity.

The **first wave** of research was generated from studies reporting descriptive characteristics of youngsters who seemed to develop well despite their genetic or environmental risk. These correlates of good adaptation included a wide array of personal attributes and skills, such as self-efficacy and positive peer relationships, which are substantiated in reducing risk and exhibiting strength-based behaviors (Carver 1998; Garmezy, 1993; Werner, 1995; Windle, 2010). Consistent with this first wave approach, identifiable characteristics which underpin gender-specific types of resilience have been proposed. Females may prefer adaptive behavior which involves mutual support and "tend and befriend" responses termed *relational resilience* (Taylor et al., 2000). Males tend to project external confidence and attribute failure externally to preserve an image of self-reliance or *pseudo-resilience* (Hartling, 2003; Pollack, 2006).

The **second wave** of research focuses on the systematic "individual x environment interactions" that promote mastery of developmental tasks such as positive peer relationships, appropriate conduct, and academic achievement (Luthar, 2006). Hence, resilience here is not viewed as a general quality or trait which can be applied to all across all risk contexts (Heller et al., 1999). Rather, resilience represents a multidimensional interactive construct which may be innate and/or learned which enable people to lead more productive lives despite being at greater risk than average for serious problems (Brooks, 2006; Rutter, 2006).

In the **third wave**, resilience-building is the focus of theory-driven interventions targeted on influencing developmental pathways (e.g. Weissberg, Klumpfer & Seligman, 2003). It is proposed that as multiple risk factors increase across the life course, there should be multiple, plausible routes to

Resilience 67

intervention which are timed to protect against salient risks and promote developmental competencies.

A contemporary **fourth wave** aims to gain a deeper understanding of how biobehavioral processes work (including genes, adaptive brain functioning, and development) in responding to stress (e.g. Mata, Thompson & Gotlib, 2010). Contrary to previous understanding that brain capacity is fixed and finite, emerging evidence has confirmed the immense malleability of the brain across the lifecycle; able to adapt its structure (growth of new cells) and function (rewiring of existing cells) directly in response to environmental exposure.

These waves of research have led to suggestions of the presence of two aspects of behavioral adaptation in human development: (i) a dynamic interactive *process* of adaptation between both risks and protective factors which act to modify the effects of an adverse life event; and (ii) psychosocial *outcomes* characterized by relative effective functioning within a particular risk setting. Individuals generally respond to disruption through a process of reintegration from a position of homeostasis. Within reintegration, a range of possible outcomes exist. An individual may (i) reintegrate back to a baseline state, (ii) reintegrate with loss, and (iii) dysfunction or demonstrate resilience. Resilient reintegration represents the development of growth as a result of the disruption (Richardson, 2002). Knowledge of this process may empower individuals to develop choices in responding to adversity and help them recognize that facilitated exposure to challenges may serve to catalyze this process.

6.4 Resilience: A Framework of Positive Youth Development

The similarity of risk and protective factors across the domains of the home, health, education, and wider society provides resilience with the potential to be an organizing concept for interventions to combat mental illness in young people. Interest in the conceptualization, measurement, and promotion of young people's wellbeing has become a prominent theme across many spheres of policy resulting in a plethora of new initiatives across governments and charities (Ager, 2013). Emphasis is increasingly being placed on character-building and development of emotional strengths in young people not only to provide long-term protection from risks to mental health, but to enable effective transitions into adulthood, promote social mobility, and underpin educational attainment (Care, Griffin & Wilson, 2018).

Such strategies have not been without their critics, leaving gaps for the development of more nuanced, targeted resilience-building interventions. Firstly, resilience has often been criticized due to ambiguities in both definitions and terminology (Earvolino-Ramirez, 2007; Vanderbilt-Adriance & Shaw, 2008) casting some doubt on the utility of resilience as

68   *J.F. Allan*

a consistent theoretical construct (Bodin & Winman, 2004; Davydov et al., 2010). Debate continues concerning what constitutes the attributes, personal meaning, and the level and type of adversity experienced for someone to be termed resilient and how best to measure successful adaptation to hardship. Very different constellations of psychosocial processes may be antecedent to a range of resilient outcomes within individuals. From this understanding, interventions need to investigate the transactional processes for promoting resilience across adolescent domains and contexts on the path to normative development. (Ungar & Teram, 2005). Specifically, it may be more productive to identify assets and resources that have been found to promote healthy functioning in groups of young people at certain levels of development or in a particular context (Ungar, 2013).

6.5 Nature-based and Adventurous Physical Activity (APA) Builds Resilient, Healthy, and Happy Youngsters

In the context of outdoor adventure learning, there is an apparent fit between the stated goals of APA and experiences that may generate resilience in young people. Supported exposure to risk through APA subscribes to principles adopted by adolescent models of resilience, whereby moderate levels of risk provide situational and ongoing protective resistance, constituting a "steeling effect" for later stress (Olsson et al., 2003; Rutter, 2013). Idealized, residential nature-based APA programmes represent a microcosm of the challenges facing students in transitions, including establishing peer connections, becoming familiar with new routines, and managing increasing levels of cognitive and affective complexity (Allan & McKenna, 2019). Previously, following participation in APA, students have reported increases in resilience equating to effect sizes (magnitude of change) ranging from 0.20 (small) to 1.10 (large) compared to non-attendees (Beightol et al., 2012; Hayhurst et al., 2013; Kelly, 2019; Neill & Dias, 2001; Overholt & Ewert, 2015; Scarf et al., 2016; Wittington & Budbill, 2015). Under the premise of optimizing student integration into a new environment, US universities implement one-week Outdoor Orientation Programmes (OOPs) with variable success reporting greater levels of emotional and social development, positive attitudes toward the institution and increases in academic performance in the short-term and over time (e.g. Bell & Chang, 2017; Davidson & Ewert, 2020; Micheal, Morris-Duerr & Reichert, 2017; Schwartz & Belknap, 2017).

Notwithstanding these findings, the dynamic interplay between APA exposure, increased psychosocial functioning, and resilient outcomes in young people are largely unclear. Methodological limitations (e.g. over-reliance on anecdotal evidence, small sample sizes, lack of control groups and follow-up data, and singular measurement) have made it difficult to validate short-term benefits. There remains a strong requirement to investigate the mediating effects of gender and evaluations of personal competencies combined with environmental (programme) conditions which may build resilience. Understanding the appropriate dose or level of immersion within APA experiences is necessary to develop efficacious programmes which promote healthy adaptive changes whilst avoiding maladaptive responses. Until these issues are addressed, critics will continue to argue that positive outcomes emanating from APA are largely based upon intuitive belief systems and untested assumptions rather than being derived from a broad empirical evidence base (Brookes, 2003a, b; Sheard & Golby, 2006).

6.6 Research Endeavours: Psychological Resilience and APA Programming in Student Populations

Our research responds directly to the prevailing gaps in literature. We have delivered large-scale, empirically robust studies investigating *if*, and *how*, nature-based and APA residential programmes reveal and strengthen the adaptive capabilities of young people. The four progressive waves of resilience research identified earlier in the chapter have provided a focus for our research aims and objectives.

6.6.1 Wave 1: Descriptive Characteristics of Students' Resilience Before, During, and Following Exposure to Nature-based APA Programmes

The adaptive capabilities of over 2,500 university inductees from 16 courses across 5 years have been profiled. This represents the largest, most unique study of its kind. Trajectories of individuals' adaptive functioning across three data-capture points have symbolized the immediate and longer-term impacts of APA experiences upon students' wellbeing and educational attainment. From such extensive analyses, a gold-standard inventory of strength-based instrumentation has been established for use with students. This includes valid and reliable measures of psychological resilience (e.g. Connor & Davidson, 2003), hardiness, mindset, self-determination, sense of mastery, and positive affect.

6.6.2 Wave 2: Nature-based APA Interactions that Promote Strength-based Functioning in Students

We have identified the most powerful active ingredients of change in APA which builds psychological resilience and predicts wider adaptive functioning in new students. Such embodied, meaningful challenges – which require inductees to realign their perceived capabilities – may help normalize difficulties that all learners face in HE. These correlates of positive behavior enable students to readjust, grow, and succeed in their academic studies.

70   J.F. Allan

6.6.3 Wave 3: APA as an Effective Resilience-building Intervention for Young People

Powerful, multilevel statistical analyses have evidenced efficacious, positive change in strength-based functioning across student populations and subgroups (e.g. annual cohorts, gender, and socioeconomic status). This affords meaningful depth *and* breadth of research outcomes.

6.6.4 Wave 4: Nature-based APA Builds Brain Resilience

Precise, objective analyses of unconscious neurobiological processes have questioned assumptions that there are common processes across all APA programmes generating intuitively appealing outcomes.

6.7 The First Wave: Characteristics of Students' Resilience

6.7.1 Psychologically Vulnerable, Poor University Readiness

Our research confirmed that new students are psychologically vulnerable on entry into HE, necessitating a greater emphasis of universities to diagnose and address the evolving needs of their inductees (Allan, McKenna & Dominey, 2013). Data revealed that inductees' incoming resilience was akin to that of a group possessing lower levels of mental health and similar to students' resilience reported across a range of international studies. This provides support for the idea that students disproportionately experience mental illness, poor resilience, and/or problematic transitions into HE. It adds credence to UK and international concerns for the mental health problems and poor HE readiness of new students (e.g. Institute for Employment Studies, 2016) and provides justification for the use of interventions to build their resilience.

6.7.2 Complex, Unpredictable

We confirmed resilience as a complex and unpredictable concept, revealing that there are many variations in the resilience required for students to progress. For example, our female students' more "relational" forms of resilience were more facilitative of their subsequent academic outcomes than males' resilience. Bucking a conventional understanding that "more resilience helps performance," for males, high resilience was linked with poorer prospective academic performance. These findings convey that self-reporting of high resilience may not be universally virtuous. Further, it is the functional use of resilience (how best this is employed and not necessarily the outcomes) which is important to promote an array of adaptive responses.

6.7.3 Distinctive, Amenable to Change

Although resilience is undoubtedly complex, we found highly distinctive, modifiable patterns of resilient behavior in young people. Throughout our research, students' adaptive behaviors were similarly aligned from a wide range of psychometric instrumentation. These findings validated our data capture methods and confirmed the amenability of students' resilience to our forms of intervention. None of our intervention strategies appeared to worsen inductees' perceived fragility. Rather, data reported the presence of learned skill sets in HE (communication skills, adaptive problem-solving, and self-management/self-development) recognized as necessary for young people to navigate themselves throughout university and beyond.

6.7.4 Inclusive

Our interventions impacted most positively upon students who may have been the most vulnerable on entry into HE. Inductees with the lowest initial levels of resilience achieved the greatest increases and retention of resilience (Allan, 2017). This outcome upholds findings from our previous work which involved evaluating the impact of APA programming upon the self-determination of schoolchildren in transition from primary to secondary school (Allan et al., 2014). More importantly, it suggests that AP experiences which are stimulating and offer room to grow, offer students identified as vulnerable relatively better outcomes than those with higher initial adaptive qualities (Boffey, 2013).

6.7.5 Support for Academic Achievement

Resilience plays an important role for new students acquiring academic success in HE. Logistic regression modelling within our research reported that higher resilience on entry and following the APA programme predicted more favorable academic outcomes (Allan, 2019). Crucially, subdomains of resilience which contributed to this prospective academic success (i.e. close and dependable relationships, dealing effectively with change, taking control of difficult situations) were all heightened through, and predicted by, frequent exposure to distinct APA experiences and practices. This supports the use of APA to generate skill sets which could readily convert into teachable behaviors and approaches, many of which have proven worth for promoting retention and achievement in HE (e.g. Johnson et al., 2014).

6.8 The Second Wave: Nature-based APA Interactions that Promote Strength-based Functioning in Students

Predictive modelling in our research identified the types of experiences and degree of exposure which generated participants' resilience during APA programming in HE. Two validated bespoke instruments captured participants' self-perceptions of their (i) level of immersion within APA components of the programme (Camp Rating Scale, CRS) (Figure 6.1), and (ii) competencies acquired associated with adaptive functioning

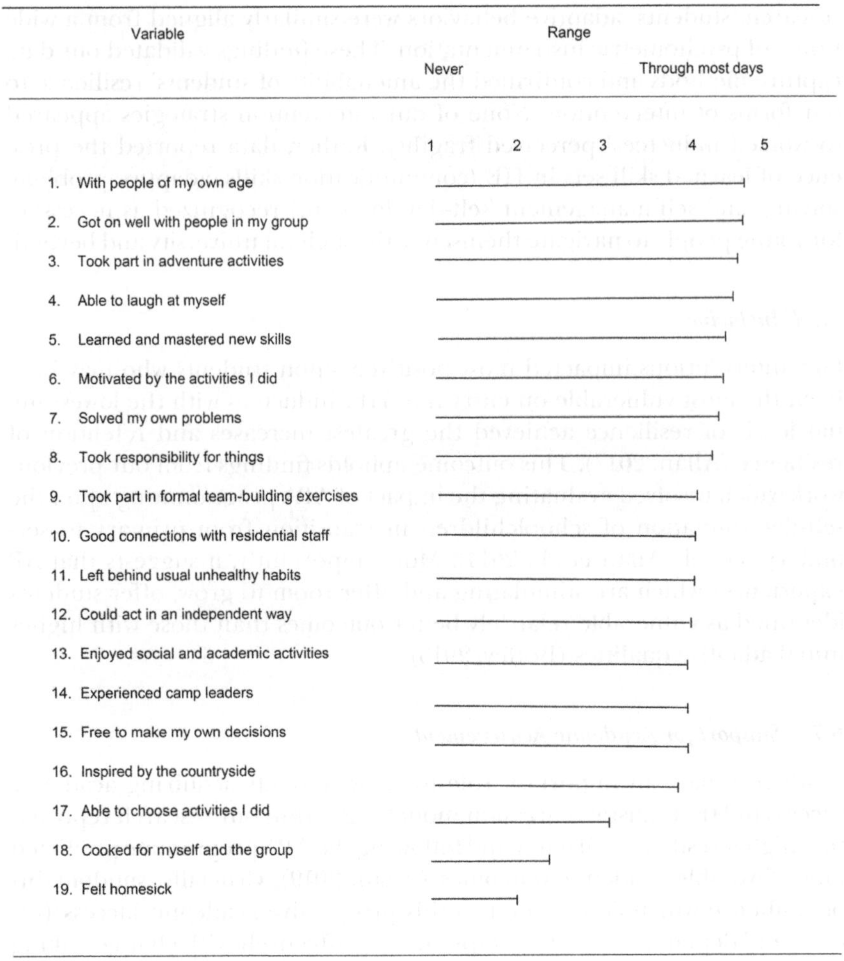

72   J.F. Allan

Variable	Range
	Never .... Through most days
	1 2 3 4 5
1. With people of my own age	
2. Got on well with people in my group	
3. Took part in adventure activities	
4. Able to laugh at myself	
5. Learned and mastered new skills	
6. Motivated by the activities I did	
7. Solved my own problems	
8. Took responsibility for things	
9. Took part in formal team-building exercises	
10. Good connections with residential staff	
11. Left behind usual unhealthy habits	
12. Could act in an independent way	
13. Enjoyed social and academic activities	
14. Experienced camp leaders	
15. Free to make my own decisions	
16. Inspired by the countryside	
17. Able to choose activities I did	
18. Cooked for myself and the group	
19. Felt homesick	

Figure 6.1 Camp Rating Scale (CRS), Mean (SD) responses.

(Perceived Competencies Scale, PCS) (Figure 6.2). On the CRS, inductees were much more likely to increase their resilience if they engaged within experiences whereby they "learned and mastered new skills" (most dominant predictor of change), were "free to make decisions," "got on well with people in my group," and "left behind usual unhealthy habits." On the PCS, "my social relationships", "my mental strength," "my level of optimism," and "manage life's ups and downs" were the dominant competencies most likely to heighten resilience. In one regression model, females were 35% more likely to be in a group of students with the highest improvement in resilience compared to males (Allan & McKenna, 2019).

This research was based on clear chains of inferential reasoning supported and justified by rigorous, objective practices across five years.

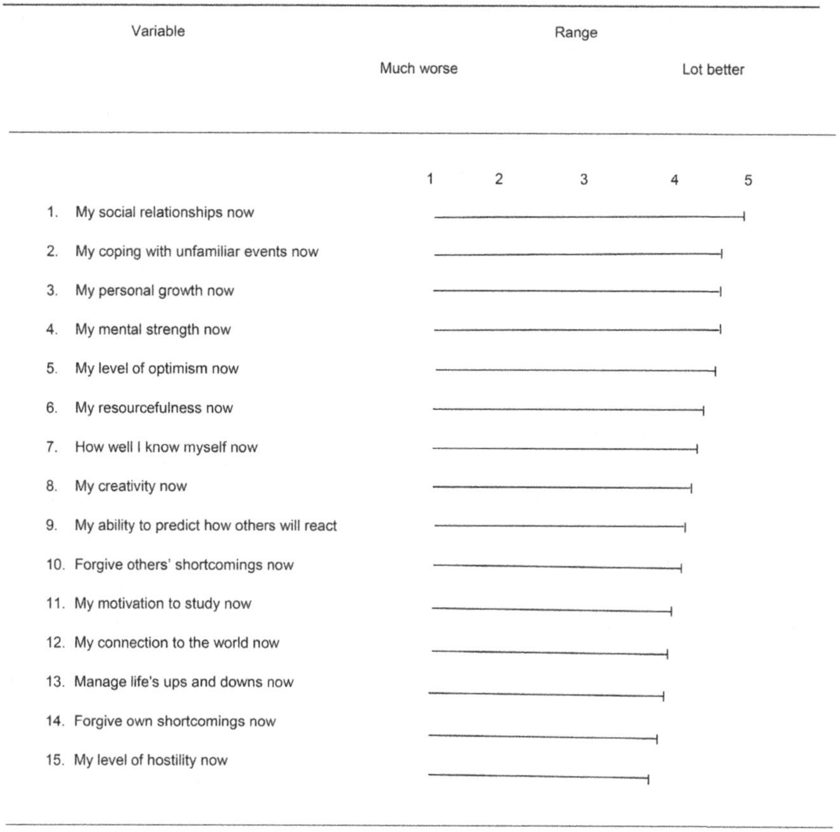

Variable	Range				
	Much worse				Lot better
	1	2	3	4	5

1. My social relationships now
2. My coping with unfamiliar events now
3. My personal growth now
4. My mental strength now
5. My level of optimism now
6. My resourcefulness now
7. How well I know myself now
8. My creativity now
9. My ability to predict how others will react
10. Forgive others' shortcomings now
11. My motivation to study now
12. My connection to the world now
13. Manage life's ups and downs now
14. Forgive own shortcomings now
15. My level of hostility now

Figure 6.2 Perceived Competencies Scale (PCS), Mean (SD) responses.

These findings provide powerful evidence for how enhanced resilience is predicted by manageable combinations of enabling processes and programme approaches. It shows that resilience was derived from actively confronting challenges; indicating a purposeful compatibility between participants needs and the dynamics of known components of APA programming. Arguably, these components constitute a broad set of readily available assets and resources to any community of practice intent on building individual and collective agency to protect against stress and support the healthy development of young people.

6.9 The Third Wave: APA as an Effective Resilience-Building Intervention for Young People

Nature-based APA residential programmes within our research enabled significant heightened adaptive capabilities of young people in the short term and across time. In our largest study, a significant 6.29% increase

74 *J.F. Allan*

(effect size = 0.38) was reported in the psychological resilience of over 2500 university inductees attending in excess of forty APA residential programmes. These students achieved an 8.35% greater increase in resilience compared to similar inductees who reported negative outcomes following a university-based induction programme (ES difference = −0.526). To substantiate these increases in resilience, APA programme inductees also experienced immediate positive changes in additional measures of adaptive capacity (e.g. The Mindset Scale, Dweck, 2006; and Modified Differentiated Emotions Scale, Fredrickson, 2004). The magnitude and direction of changes in resilience (ES) exceeded the educationally significant ESs of similar smaller studies and represented therapeutic value for young people (Allan & McKenna, 2019). These findings provide a powerful justification for using APA residential programming for developing immediate increases in the resilience of HE inductees.

A further study investigated the sustainability of the inductees' adaptive capabilities three months following the APA programme. A significant decrease in students' resilience portrayed limited retention of adaptive capacity and/or a realignment of their resilience to pre-programme levels. In line with theoretical understanding, inductees' resilience reflected a healthy, harm-reducing 'bounce-back' recovery following stress. Over two-thirds of students increased, retained or incurred only a small deficit in resilience at three months. Both genders reported comparable resilience profiles before, immediately following the APA and at three months. However, greater scrutiny of the data revealed females' resilience was more enduring and aligned with better prospective academic outcomes. Crucially, inductees who began APA programmes with the lowest resilience, and arguably the greatest need, made a "moderate" effect size gain across time (Allan, 2020). Given the nonuniformity and complexity of resilience, it is naive to expect that natural settings will routinely generate sustainable life experiences for students. Nonetheless, this study contends APA experiences which are structured to meet their transitional needs will act as an effective bridging effect across contexts to underpin students' ongoing wellbeing.

We have also reported immediate and sustained increases in the adaptive capabilities of school children resulting from their purposive exposure to APA programming. In direct comparison to generic APA programmes and schools-based inductions, "tailor-made" nature-based APA programmes have acted as the most significant catalyst for the development of self-determined behaviors and psychological wellbeing of students during educational transitions (Allan et al., 2014; Allan, Slee & Bell, 2017; Slee & Allan, 2019). Directly addressing the transitional needs of young people from disadvantaged households, students in our research studies have been systematically empowered to build skill sets needed to successfully assimilate into secondary school. Using the three subcomponents of the Self-Determination Theory (SDT) (Deci & Ryan, 2012), these skills

Resilience 75

include *Competence* (the ability to complete tasks), *Autonomy* (the capacity to self-direct learning), and *Relatedness* (how well a person can connect with others). Within our "tailor-made" programmes, APA facilitators and schoolteachers have successfully collaborated to embed SDT practices into their bespoke programme design; allowing children to plan their activities and connect learning to curriculum subjects, undertake independent risk-taking, and review naturally emerging experiences. To consolidate learning, children have been encouraged to move from describing outcomes and applying basic problem-solving (primary learning) to selecting, appraising, and presenting an understanding of skills needed to achieve in secondary school. Mixed methods data generated from these studies provide encouragement for schools delivering active programmes to smooth the transitions of incoming school children, particularly those targeted at more vulnerable groups.

6.10 The Fourth Wave: Nature-based APA Builds Resilient Brains

Human resilience can be explained by the brain's innate capability to adapt its structure (growth of new cells) and function (rewiring of existing cells) directly in response to environmental exposure. In our conceptual paper (Allan, McKenna & Hind, 2012), we argue that adventure-based behavioral responses are underpinned by each of these changes in brain functioning. To formulate our argument, we evaluated each of the active components of APA programming through a neurobiological lens. These included *the physical outdoor environment, facilitators, processes of learning, groups*, and the *participant*. For example, the dynamic nature of the *outdoor physical environment* supports elaborate neural adaptation which allows people who learn in multisensory environments to perform better than those in unisensory settings. The use of the brain's mirror neurons, whereby individuals are able to respond to expressions in the face of others, allows *facilitators* to develop intuitive insight into the fears and aspirations of participants, which promotes trust. The *processing* of information in APA learning is enhanced through the brain actively seeking and responding to biologically rewarding and meaningful stimuli. The *group* uses specially adapted neural structures and capacities which empower growth-fostering connections in testing conditions. Remarkable differences in the brain biology of the *participant* create the opportunity for effort-driven, custom-built challenges which build strong and enduring neural pathways which we recognize as personal growth.

We continue to undertake neurobiological research into APA and resilience to deepen our understanding of the attainment of personal growth objectives which are less prone to chance. It is envisaged that shining a scientific light into the fundamental processes of "stress and recovery" in APA will reveal a structure and order of human adaptive behavior that

76 *J.F. Allan*

is present in all of us. A growing scientific awareness of what is known, and of understanding what is now emerging, will help develop more credible insights and refine both practice-based evidence and deliver evidence-based practices.

6.11 Conclusion

In wider society, change is happening faster than can be understood or managed – from our ecological concern for the planet to welfare and education. To survive and prosper in such potentially destructive times, young people need the flexibility and self-awareness that resilience can provide. Addressing widespread evidential gaps, the intention of our research has been to investigate the purposive use of nature-based APA for building the resources needed for young people to meet the demands of educational transitions. The complex nature of this work has ensured both strengths and caveats attributed to our findings. The strengths center upon the robust methodologies which established resilience emanating from APA programming as an efficacious mechanism whereby students could succeed across adolescent domains and contexts. Limitations include the lack of qualitative, indepth understanding of inductees' experiences which may have revealed naturally emergent variables of interest within APA programmes.

On balance, many new important findings have resulted from our empirical investigations, many of which inform professional practice. We confirmed that university inductees comprised a vulnerable group of young people susceptible to poor adaptability and mental health. This signifies the importance of early induction practices which should be designed to reverse societal practices (risk-aversion, reductive education) attributed to students' low incoming adaptive functioning. Carefully aligned induction practices enable young people to realign their personal and collective capabilities to cope with the realities of student life. Our detailed statistical analysis reveals that inductees' resilience is complex, unpredictable, gender-specific, and yet, portrays characteristic patterns of positive cognitive and affective skills which support academic attainment. Most importantly, inductees' resilience was highly modifiable; exposure to continually refined APA programming was able to maximize the potential for immediate and lasting biopsychosocial benefits for a wide range of young people. These findings should reassure APA advocates about the impacts of outdoor adventure upon students' adaptive functioning. At the same time, they can help others design pedagogy and/or formulate any effective personal development programme across educational contexts. In future, we need to increase our knowledge of transactional processes within and between APA components and participants. This will allow for a greater critical use of strength-based practices with even more prescribed outcomes. Notably, emphasis should be placed upon the value of developing inductees' self-reliance, mastery learning, freedom to fail, problem-solving, learning through natural, multisensory stimulation, collaborative learning in testing conditions, and effort-driven, custom-built challenges.

References

Ager, A. (2013). Annual research review: Resilience and child well-being – public policy implications, Journal of Child Psychology and Psychiatry, 54(4), pp. 488–500.

Aljohani, O. (2016). A review of the contemporary international literature on student retention in higher education. International Journal of Education and Literacy, (4) 1; doi:10.7575/aiac.ijels.v.4n.1p.40.

Allan J. F., & Charura D. (2018). Spiritual development, meaning making, resilience and potential for post-traumatic growth among asylum-seekers and refugees: An interpretative phenomenological analysis, qualitative methods in psychology. UK: Aberystwyth University, The British Psychological Society. www.bps.org.uk/qmip2017.

Allan, J. F., & McKenna, J. (2019). Outdoor adventure builds resilient learners for higher education: A quantitative analysis of the active components of positive change, Sports, 7, 122; doi: 10.3390/sports7050122.

Allan, J. F., & McKenna, J. (2021). From Surviving to Thriving; Trajectories of Resilience in University Inductees Following Outdoor Adventure (OA) Residential Programmes Adolescent Psychiatry (in press).

Allan, J. F., Kay, H., Peacock, C., Hart, S., Dillon, M., & Brymer, E. (2020). Health and wellbeing in an outdoor and adventure sports context, Sports, 8, 50; doi: 10.3390/sports8040050.

Allan, J. F., McKenna, J., & Dominey, S. (2013). Degrees of resilience: Profiling psychological resilience and prospective academic achievement in university inductees, British Journal of Guidance & Counselling, 42(1), pp. 9–25.

Allan, J. F., McKenna, J., & Hind, K. (2012). Brain resilience: Shedding light into the black box of adventure processes. Australian Journal of Outdoor Education, 16(1), pp. 3–14.

Allan, J. F., McKenna, J., Buckland, H., & Bell, R. (2014). Getting the Right Fit: Tailoring Outdoor Adventure Experiences for the Transition of Schoolchildren, Physical Education Matters, Spring Edition.

Allan J. F., Slee V., & Bell R. (2017). Schools Transition Outdoor Project Report Leeds Beckett University, Nell Bank Adventure Education Centre and Bradford Adventure Development Unit, Bradford Metropolitan District Council, 2017 (Report).

Ayala, J. C., & Manzano, G. (2018). Academic performance of first-year university students: The influence of resilience and engagement, Higher Education Research & Development, doi: 10.1080/07294360.1502258.

Beightol, J., Jevertson, J., Carter, S., Gray, S., & Gass, M. (2012). Adventure education and resilience enhancement, Journal of Experiential Education, 35(2), pp. 307–325.

Bell, J., & Chang, H. (2017). Outdoor orientation programs: A critical review of program impacts on retention and graduation, Journal of Outdoor Recreation, Education, and Leadership, 9(1), pp. 56–68.

Bodin, P., & Wiman, B. (2004). Resilience and other stability concepts in ecology: Notes on their origin, validity and usefulness. ESS bulletin, 2, pp. 33–43. In Fletcher, D., & Sarkar, M. (2013), Psychological resilience: A review and critique of definitions, concepts and theory, European Psychologist, 18(1), pp. 12–23.

78 J.F. Allan

Boffey, D. (2013). State School Graduates Failing to Reach Job Potential Despite Outperforming Their Private School Counterparts at University, State-Educated Students Do Less Well After College, Higher Education, The Observer, <www.the guardian.com> [Accessed 23 January 2013]

Bonanno, G. (2004). Loss, trauma, and human resilience: Have we underestimated the human capacity to thrive after extremely aversive events?, American Psychologist, 59(1), pp. 20–28.

Brookes, A. (2003a). A critique of neo-Hahnian outdoor education theory, Part one: Challenges to the concept of 'character building', Journal of Adventure Education and Outdoor Learning, 3(1), pp. 49–62.

Brookes, A. (2003b). A critique of neo-Hahnian outdoor education theory, Part two: The fundamental attribution error in contemporary outdoor education discourse, Journal of Adventure Education and Outdoor Learning, 3(2), pp. 119–132.

Brooks, J. E. (2006). Strengthening resilience in children and youths: Maximising opportunities through the schools, Children and Schools, 28(2), pp. 69–76.

Bryan, J. (2005). Fostering educational resilience and achievement in urban schools through family-community partnerships, Professional School Counselling, 8(3), pp. 219–228.

Calhoun, L. G., & Tedeschi, R. G. (2004). The foundations of posttraumatic growth: New considerations, Psychological Inquiry, 15(2), pp. 93–102.

Care, E., Griffin, P., & Wilson, M. (Eds.) (2018). Assessment and teaching of 21st Century skills: Research and applications. Dordrecht: Springer.

Carver, C. (1998). Resilience and thriving: Issues, models, and linkages, Journal of Social Issues, 54(2), pp. 245–266.

Cassidy, S. (2015). Resilience Building in Students: The Role of Academic Self-Efficacy, Frontiers in Psychology. <http://dx.doi.org/10.3389/fpsyg.2015.01781> [Assessed December 2015].

Challen, A. R., Machin, S. J., & Gillham, J. E. (2014). The UK Resilience Programme: A school-based universal nonrandomized pragmatic controlled trial, Journal of Consulting and Clinical Psychology, 82(1), pp. 75–89.

Connor, K. M., & Davidson, J. (2003). Development of a new resilience scale: The Connor-Davidson Resilience Scale (CD-RISC), Depression and Anxiety, 18(4), pp. 76–82.

Craig, C. (2009). The Curious Case of the Tail Wagging the Dog and Well-being in Schools, Centre for Confidence and Well-being, February 2009.

Davidson, C. & Ewert, A. (2020). College student commitment and outdoor orientation programming, Journal of Experiential Education, doi.org/10.1177/1053825920923709.

Davydov, D., Stewart, R., Ritchie, K., & Chaudieu, I. (2010). Resilience and mental health, Clinical Psychology Review, 30(5), pp. 479–495.

DeBerard, M., Spielmans, S., Glen I., & Julka, D. L. (2004). Predictors of academic achievement and retention among college freshmen: A longitudinal study, College Student Journal, 38(1), p. 66.

Deci, E. L., & Ryan, R. M. (2012). Self-determination theory. In P. A. M. Van Lange, A. W. Kruglanski, & E. T. Higgins (Eds.), Handbook of theories of social psychology, pp. 416–436, Sage Publications Ltd. New York https://doi.org/10.4135/9781446249215.n21.

Deieso, D. & Fraser, B. J. (2019). Learning environment, attitudes and anxiety across the transition from primary to secondary school mathematics. Learning Environment Research, 22, pp. 133–152, https://doi.org/10.1007/s10984-018-9261-5.

Dweck, C. (2006). Mindset: The new psychology of success. New York: Random House.

Earvolino-Ramirez, M. (2007). Resilience: A concept analysis, Nursing Forum, 42(2), pp. 73–82.

Elizondo-Omana, R. E., Garcia-Rodriguez M., & Guzman Lopez S. (2007). Resilience in medical students, FASEB Journal, 21(5), pp. 214.

Esquivel, G. B., Doll, B., & Oades-Sese, G. V. (2011). Introduction to the special issue: Resilience in schools, Psychology in the Schools, 48(7), pp. 649–651.

Ewert, A. & Tessneer, S. (2019). Psychological resilience and posttraumatic growth, Journal of Experiential Education, doi.org/10.1177/1053825919859027.

Ewert, A., & Yoshino, A. (2011). The influence of short-term adventure-based experiences on levels of resilience, Journal of Adventure Education and Outdoor Learning, 1(1), pp. 35–50.

Fletcher, D., & Sarkar, M. (2013). Psychological resilience, European Psychologist, 18(1), pp. 12–23.

Fredrickson, B. L. (2004). The broaden-and-build theory of positive emotions, Philosophical Transactions of the Royal Society London Biological Sciences, 359, pp. 1367–1377.

Fuller, C., Powell, D. & Fox, S. (2017). Making gains: The impact of outdoor residential experiences on students' examination grades and self-efficacy, Educational Review, (69) 2, pp. 232–247.

Galante, J., Dufour, G., Vainre, M., Wagner, A. P., Stochl, J., Benton, A., Lathia, N., Howarth, E., & Jones, P. B. (2018). A mindfulness-based intervention to increase resilience to stress in university students (the mindful student study): A pragmatic randomised controlled trial, Lancet Public Health, 3(2), pp. 72–81.

Garmezy, N. (1993). Vulnerability and Resilience. In: Funder, D.C., & Parke, R.D. (Eds.), Studying lives through time: personality and development. Washington DC: American Psychological Association, pp. 377–398.

Gartland, D., Bond, L., Olsson, C., Buzwell, S., & Sawyer, S. (2011). Development of a multi-dimensional measure of resilience in adolescents: The adolescent resilience questionnaire, BMC Medical Research Methodology, 11(1) pp. 1–10.

Glass, M. (2010). College Transition Experiences of Students with Mental Illness, Doctoral Dissertation. Virginia Polytechnic Institute, Blacksburg, Virginia.

Hartling, L. (2003). Strengthening resilience in a risky world, it's all about relationships. Women in therapy, The Howarth Press, 2(31), pp. 51–70.

Harvey J., & Delfabbro, P. H. (2004). Psychological resilience in disadvantaged youth: A critical overview, Australian Psychologist, 39(1), pp. 3–13.

Hayhurst, J., Hunter, J., Kafka, S., & Boyes, M. (2013). Enhancing resilience in youth through a 10-day developmental voyage, Journal of Adventure Education and Outdoor Learning, 15(1), pp. 40–52.

Heller, S. S., Larrieu, J. A., D'Imperio, R., & Boris, N. W. (1999). Research on resilience to child maltreatment: Empirical considerations, Child Abuse and Neglect, 23, pp. 321–338.

Higher Education Policy Institute (2019). Male and female participation and progression in higher education. Higher Education Policy Institute, UK.

80 J.F. Allan

Holloway, D., Green, L., & Livingstone, S. (2013). Zero to Eight: Young Children and their Internet Use, LSE, London and EU Kids Online, pp. 10–13.

Hubble, S., & Bolton, P. (2019). Support for Students with Mental Health Issues in Higher Education in England, House of Commons Library, Number 8593.

Hussain, R., Guppy, M., Robertson, S., & Temple, E. (2013). Physical and mental health perspectives of first-year undergraduate rural university students, British Medical Council Public Health, 13(1) pp 2–11.

Hutchings, M. (2015). Exam factories? The impact of accountability measures on children and young people. The National Union of Teachers, London Metropolitan University, UK.

Institute for Employment Studies (2016). IES Annual Review, December 2016, UK.

Johnson, J., & Crenna-Jennings, W. (2018). Prevalence of mental health issues within the student-aged population. Education Policy Institute, London UK.

Johnson, M., Taasoobshirazi, G., Kestler, J., & Cordova, J. (2014). Models and messengers of resilience: A theoretical model of college students' resilience, regulatory strategy use, and academic achievement, Educational Psychology, 35(7), pp. 869–885.

Kelly, J. (2019). Influence of outdoor and adventure activities on subjective measures of resilience in university students, Journal of Experiential Education, 42(3), pp. 264–279.

Kessler, R. C., Berglund, P., Demile, O., Jin, R., Merikangas, K. R., & Walters, E. E. (2012). Lifetime prevalence of onset distributions of DSM-IV disorders in the national comorbidity survey replication, Archives of General Psychiatry, 62, pp. 593–603.

Layhard, R., & Hagell, A. (2015). Transforming the Mental Health of Children, Report of the WISH Mental Health and Wellbeing in Children Forum, 2015. World Innovative Summit for Health, Qatar Foundation Imperial College, London, UK.

Lukianoff, G., & Haidt, J. (2019). The Coddling of the American Mind: How Good Intentions and Bad Ideas Are Setting Up a Generation for Failure, UK, Penguin Books.

Luthar, S. S. (2006). Resilience in development: A synthesis of research across five decades. In: Cicchetti, D., & Cohen D. J. (Eds.) (2006), Developmental Psychopathology (2nd Ed.), Risk, Disorder and Adaptation. New York: Wiley, pp. 739–795.

Masten, A. S. (2014). Global perspectives on resilience in children and youth, Child Development, 85, pp. 6–20.

Mata, J., Thompson, R. J., & Gotlib, I. (2010). BDNF genotype moderates the relation between physical activity & depressive symptoms, Health Psychology, 29, pp. 130–133.

McIntosh, E., & Shaw, J. (2017). Student Resilience: Exploring the positive case for resilience. Unite Students, Bristol UK

Micheal, J. M., Morris-Duerr, V., & Reichert, M. S. (2017). Differential effects of participation in an outdoor orientation program for incoming students, Journal of Outdoor Recreation, Education, and Leadership, 9(1), pp. 42–55.

Murphey, D., Barry, M., & Vaughn, B. (2013). Positive mental health: resilience. Child trends adolescent health highlight. Bethesda, Maryland: Child Trends.

Neill, J. T., & Dias, K. L. (2001). Adventure education and resilience; The double-edged sword, Journal of Adventure Education and Outdoor Learning, 1(2), pp. 35–42.

Norris, F. H., Tracy, M., & Galea, S. (2009). Looking for resilience: Understanding the longitudinal trajectories of responses to stress, Social Science and Medicine, 68, pp. 2190–2198.

Olsson, C., Bond. L., Burns, D. A., Vella-Broderick, S. M., & Sawyer, S.M. (2003). Adolescent resilience: A concept analysis, Journal of Adolescence, 26(2), pp. 1–11.

Overholt, J., & Ewert, A. (2015). Gender matters: Exploring the process of developing resilience through outdoor adventure, Journal of Experiential Learning, 38(1), pp. 41–55.

Paterson, C., Tyler, C., & Lexmond, J. (2014). Character and Resilience Manifesto, The All-Party Parliamentary Group on Social Mobility, with Centre Forum and Character Counts.

Pereira, S., Reay, K., Bottell, J., & Walker, L. (2019). University Student Mental Health Survey, 2018; A large-scale study into the prevalence of student mental illness within UK universities, Insight Network, London UK.

Pidgeon, A., McGrath, S., Magya, H., Stapleton, P., & Lo, B. (2014). Psychosocial moderators of perceived stress, anxiety and depression in university students: An international study, Open Journal of Social Sciences, 2, pp. 23–31.

Pidgeon, A., Rowe, N., Stapleton, P., Magyar, H., & Lo, B. (2014). Examining characteristics of resilience among university students: An international study, Open Journal of Social Sciences, 2, pp. 14–22.

Pollack, W. S. (2006). Sustaining and reframing vulnerability & connection, creating genuine resilience in boys and young males. In: Goldstein S., & Brookes, R. B. (Eds.) (2006), Handbook of resilience in children. New York: Springer Science and Business Media, pp. 65–77.

Provencher, H., & Keyes, C. (2011). Complete mental health recovery: Bridging mental illness with positive mental health, Journal of Public Mental Health, 10(1), pp. 57–69.

Richardson, G. E. (2002). The metatheory of resilience & resiliency, Journal of Clinical Psychology, 58(3), pp. 307–321.

Royal College of Psychiatrists (2011). The mental health of students in higher education. London: Royal College of Psychiatrists, CR166.

Rutter, M. (2006). Implications for resilience concepts for scientific understanding, New York, Annals of Academic Science, 1094, pp. 1–12.

Rutter, M. (2013). Annual research review: Resilience – clinical implications, The Journal of Child Psychology and Psychiatry, 54, pp. 474–487.

Scarf, D., Moradi, S., McGaw, K., Hewitt, J., Hayhurst, J. G., Boyes, M., Ruffman, T., & Hunter, J. A. (2016). Somewhere I belong: Long-term increases in adolescent's resilience are predicted by perceived belonging to the in-group, British Journal of Social Psychology, 55, pp. 588–599.

Schwartz, F., & Belknap, C. J. (2017). Effects of a college orientation program on trait emotional intelligence, Journal of Outdoor Recreation, Education, and Leadership, 9(1), pp. 69–82.

Sheard, M., Golby, J. (2006). The efficacy of an outdoor adventure education curriculum on selected aspects of positive psychological development, Journal of Experiential Education, 29(2), pp. 187–209.

Slee, V., & Allan, J. (2019). Purposeful outdoor learning empowers children to deal with school transitions, Sports, 7, 134, pp. 1–14.

82 *J.F. Allan*

Storrie, K., Ahern, K., & Tuckett, A. (2010). A systematic review: Students with mental health problems: A growing problem, International Journal of Nursing Practice, 16, pp. 1–6.

Taylor, S., Charura, D., Williams, G., Allan, J., Cohen, E., Meth, F., & Shaw, M. (2018). Loss, grief and growth: An interpretative phenomenological analysis of experiences of trauma in asylum-seekers and refugees, Traumatology, https://doi.org/10.1037/trm0000250.

Taylor, S. E., Klein, L. C., Lewis, B. P., Greuenwarld, T. C., Gurney, R. A., & Upfdegraff, J. A. (2000). Bio-behaviourial responses to stress in females: Tend-and-befriend, not fight-or-flight, Psychological Review, 102(3), pp. 411–429.

The Children's Society (2014). The Good Childhood Report, 2014, London, UK, The Children's Society.

The Children's Society (2015). The Good Childhood Report, 2015, London, UK, The Children's Society.

Thorley, C. (2017). Not by degrees, improving students' mental health in UK universities, Institute for Public Policy Research, London UK.

Tillmann, S., Tobin, D., Avison, W., & Gilliland, J. (2018). Mental health benefits of interactions with nature in children and teenagers: A systematic review, Journal of Epidemiology and Community Health, 72(10), pp. 958–966.

Ungar, M. (2013). Resilience, trauma, context, and culture, Trauma, Violence, and Abuse, 14, pp. 255–266.

Ungar, M., & Teram, E. (2005). Qualitative resilience research: Contributions and risks. In: M. Ungar (Ed.), Handbook for working with children and youth, pathways to resilience across cultures and contexts. Thousand Oaks, CA: Sage Publications, pp. 149–164.

van den Berg, M., et al. (2015). Health benefits of green spaces in the living environment: A systematic review of epidemiological studies, Urban Forestry & Urban Greening, 14(4), pp. 806–816.

Vanderbilt-Adriance, E., & Shaw, D. (2008). Conceptualizing and re-evaluating resilience across levels of risk, time, and domains of competence, Clinical Child and Family Psychology Review, 11(1–2), pp. 30–58.

Weissberg, R. P., Kumpfer, K. L., & Seligman, M. E. P. (2003). Special issue, prevention that works for children and youth: An introduction, American Psychologist, 58, pp. 425–432.

Werner, E. E. (1995). Resilience in development. Current Directions in Psychological Sciences, 4, pp. 81–85.

Windle, G. (2010). What is resilience? A review and concept analysis. Reviews in Clinical Gerontology, 21(2), pp. 152–169.

Wittington, A., & Budbill, N. W. (2015). Promoting resiliency in adolescent girls through adventure programming, Journal of Adventure Education & Outdoor Learning, 16(1), pp. 1–15, doi: 10.1080/14729679.2015.1047872.

World Health Organization (2014). Health for the World's Adolescents. World Health Organization.

World Health Organization, (2015). Mental Health Atlas 2014. World Health Organization.

World Health Organization, (2020). World Health Statistics 2020: Monitoring health for the SDGs. World Health Organization.

7 Phenomenology and Human Wellbeing in Nature: An Eco-phenomenological Perspective

*Robert D Schweitzer, Eric Brymer,
and Harriet Louise Glab*

The concept of wellbeing, though increasingly a focus of research, continues to elude a clear definition. In this paper, wellbeing is defined as a state of balance or equilibrium between resources and demands – psychological, physical, and social – within an individual's life and community. There is now a resounding consensus that engagement with, and physical activity in, the natural world affords a range of benefits (Brymer, Freeman & Richardson, 2019) including improved cognitive functioning (Taylor, Kuo & Sullivan, 2001; Wells, 2000), enhanced life skills (Mayer & Frantz, 2004), accelerated recovery from illness (Crimpach & Ronis, 2003; Ulrich, 1984), increased capacity to cope with pain (Diette et al., 2003), a sense of community belonging (Kingsley & Townsend, 2006), promotion of a sense of self-control and peace (Faber et al., 2002), decreased stress levels (Lawton et al., 2017), and simultaneous promotion of positive, and reduction of negative, affect (Berg, Koole & Wulp, 2003; Hartig et al., 2003; Pretty et al., 2005). Increasingly, hospitals, educational institutions, and mental health practitioners are prescribing nature for the treatment of a range of stress and mood-related disturbances.

7.1 The Relationship Between Humans and the Rest-of-Nature

Within the last three decades, researchers and philosophers from a variety of fields have attempted to explain the ways in which we experience the natural world as beneficent. Traditional theoretical frameworks have been critiqued as insufficient (Araujo et al., 2019; Joye & van den Berg, 2011) not only because of the bias toward modern Western researchers and Western conceptualizations of the natural world but also because the language and assumptions underpinning traditional frameworks are not able to conceptualize the full range of experiences in nature and, importantly, do not fully explicate how nature supports wellbeing (Berto, 2014; Brymer et al., 2014). In this chapter, we reject a more traditional reductionist paradigm in favor of an eco-phenomenological paradigm in which all elements are interdependent and contribute to wellbeing as an emergent way-of-being in the world.

DOI: 10.4324/9781003154419-9

7.2 Phenomenology, Eco-phenomenology, and Lived Experience

Phenomenology refers to "the direct investigation and description of phenomena as consciously experienced, without theories about their causal explanations and as free as possible from unexamined preconceptions and presuppositions" (Spiegelberg, 1970, p. 810). Wertz describes phenomenology, as "not a doctrine or fixed body of knowledge, but a core method of investigation" (Wertz, 2015, p. 85) aimed at understanding consciousness and lived experience, often termed the life world independent of any assumptions, as far as that is possible.

Eco-phenomenology, drawing upon the writings of Husserl, Merleu-Ponty, and Levinas, expands phenomenological principles to include cross-disciplinary perspectives extending beyond anthropocentric assumptions to also address environmental issues. More generally, this approach seeks to "reflect on the visceral texture of experience, the sensuous perceiving of life," as "given" to the experiencer," (Finlay, 2011, p. 4).

Phenomenology in its anthropocentric form gives primacy to the notion of intentionality, that is human consciousness directed toward the other. Human wellbeing is thus conceived, not simply as an expression of bodiliness and the absence of disease, but refers to those relationships and the ways in which we construct meaning which lies at the core of our humanness. Drawing upon an eco-phenomenological perspective, phenomenology allows us to consider the notion of intentionality in the context of the rest-of-nature and relationships involving both self and nature as co-constituted. The notion of "returning to things themselves", from an eco-phenomenological perspective, offers us an opportunity:

> ... to return to that world which precedes knowledge, of which knowledge always speaks, and in relation to which every scientific schematization is an abstract and derivative sign-language, as is geography in relation to the countryside in which we have learnt beforehand what a forest, a prairie or a river is (Merleau-Ponty, 1962, p. viii)

The notion of *lifeworld* features prominently in the context of phenomenological research on lived experience. *Lebensweldt* or *lifeworld* was proffered by Husserl (1960) and refers to the rhythms and patterns that characterize everyday life but that are beyond conscious awareness. The lifeworld may be seen as "the unstated, implicit commitment to, or unnoticed in the world as there, existing independently of us in all of its complexity" (Zayner, 1973, p. 35). A phenomenological exploration of lived human experience of the natural world is critically important, particularly in the context of our deteriorating health and wellbeing. In this chapter notions of the life world are explored in the phenomenological sense of lived time, lived other, lived space and lived body. These notions are derived from research involving in-depth interviews undertaken as part of a phenomenological study of peoples experience of nature (Glab, 2017; Schweitzer, Glab & Brymer, 2018). The study, utilizing snowball sampling technique, comprised 9 people, (males n=2, and females n-7) aged between 25 and 60 years with most in their late 20s or early 30s and residing in South East Queensland, Australia. The inclusion criterion was that participants identified as having lived experience of the phenomenon, and also identified the rest of the natural world as being significant to their wellbeing (Giorgi, 2009). Participant interviews inform the sections following.

7.3 Lived Experience of the Natural World

Human lived experience of the natural world can be described as visceral and multifaceted. At its core it involves the interaction between the world and an embodied active agent. People who report wellbeing through nature experiences describe sensory, interpersonal, and intrapsychic experiences with the natural world, which illuminate key aspects of the lived experience of the natural world. The experience of self and world are inextricably connected with phenomenological notions of lived time, lived other, lived body and lived space. Wellbeing resulting from relationships between humans and the rest-of-nature can be thought about in terms of both natural world intersubjectivity and intrasubjectively; in this way, people who make a conscious effort to reflect upon their experience of nature, experience self as part of the natural world. The eco-phenomenological interpretation goes one step further in its recognition of relationships in a nonhierarchical manner.

Those interviewed for the study revealed that early embodied experiences of *being with* the rest-of-nature in various forms translated into a sense of belonging. Embodied experience of belonging to the rest-of-nature was illuminated as being fundamental to the sense of wellbeing. The significance of relating to the rest-of-nature was manifest in descriptions of profound longing for experiences of immersion in specific natural contexts when suffering from what may be described as urban claustrophobia – a sense of being trapped in urban environments.

From an eco-phenomenological perspective, this relational notion goes beyond human interconnection and human-rest-of-nature interconnection. Rather than fostering the notion of the individual, competition, and hierarchy, this stance is affirming of human energy being based upon an awareness and understanding of self within a larger context.

Although an individual's lived experience of the rest-of-nature is superficially unique in many respects, understanding these essential components may help explain how contact with the rest-of-nature enhances human health and wellbeing.

7.4 Lived Time

The notion of lived time (temporality) is located in past, present, and future (Husserl, 1960), beyond a mathematical abstract understanding of time (Bollnow, 1961). In phenomenological language, all events are connected. In these terms, the lived experience of wellbeing in relation to the rest-of-nature is in one sense a moving toward an experience and transformation. Early experiences of the natural world continue to be part of human consciousness in the present. Interviews were conducted with people who report their lived experience of wellbeing in relation to the rest-of-nature. They furthermore contend that their wellbeing stems from profound experiences related to childhood memories of play, adventure, and learning in the natural world. Childhood experiences are entwined with the rest of the natural world. The earliness of experience with the rest-of-nature gives expression to the experience of self and world as being inextricable.

A traditional phenomenological interpretation of these experiences frames lived time as a future-oriented activity that is bound by past experiences. That is, time loses its traditional, linear systematic process as defined by the external and changes shape. The interval moment that is present (Le Poidevin, 2000) is suddenly stretched, past and future slip by as expected in the mundane attitude but the now of time seems to hover for a while. This description is reminiscent of descriptions of mindfulness, a much discussed quality associated with the promotion of wellbeing. The eco-phenomenological perspective, routed in the self-rest-of-nature relationship, provides for the potential for time to be timeless and the lived experience of time in this manner to evoke wellbeing.

7.5 Lived Other

Lived other in the context of wellbeing and the human-rest-of-nature relationship has been described in two particular ways: other as anthropocentric and interpersonal, and other as ecocentric and in relation to the rest-of-nature. In addition to the earliness of experiences with the rest-of-nature, people described the importance of the experience being shared with significant others. In particular, the influence of parental attitudes toward the rest-of-nature emerged as a central feature shaping participants' experiences. For example:

> *I just thought of my family… we used to have a veggie garden and we'd all spend days out, you know, Dad would be putting in the tanks for the tomato plants and Mum would be pruning the squash plants and I guess we would have the time to be together… My parents enjoy being outdoors and my sister and I enjoy being outdoors, and a lot of our family time is spent in activities that are outdoors* (Josie, 25 years old).

Reports by people interviewed suggested that their early experience with parents and family members served to cultivate an affinity for the rest of the natural world through setting examples through attitudes and relationships, and/or through encouraging time spent outdoors and engaging with the rest-of-nature.

The second dimension of lived other relates to the other as nature. Merleau-Ponty pointed to an extended notion of alterity beyond the anthropocentric focus to include the lived experience of alterity within selfhood and with nature (Johnson & Smith, 1990). This notion suggests a return from the dialectic alienated view of "the natural world" as out-there and different to humanity to an embracement of the self-nature relationship which, in turn, restores interconnectedness (Langer, 1990) and re-establishes intimacy and humility. From this perspective, the rest-of-nature can be described as a genuine "other" beyond the anthropocentric view of what constitutes the other and characterized by traditional phenomenology. An eco-phenomenological perspective is open to an appreciation of the richness, complexity, and beauty of the rest-of-nature. The experience of *nature* as "the other," is an experience of a genuine intimate relationship which, in reciprocity, reveals that which is within the human embodied experience. The lived experience of wellbeing in relation to the rest-of-nature is linked to the restoration of the "squirrel self" (Zimmerman, 1992, p. 269) which, in turn, restores our true humanity. This relationship is given form in the sculptor, Dylan Lewis' shamanic figures (see Figure 7.1).

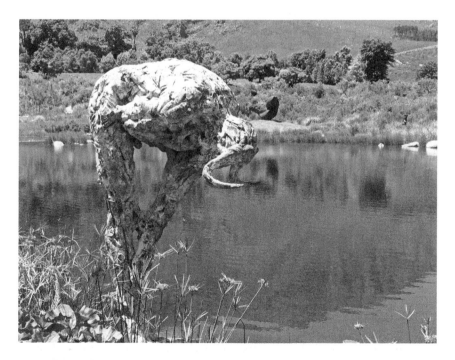

Figure 7.1 Sculpture by Dylan Lewis representing a shamanic figure.

88   E. Brymer, R.D. Schweitzer, and H.L. Glab

The powers of the shaman are believed to arise through the shaman's contact with another world, which may well relate to his or her own ancestors and those of the group, which, in turn, are experienced as embodied and immediate. This centuries-old tradition is thus the result of an intimate relationship in which the self and rest-of-nature merge with little demarcation.

An experience of the integration of self-as-other and natural-world-as-other reveals a belonging to the world as it is calling toward the primordial Being which, in turn, is fundamental to human wellbeing and liberates the need to dominate and control.

In our research, participants articulated that early experiences with the rest of the natural world were fundamental in the development of an embodied experience of being part of nature. Participants described awareness of the natural world being powerful and unpredictable, but somehow enlivening at the same time. A sense of longing was a common characteristic, amplified in urban settings. In particular, work environments characterized by fluorescent lighting, scarce windows, and limited opportunity to experience self as with or of nature, were associated with feelings of entrapment, as articulated in the below excerpt:

> *I do struggle already, I struggle in this house, and I struggle in the office that I'm in, like you know for a case conference we are in a room that has fluorescent lighting and no windows and I find that environment incredibly hard to endure for more than three hours. Well, it's hard to concentrate, it is, it makes me feel trapped like I need to get out of there, and yeah I start to feel tense and stressed, like kind of suffocated on a mild level* (Kate, 34 years old).

At surface level, participants experienced the natural world as an antidote to urban modernity. Several participants described a personal threshold at which prolonged absence from the natural world became unbearable. Time spent with specific aspects of the rest-of-nature affords a holistic restoration that is unparalleled by other interactions or experiences.

An important constituent of an eco-phenomenological perspective (i.e. dual experience of vulnerability and safety in the natural world) shares similarities with previous explications whereas experiences of fear are generally regarded as aversive and as needing to be avoided. The experiences of vulnerability and fear in the context of health are seen as promoting growth, enhancing self-efficacy, and affording positive experiences of self (Brymer & Schweitzer, 2013).

While experiences of wellbeing are often characterized by feelings of vitality and flourishing on other occasions wellbeing is related to sadness and even grief and loss. Common to all participants in our study were experiences of grief and loss at the destruction of the natural world – reflecting a sense of belonging to, and with, the natural world and their immersion within this world. Grief and loss at the destruction of the

Phenomenology and Human Wellbeing 89

natural environment are consistent with research in which environmental activists gave witness to the destruction of the natural world (Cianchi, 2015). Participants' experiences of grief in response to destruction of the natural world are in harmony with the notion of *solastalgia*, described by philosopher Glenn Albrecht et al, 2007) as feelings of grief, health threat, and powerlessness in response to environmental degradation, underpinning the relationship between nature and wellbeing.

7.6 Lived Body

Corporeality or lived body describes the notion that sentient beings experience the world through their bodies (van Manen, 2014). Bodily energy is enhanced and wellbeing taken forward to the future. The experience is also about moving beyond the bodily experience as conventional through body experience as primal and into unity and harmony as if the boundary role of skin disappears or merges with the external. From an eco-phenomenological perspective, experience moves beyond "human" experience to "raw," primordial experience uncluttered by thought and emotion.

Participants described somatic experiences of vulnerability and safety and containment with the rest-of-nature:

> *I guess there's a lot of unknowns when you're walking through a forest and you're sort of entrusting in your surroundings and there's some freedom in that. Pretty much everything is out of your control, you're just walking through a forest and anything can happen but at the same time, I experience safety in that* (Josie, 25 years old).

The paradox of relinquishing control over surroundings and allowing for uncertainty in terms of safety and survival was common:

> *Well, we know that nature is forceful and cruel and capable of incredible destruction. It can be furious and relentless and hostile. And while we cannot predict the onslaught of destruction... we know that it's always a possibility. And there is a collective acceptance I think, that nature can be all of these things. (Daisy, 27 yrs old).*

The participant continued and made a link to wellbeing with her assertion that:

> *But it is also entirely life-giving and life-sustaining. It makes me think of the idea of rupture and repair as in psychodynamic therapy – nature is this beautiful, steady parent with the capacity for anger. And even though the anger can be awful, fatal in some cases, there is always repair, in that it returns to being a beautiful, sustaining, and containing other* (Hannah, 28 years old).

90   *E. Brymer, R.D. Schweitzer, and H.L. Glab*

Being part of the natural world offers a richness of felt experience, ranging from intense fear and vulnerability to safety and comfort which underpins the sense of wellbeing and a sense of containment:

> *I experienced a range of feelings in nature, it wasn't always like joy. Now I seek it out because I need some more joy, but before it was like everything… It was where I played, it was where I fought with my brother, it was where I went with my dog, it was where I saw scary things, where I ventured alone and like, got a bit of independence, like tested my independence* (Jen, 30 years old).

Such experiences that may be regarded as opposite to one another offer a richness of emotion ranging from joy and delight to play and exploration and to fear that the self is experienced as capable of autonomy and perhaps even survival.

> *"We are the play things of the forces that laid out the oceans and chiselled the mountains. Sublime places gently move us to acknowledge limitations that we might otherwise encounter with anxiety or anger in the ordinary flow of events."* (de Botton, 2002 p. 176).

Lived body in the context of wellbeing when in relationship to the rest-of-nature experience is both about external extremes and inner extremes. Integration transforms as awareness is expanded and previously assumed boundaries dissolve.

7.7 Lived Space

Lived space is defined as felt space (van Manen, 2014). On the surface, the experience of being with the rest-of-nature takes place within the observable dimensions of space as outdoor physical space. However, the nature and wellbeing experience would seem to be beyond this. Lived space would seem to be about moving beyond the predictable and into a space that is experienced as a returning home to inner space (Bollnow, 1961). At some point in the experience, boundaries dissolve as attachment to the physical body is lost and both inner and outer space seem to be experienced as one space. This perspective is consistent with the eco-phenomenological stance in which there is a dissolution of self and other, so characteristic of Western empiricism.

7.8 Integration and Conclusions

An eco-phenomenological approach, wonderfully articulated in the title of a book, "Eco-Phenomenology: Back to the Earth Itself," encapsulates perspectives on the relationship between humans and the rest-of-nature (Brown & Toadvine, 2003). Eco-phenomenology offers a depth of

Phenomenology and Human Wellbeing 91

understanding not possible to achieve through traditional empirical methodologies or anthropocentric phenomenological approaches. The notions of lived time, body, other, and space are given expanded meaning when drawn from an eco-phenomenological perspective.

Wellbeing is revealed through the lived experience of being in relation with the rest-of-nature. The experience is characterized by immense feeling and meaning, extending beyond an evolutionary or genetic instinct, or positive response to replenishment of cognitive resources. Positive experiences with the rest of the natural world reveal that human experience of the natural emerges as determining our sense of wellbeing, our experiences of belonging and oneness, and experiences of fear, vulnerability, grief, loss, and longing. It is in this sense that the rest of the natural world affords fundamental wellbeing.

On a phenomenological level, the experience of self in relationship with the rest-of-nature incorporates natural landscapes and aesthetic dimensions. This relationship is particularly well represented in the metaphorical work of sculptor, Dylan Lewis, See Figure 7.2. These relationships are reflected in the placement of his work in the vast expanses of nature, and as engaging with nature.

The work of Dylan Lewis is particularly salient in reflecting the changes experienced by humans over the past millennia in his statement that:

> *"All my sculpture … has been inspired by the natural wild places of Southern Africa …Humans have largely tamed the wilderness, we've fenced out the wild lands, cut down the forests and exterminated the lions and tigers. I believe we have so rapidly disconnected ourselves from the wild natural places in which we evolved over millennia that we are struggling to make sense of that separation. We're disturbed, we're in transition. My sculpture is an attempt to find the image in the emotion exploring wild untamed aspects of the human psyche."* (Dylan Lewis: Shapeshifting 2019. ARTAFRICA. https://artafricamagazine. org/dylan-lewis-shapeshifting/)

The interplay between human beings and engagement with the rest of the natural world contributes to human wellbeing. First, experience of the rest of the natural world is layered and multifaceted. Human lived experience, or being part of the natural world, is characterized by emotional-relational memory with deep and primitive origins in childhood. The ways in which people make sense of their experiences contribute to our current understanding of the relationship between humans and the rest-of-nature as revealed by an eco-phenomenological explication. Lived experience of the rest of the natural world has significant import for our understanding of wellbeing. The richness of this experience illuminates the limitations of our current understanding of the interplay between each element of our very existence.

Our motivation in adopting an eco-phenomenological perspective is related to the observation of decreasing consciousness of our being part of

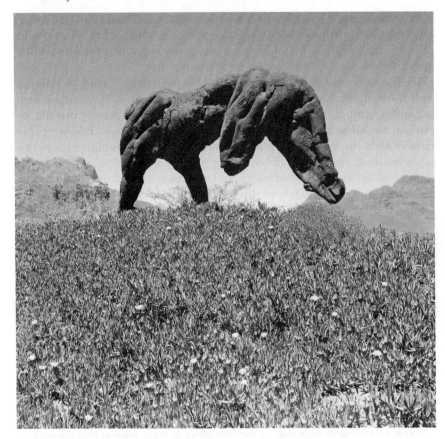

Figure 7.2 The sculptures of Dylan Lewis give expression to the self in relation to the rest of nature. In this image, he reflects the link between self and nature, highlighting both form and disintegration in a natural setting.

the rest of the natural world arising through processes of modernization and urbanization, impacting upon multiple metrics of wellbeing. These are well documented. Future research would benefit through greater recognition of the human experience of the rest of the natural world – and the ways in which this relationship is primal to other understandings of the physical world. These may incorporate art and also Indigenous people's lived experience for whom relationship with the land represents a significant part of life.

It is implicit in our argument that we have a continued need to integrate theory, philosophy, and methodological paradigms to gain a richer understanding of human experience. The impact of this perspective goes beyond the human-nature relationship and requires radical changes in the ways in which we think about multiple contexts, including urban planning, health, education, business, and resource allocation in a contemporary technologically driven global society.

References

Albrecht, G., et al. (2007). Solastalgia: The distress caused by environmental change. Australasian Psychiatry, 15, S95–S98. Retrieved from http://www.ncbi.nlm.nih.gov/pubmed/18027145

Berto R. (2014) The role of nature in coping with psycho-physiological stress: a literature review on restorativeness. Behav Sci (Basel). 2014 Oct 21;4(4):394–409. doi: 10.3390/bs4040394. PMID: 25431444; PMCID: PMC4287696.

Bollnow, O. F. (1961). Lived-space. Philosophy Today, 5, 31–39.

Brown, C. S., & Toadvine, T. (2003). Eco-phenomenology: Back to the earth itself. Albany, NY: Suny Press.

Brymer, E., & Schweitzer, R. (2013). Extreme sports are good for your health: A phenomenological understanding of fear and anxiety in extreme sport. Journal of Health Psychology, 18, 477–487. doi: 10.1177/1359105312446770

Brymer, E., Freeman, E., & Richardson, M. (2019). One Health: The wellbeing impacts of human-nature relationships, Frontiers.

Cianchi, J. (2015). Grief from the destruction of nature. In Cianchi, J (Ed.), Radical Environmentalism (pp. 141–153). London: Palgrave Macmillan.

Crimpach, B., & Ronis, D. (2003). An environmental intervention to restore attention in women with newly diagnosed breast cancer. Cancer Nursing, 26, 284–291. doi: 10.1097/00002820-200308000-00005

de Botton, A. (2002). The art of travel. London: Penguin.

Diette, G. B., Lechtzin, N., Haponik, E., Devrotes, A., & Rubin, H. R. (2003). Distraction therapy with nature sights and sounds reduces pain during flexible bronchoscopy. Chest, 123, 941–948. doi:10.1378/chest.123.3.941

Faber Taylor, A., Kuo, F. E., & Sullivan, W. C. (2001). Coping with ADD: The surprising connection to green play settings. Environment & Behaviour, 33, 54–77. doi: 10.1177/00139160121972864

Finlay, L. (2011). Phenomenology for therapists: Researching the lived world. Oxford: Wiley-Blackwell.

Giorgi, A. (2009). The descriptive phenomenological method in psychology: A modified Husserlian approach. Pittsburgh, PA: Duquesne University Press.

Glab, H. L. (2017). A phenomenological exploration of lived human experience of the natural world: Unpublished Thesis, Queensland University of Technology.

Hartig, T., Evans, G. W., Jamner, L. D., Davies, D. S., & Gärling, T. (2003). Tracking restoration in natural and urban field settings. Journal of Environmental Psychology, 23, 109–123. doi:10.1016/S0272-4944(02)00109-3

Husserl, E. (1960). Cartesian meditations. The Hague: Martinus Nijhoff.

Joye, Y., & van den Berg, A. (2011). Is love for green in our genes? A critical analysis of evolutionary assumptions about restorative environments research. Urban Forestry & Urban Greening, 10, 261–268. doi: 10.1016/j.ufug.2011.07.004

Kingsley, J. Y., & Townsend, M. (2006). 'Dig in' to social capital: Community gardens as mechanisms for growing urban social connectedness. Urban Policy and Research, 24, 525–537. doi: 10.1080/08111140601035200

Langer, M. (1990). Merleau-Ponty and deep ecology. In G. A. Johnson & M. B. Smith (Eds.), Ontology and alterity in Merleau-Ponty (pp. 115–129). Evanston, Ill.: Northwestern University Press.

Le Poidevin, R. (2000). The experience and perception of time. Retrieved 8th April, 2004, from http://plato.stanford.edu/archives/fall2000/entries/time-experience/

Mayer, F. S., & Frantz, C. M. (2004). Connectedness to nature scale: A measure of individual's feeling in community with nature. Journal of Environmental Psychology, 24, 503–515. doi: 10.1016/j.jenvp.2004.10.001

Merleau-Ponty, M. (1962). Phenomenology of perception. Routledge: London.

Pretty, J., Peacock, J., Sellens, J., & Griffin, M. (2005). The mental and physical health outcomes of green exercise. International Journal of Environmental Health Research, 15, 319–337. doi: 10.1080/09603120500155963

Schweitzer, R. D., Glab, H. L., & Brymer, E. (2018). The human-nature experience: A phenomenological-psychoanalytic perspective, frontiers in psychology, section environmental psychology. Frontiers in Psychology, 14;9:969. https://doi.org/10.3389/fpsyg.2018.00969

Seamon, D. (1982). The phenomenological contribution to environmental psychology. Journal of Environmental Psychology, 3, 119–140. doi: 10.1016/S0272-4944(83)80031-0

Spiegelberg, H. (1975). Doing phenomenology: Essays on and in phenomenology. The Hague: Martinus Nijhoff.

Taylor, A. F., Kuo, F. E., & Sullivan, W. C. (2001). Coping with ADD: The surprising connection to green play settings. Environment & Behaviour, 33, 54–77. doi: 10.1177/00139160121972864

Ulrich, R. S. (1984). View through a window may influence recovery from surgery. Science, 224, 420–421.

van den Berg, A., Koole, S. L., & van der Wulp, N. Y. (2003). Environmental preference and restoration: How are they related? Journal of Environmental Psychology, 23, 135–146. doi: 10.1016/S0272-4944(02)00111-1

van Manen, M. (2014). The phenomenology of practice: Meaning-giving methods in phenomenological research and writing. Walnut Creek, California: Left Coast Press.

Wertz, F. (2015). Phenomenology: Methods, historical development, and applications in psychology in the Wiley Handbook of Theoretical and Philosophical Psychology, Edited by Jack Martin, Jeff Sugarman, and Kathleen L. Slaney. Burnaby, Canada: Simon Fraser University.

Zayner, R. M. (1973). Solitude and sociality: The critical foundations of the social sciences. In G. Psathas (Ed.), Phenomenological Sociology. New York: Wiley.

Zimmerman, M. E. (1992). The blessing of otherness: Wilderness and the human condition. In M. Oelschlaeger (Ed.), The Wilderness Condition: Essays on Environment and Civilization. San Fransisco: Sierra Club Books.

8 Developing Integrated Conceptual Green Exercise Models

Claire Wicks, Jo Barton, and Mike Rogerson

8.1 Introduction

Within green exercise literature, theories such as Attention Restoration Theory (Kaplan & Kaplan, 1989) and Stress Reduction Theory (Ulrich et al., 1991) provide hypotheses about how engagement with the natural environment enhances physical and mental health outcomes. However, these theories do not consider the multiple factors, variables, and possible causal pathways that lead to improved health outcomes. Conceptual models, however, use key factors and variables drawn from scientific evidence and the interaction between these components to establish real-world pathways between exposure and health outcomes.

This chapter discusses a range of models, highlighting variation in the components, complexity, and terminology used. We will discuss how the purpose of the model (i.e. the relationship it is trying to understand) can influence these features. After briefly reviewing findings from green exercise research, we focus first on models illustrating the nature and health relationship, which demonstrate casual pathways between exposure to green space and health outcomes. Such models suggest that benefits to human health are derived through nature acting upon an individual. Second, we look at models of green exercise and health, which focus more on the complexities between human behaviors and health outcomes. Green exercise models propose that it is the human behavior that occurs when individuals and the environment interact that determines the health benefits gained. As the purpose of public health interventions is most often to shape our behavior, whether to prevent behavior (i.e. smoking cessation), or to enhance behavior (i.e. increasing physical activity), understanding human behavior is essential to ensuring interventions are effective. As such, models can provide a blueprint for researchers and health care professionals to guide and develop public health research and interventions.

8.2 Brief History of Green Exercise Research

Green exercise research has continually drawn on adjacent areas of research and knowledge, such as mainstream psychologies and exercise

DOI: 10.4324/9781003154419-10

science, which is evident through the methodologies and experimental designs used within green exercise research. The focus of much early green exercise research was on establishing whether engaging in green exercise was beneficial for health and wellbeing outcomes. Researchers manipulated environmental settings and compared outcomes of physical activity undertaken in nature with those from other settings, including indoor (Calogiuri et al., 2016; Focht, 2009; Ryan et al., 2010) and urban environments (Bodin & Hartig, 2003; Song et al., 2015). Such research sought to identify the additional benefits that might be gained through exposure to the natural environment. As interest in this area of research developed, so too did the number of studies reporting results in favor of the health-enhancing benefits of the natural environment. Reviews reported that greater improvements in mood and other wellbeing-related measures were associated with performing physical activity in natural environments compared to more synthetic indoor and outdoor environments (Bowler et al., 2010; Thompson Coon et al., 2011). With a growing evidence base supporting the benefits of green exercise, the type of research being conducted evolved and the focus developed to understanding not only if, but also *how* green exercise benefitted health. To investigate this, researchers sought to identify which specific characteristics of the environment, populations, and physical activity might be responsible for enhanced health outcomes. For example, the research of White et al. (2010) investigated whether the proportion of the environment dominated by green, blue, or urban elements influences preference, affect, and perceived restoration. While Rogerson et al. (2016) examined the role of environmental, exercise, and personal factors in generating psychological outcomes of green exercise, and Wooller et al. (2018) investigated whether the visual or audio stimuli experienced in natural environments was more effective for recovery from stress. Such research has advanced our understanding of the relationship between green exercise and enhanced health outcomes and has underpinned and driven the development of the conceptual models that have emerged in recent years.

8.3 Nature and Health Models

Several different models have been proposed to explain the relationship between exposure to the natural environment and health. Here we discuss some features of these models, which although focus more broadly on impacts of natural environments rather than green exercise specifically, provide a useful starting point for understanding and developing green exercise models.

Typically, models designed to represent the effect of nature on health offer a mechanistic account of how the relationship might operate. They tend to begin with exposure to nature and demonstrate a linear and sequential pathway through one or more variables, which ultimately result

Developing Integrated Conceptual 97

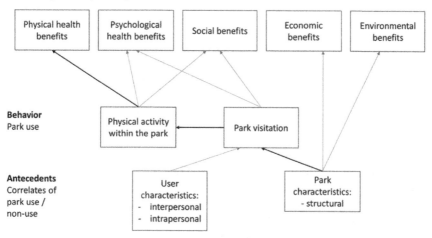

Figure 8.1 The hierarchical model proposed by Bedimo-Rung et al. (Bedimo-Rung et al., 2005) as redrawn by Lawrence, Forbat and Zufferey (2019).

in a change in health outcomes. For example, the hierarchical model proposed by Bedimo-Rung, Mowen and Cohen (2005) (Figure 8.1) describes a pathway between park use and health outcomes through three consecutive levels: antecedents, behavior, and outcomes. Interpreting the relationship between nature and health in a linear manner partly results from the epidemiological evidence upon which the models are based. This evidence offers a limited understanding of the relationship by measuring only the effect of an independent variable by the change in a dependent variable. However, this relationship is likely to be much more complex, with mutual interaction between variables, rather than a sequence of cause and effect relationships. Although more linear models are clear and relatively testable, they do not allow for any interaction within or between individual variables or levels.

We know that the natural environment does not just shape human behavior, but that human behavior also shapes the natural environment, for example, through building developments and conservation work. The diagram in Figure 8.2, developed by Lawrence, Forbat and Zufferey (2019), demonstrates how research to date has shaped our understanding of nature and health relationships (left-hand side) whereby the effect of one component is tested on another. However, to advance our knowledge of the possible relationships between components, the authors call for a more integrative approach that enables interpretations of multiple causation (right-hand side).

Whilst still linear in nature, the model proposed by Lachowycz and Jones (2013) (Figure 8.3) is more complex and indicates that the variables

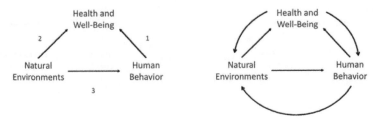

Figure 8.2 On the left, the more typical approach of nature and health research, and on the right, the proposed integrative approach (Lawrence, Forbat & Zufferey, 2019).

within their model have different roles. They also show that some interaction may occur within and between levels. Their model describes the pathway between access to greenspace and psychological and physiological health outcomes, and identifies variables as potential moderating factors, mechanisms of moderation, or potential mediators.

That the variables within a model can have different functions is critical to our understanding of how improved health outcomes can be achieved and to fully harness the benefits of the natural environment for health. For example, Barton and Pretty (2010) report that males experienced slightly larger improvements in mood following green exercise than

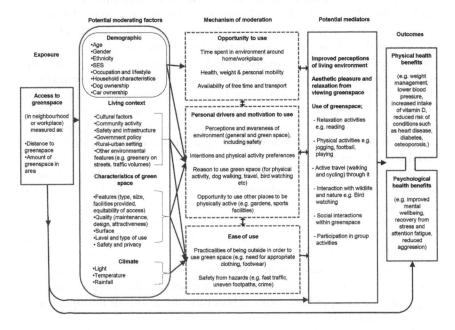

Figure 8.3 Lachowycz and Jones' socioecological framework for the relationship between greenspace access and health.

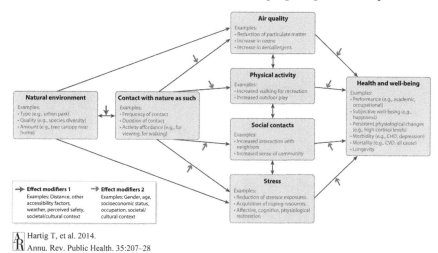

Figure 8.4 Hartig et al.'s model.

females, suggesting gender may be a moderating variable for mood-related outcomes. However, within Lachowycz and Jones' model, the moderating and mediating variables are suggested to influence health only at specific points in the pathway. Conversely, Hartig et al. (2014) propose that the roles of moderators operate at three different stages within their model of natural environments and health and wellbeing (Figure 8.4). Bass, Ewert and Chavez (1993) investigated the role of ethnicity and race in perception, use, and recreation behavior in an outdoor recreation setting. They reported that ethnicity significantly influenced the perception of the environment, activity participation, and the communication channels through which participants learned of the specific recreational area. Findings such as these support the proposition that moderators can have multiple points of influence. Hartig et al.'s model links environment and health along four central pathways, namely air quality, physical activity, social contacts, and stress.

Whilst a plethora of factors and pathways function in a variety of ways to link nature to human health and wellbeing, central pathways are those thought to play the most significant and influential roles. Identifying potential central pathways continues to challenge researchers. Kuo (2015) proposed that a central pathway should meet three criteria: (1) account for the size of nature's impact on health, (2) account for the specific outcomes tied to nature, and (3) subsume other pathways between nature and health. In their model, immune function is identified as a central pathway, which the authors test against the three criteria described (Figure 8.5). As stated by Hartig et al. (2014), exposure to nature often involves one or more of these central pathways and it is likely that multiple pathways are engaged simultaneously, thereby adding a further layer of complexity

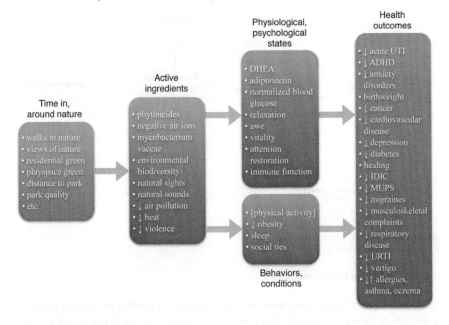

Figure 8.5 Kuo's model.

to understanding and modeling environment-health and wellbeing relationships. It is evident that the nature-health relationship is perceived to be dynamic, variable, and context-dependent, informed by a number of biopsychosocial factors.

8.4 Etiology

As discussed already, researchers face many challenges when trying to map nature–health relationships into models. Further considerations such as the discipline(s) of the research team, and any underpinning theories of interest, can also influence the development of a model. For example, the multidisciplinary team behind the model proposed in Markevych et al. (2017) (Figure 8.6) states that the three domains specified (reducing harm, restoring capacities, and building capacities) are "*not intrinsic to the subject matter but rather reflect the different concerns of particular research fields.*" Lachowycz and Jones (2013) used a socioeconomic framework to underpin their model. Their approach ultimately influenced both the variables included and the structure of the model, therefore shaping how it presents the nature and health relationship. The diversity of models informed by a range of disciplines suggests there may be a role for a new discipline to advance this research agenda. Furthermore, the different definitions of green space within models may also determine the variables included. For example, whereas

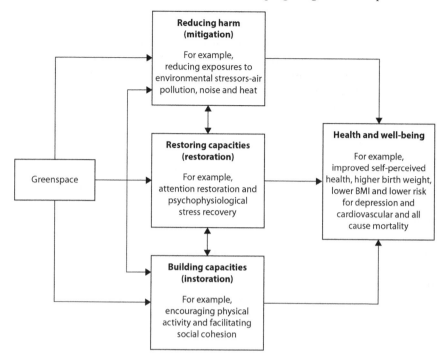

Figure 8.6 Merkevych et al.'s model.

Bedimo-Rung et al. (2005) discuss their model in relation to park use, Tzoulas et al. (2007) consider influences of urban and periurban green infrastructure, which encompasses components of the ecosystem such as biodiversity, habitat provision and water purification, which are factors not explicitly included in any of the other models discussed here. Similarly, Northridge, Sclar and Biswas (2003) discuss the built environment and health, and their model contains variables relating to aspects of land development policy such as land use and zoning regulations. This point raises many questions, such as how the definition of, or type of greenspace or nature environment considered, might influence how any given model operates.

Whilst the above is not intended to be an exhaustive review of nature and health models, it demonstrates the challenge researchers are faced with when trying to conceptualize such a complex relationship. A shift toward a more coherent and integrative approach is required that acknowledges nature as the dynamic vehicle facilitating interactions, rather than a passive entity. Further, we acknowledge that relationships between environments and human health and wellbeing may be interpreted from many different discipline interests, or indeed, epistemological perspectives, resulting in heterogeneity between models.

8.5 Conceptual Models

As part of their own review of models of nature and health, Lawrence, Forbat and Zufferey (2019) present a conceptual ecological health model, based on the core principles of human ecology, applied to people–environment relationships. It was developed with researchers and professional practitioners from a range of disciplines including human ecology, land use planning, and health promotion (Figure 8.7). The model presents a broader systemic framework and model of the relationship between the natural environment and health. It details six contextual variables (physical, environmental nuisances, social, individual, activity constraints, and activity facilitators), which influence five domains (state of green public space, policies and programs, state of human health and wellbeing, state of human habitat/ecosystem, and human agency/behavior). The variables within each domain are connected through mutual interaction and feedback loops making this a fully integrative model.

Here we highlight two features of the conceptual model, which most notably advance thinking around the nature and health relationship. First, as mentioned, this model includes mutual interaction and feedback loops between components. Mutual interaction between components demonstrates how the various domains work systematically together within the

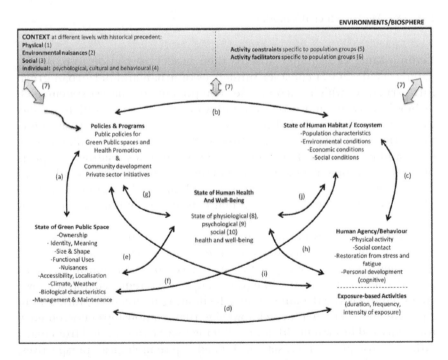

Figure 8.7 Lawrence, Forbat & Zufferey (2019).

Developing Integrated Conceptual   103

broader context, rather than working independently to influence health outcomes as seen in other models. The feedback loops display the reciprocal affects that occur when two components interact to influence each other (e.g. exposure to nature improves health outcomes and improved health can result in increased engagement with nature). Lawrence, Forbat and Zufferey (2019) state that *"Feedback causation, rather than linear causation, is the dominant driver of people–environment systems"*. Second is the domain of human agency; this model incorporates an existential view of individuals and groups in that their motivations and decisions for behavior are encompassed within the framework. This approach contrasts with the nature on health models discussed earlier, which implies that nature acts on individuals (i.e. simple causality). The human agency domain recognizes both constant states, such as motivation and lifestyle, together with temporal states, such as the lifespan and the climatic seasons. This suggests that human behavior in the natural environment is uniquely tailored by the individual and the specific moment in time that exposure occurs. As green exercise research draws on evidence and theories of human behavior derived from physical activity and psychology disciplines, human agency is essential for thinking about models of green exercise and health.

This integrative model provides a more complex and complete representation of how the nature and health relationship might operate in the real world. Understanding the relationship in this way opens a plethora of research opportunities that can enhance our understanding of nature and health relationships. The key features identified here are also evident in the two suggested models of green exercise and health, which we discuss in the following section.

8.6 Green Exercise Models

Yeh et al. (2016) utilize the theoretical framework of ecological dynamics, which integrates Gibson's ecological psychology and dynamical systems theory to understand the relationship between the natural environment, physical activity behavior, health, and wellbeing (Brymer & Davids, 2013; Gibson, 1979). Briefly, this approach is based on the perceived affordances (functional opportunities such as physical activity) that an environment offers, which are organized by an individual in relation to interacting constraints concerning the individual, task, and environment, which result in physical, psychological, or emotional behavior. That the natural environment tends to be vastly richer than indoor or urban outdoor physical activity settings not only offers individuals numerous opportunities for planned or spontaneous physical activity behavior, but also stimulates the perceptual system to a greater extent, leading to richer psychological and emotional responses (Yeh et al., 2016). For a fuller explanation of ecological dynamics perspective, please refer to Yeh et al. (2016) or Brymer, Davids and Mallabon (2014). The model presented by Yeh et al. (2016)

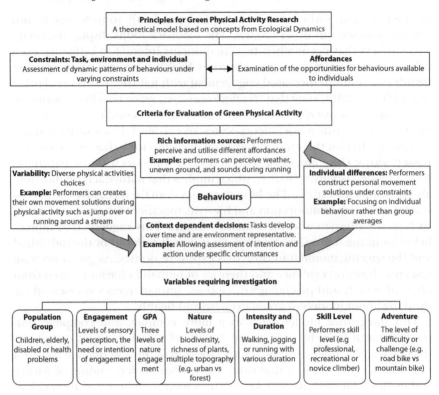

Figure 8.8 The theoretical model of principles for green physical activity research from an Ecological Dynamics perspective (Yeh et al., 2015).

demonstrates how the mutual interaction between affordances and constraints within an environment generate potential functional opportunities perceived and actioned by an individual (Figure 8.8). These opportunities arise from four criteria: rich information sources, variability, context-dependent decision, and individual differences. This model suggests that the animal-environment relationship invites behaviors including physical activity, which individuals can then choose to perform. The "variables requiring investigation" are variables that influence an individual's perception and actioning of the affordances, constraints, and evaluation criteria. For example, whereas a child may perceive the affordances of a tree as for running around, climbing, and swinging from a branch, an older adult with limited mobility may also perceive these affordances but not have the capacity (at the time) to action them, so instead action another invitation, such as to lean against the tree and rest, or to shelter from the sun or rain. The authors have separated these variables to highlight areas of research interest; however, in reality, they influence the process at each level. These variables may also moderate or mediate health outcomes resulting from green exercise.

Yeh et al.'s model emphasizes the notion that humans are not passive agents in the relationship between nature and health, but instead are active agents who continually evaluate their environment in order to make decisions about their behavior to achieve the desired outcomes. Understanding the individual as an active component in the process recognizes that affordances are unique to each person based on variables, including population group and level of adventure sought. Furthermore, the process itself is iterative and affordances or constraints may change instantaneously. This may include a change in the weather or a terrain, physiological changes within the individual, or an opportunity for a different task, such as social interaction. Such changes may initiate new affordances and is thus a continuous process of the human-environment system during green exercise. "*Through these affordances, health-enhancing physical activity in natural environments promotes mental health and well-being, through active exploration and the acquisition of skills and mastery*" (Araújo et al., 2019). Thus, the most appropriate scale of analysis is a framework that accentuates the person–environment system (Brymer, E., Crabtree, J. & King, R., 2020).

We now discuss the "Intertwining Pathways" green exercise model suggested by Rogerson et al., (2019) (Figure 8.9), which is itself partly underpinned by the ecological dynamics perspective discussed above. Like the ecological dynamics perspective, it seeks to describe both acute green exercise behaviors and experiences in great detail, and longer-term behaviors.

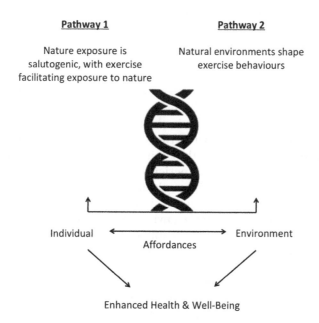

Figure 8.9 Two intertwining pathways showing how environments influence exercise and health-related outcomes (Rogerson et al., 2019).

The intertwining pathways model primarily seeks to explain how green exercise outcomes are derived (resonating with the nature-health models discussed previously). It proposes two pathways through which green exercise generates positive health and wellbeing outcomes: (1) nature exposure is salutogenic, with exercise facilitating exposure to nature; and (2) natural environments shape exercise behaviors. Importantly, this model also proposes that the two pathways interact, influencing one another (in either the acute or short term, or both), through affordances. The proposed interaction(s) of the two pathways resonates with the ecological dynamics model of green exercise and feedback loops that feature in the conceptual model presented by Lawrence, Forbat and Zufferey (2019).

Theoretical and empirical evidence is drawn upon to illustrate their model, as described briefly here. For pathway 1, theories such as Attention Restoration Theory (Kaplan & Kaplan, 1989) are cited toward explaining the psychological responses reported when humans are exposed to natural environments, which are often cited in green exercise literature. For pathway 2, cited research findings regarding environmental influences on exercise behaviors include green exercise being associated with lower perceived exertion compared to equivalent exercise indoors or in urban environments, increased levels of social interaction, and increased positive affect, also leading to greater intention to repeat the respective exercise behavior (Focht, 2009; Rogerson et al., 2016). To demonstrate interaction between, or "intertwining" of the two pathways, Rogerson et al. mapped selected findings from empirical studies onto their model. For example, evidence suggests increased social interaction occurs during green exercise (pathway 2: environment-shaping behavior), and as an additional result, both pathways are activated further; the individual is distracted from the environment, therefore reducing the potential for psychological restoration to occur (pathway 1: exposure to nature promotes benefits), whilst also experiencing social influences upon their motivation to engage in green exercise behavior again in the future (pathway 2). This example illustrates that rather than being two separate and linear pathways that operate in parallel, the two pathways interact and intertwine during and outside of the green exercise experience. We can also reason that not all instances of green exercise will result in the pathways interacting in the same manner. Instead, the nature of how these two pathways intertwine will vary due to differences in the environment, individual, and the physical activity. Rogerson et al. (2019) explain that *"the points at which the pathways link within themselves and across to one other, and what those links are, are understandably difficult to decipher, and many outcomes and shaped behaviors will not link to others."* The mapping of research findings onto a conceptual model is valuable not only to fully understand how a model operates, but also to take findings which are typically looked at in isolation and place them into a systematic framework, which helps uncover the complexities between behaviors and health outcomes.

The green exercise models featured here present human–environment systems where the dynamic interactions between and impacts on the human and natural environment drive both acute outcomes and future health-enhancing physical activity behavior. As these models focus specifically on understanding the behaviors in relation to natural environments, they do not explicitly include wider contextual issues seen in the model proposed by Lawrence, Forbat and Zufferey (2019). Rather, these green exercise models can be considered to fit within a broader framework.

8.7 Harnessing the Models

We have discussed how the nature and health models enhance our understanding of the component factors important to health and how, in addition, green exercise models offer greater scope for understanding behaviors.

Beyond guiding future research, evidence mapped to models can be used to benefit public health through many different approaches. For example, Coutts et al. (2013) reported that access to green space within one mile of residence is positively associated with self-reported levels of moderate to vigorous physical activity. While De Valck et al. (2017) reported that site characteristics influence decisions on where individuals go for outdoor recreation, and that this varies significantly depending on recreational preference. To apply this research to the conceptual models discussed, we could map evidence from these studies onto the ecological dynamics model developed by Yeh et al. (2016) as these factors relate to the individual, task, and environmental constraints, and perceived affordances discussed earlier. Combining this evidence through application to a model can be used to provide a stronger case for influencing a policy that guides environmental design. This might include ensuring that new building developments preserve or incorporate green space for residents and that adequate and appropriate facilities are available to support and encourage green exercise behavior. Another example using the intertwining pathways model might be the design of an intervention to enhance social interaction. In the intertwining pathways model, we saw that green exercise not only increased social interaction but can also lead to greater intention to repeat the health-enhancing physical activity behavior. Therefore, a green exercise-based intervention has the potential to not only increase social interaction but has the added benefit of increasing physical activity, which further enhances health and wellbeing. With public health interventions returning in the region of £14 for every £1 spent (Masters et al., 2017), green exercise interventions may increase the return on investment through addressing multiple public health issues, each of which might, in fact, further influence another, through dynamic affordances, feedback loops, or intertwining. Economic evaluation also suggests that there is a public willingness to pay for quality improvements to green and blue

108 C. Wicks, J. Barton, and M. Rogerson

spaces (Lynch, Spencer & Tudor Edwards, 2020). Together, this may make them more appealing to public health agencies and help secure funding. By mapping research onto models, we can also see how individual pieces of evidence fit together, providing a bigger and more complete picture and therefore advancing our understanding of how green exercise can be utilized for health.

We have outlined how the models of nature and health and green exercise are not unrelated entities. By integrating the knowledge from many fields of research, and by utilizing both types of models, we can begin to fully understand the physical and social characteristics of environments and experiences that can maximize the health and wellbeing outcomes of green exercise behaviors and ensure the necessary behavioral affordances can occur.

8.8 Future Directions

To confirm the validity of models, it is essential that they are rigorously tested across different populations and settings using empirical studies. However, as one study cannot test every component of a model, some coordination in the field is necessary. Different research approaches are needed in combination to best address the accuracy of models. For example, while many experimental studies control exposure variables for internal validity, they can consequently prevent individuals from utilizing the affordances of the environment. For example, studies requiring participants to walk along a path through a forest eliminate the potential for any other activity to take place. Ensuring the exercise is comparable between environmental conditions being tested allows for rigorous testing of identified variables of primary interest, but curtail acts of agency that may have demonstrated behavioral influences, which indicates that there is also need for lesser-controlled, observational studies, and qualitative approaches, for example, see Brymer, Crabtree & King (2020). With this, as we have mentioned, there may, of course, be differing levels of agreement with a model depending on the epistemology of the data used to assess it.

Researchers from empirical perspectives may also consider standardizing some aspects of experimental designs, including the types of measures used, which will help strengthen the evidence used to underpin the development of and the subsequent testing of models. While the systematic reviews of Thompson Coon et al. (2011) and Lahart et al. (2019) reported beneficial outcomes of green exercise participation, the review was limited by, amongst other factors, the considerable heterogeneity of outcome measures employed between the included studies.

While the two green exercise models discussed in this chapter can be applied to green exercise generally, researchers investigating specific areas of health or environmental settings may develop models unique to their

Developing Integrated Conceptual 109

area of research. For example, a recent study by Dzhambov et al. (2019) found that in a sample of Bulgarian university students, higher green space was associated with reduced anxiety and depression scores via intertwined capacity-building and capacity-restoring pathways. Further, the roles of suggested mediator and moderator variables, and the strength of their contribution may vary between models. As green exercise research continues to advance, we may see new models emerge that are developed for specific outcomes, populations, activity types, or environmental settings. Whilst these are legitimate and useful at their own specific level, the greatest noise can be made by larger, somehow unified, bodies of research. Indeed, this is where adoption of, or collaboration toward developing a widely accepted model, that can be engaged by researchers across a broader spectrum, can play an important role. The key message is that models need to be based on rigorous evidence, be testable and reliable, so that they can be used to inform public health policy and practice. It is through their ecological validity and application to real-world scenarios that they can make the greatest contribution to human health.

References

Araújo, D., Brymer, E., Brito, H., Withagen, R., & Davids, K. (2019). The empowering variability of affordances of nature: Why do exercisers feel better after performing the same exercise in natural environments than in indoor environments? *Psychology of Sport and Exercise, 42*, 138–145.

Barton, J., & Pretty, J. (2010). What is the best dose of nature and green exercise for improving mental health? A multi-study analysis. *Environmental Science & Technology, 44*(10), 3947–3955.

Bass, J. M., Ewert, A., & Chavez, D. J. (1993). Influence of ethnicity on recreation and natural environment use patterns: Managing recreation sites for ethnic and racial diversity. *Environmental Management, 17*(523).

Bedimo-Rung, A. L., Mowen, A. J., & Cohen, D. A. (2005). The significance of parks to physical activity and public health: A conceptual model. *American Journal of Preventive Medicine, 28*(2, Supplement 2), 159–168. doi: https://doi.org/10.1016/j.amepre.2004.10.024

Bodin, M., & Hartig, T. (2003). Does the outdoor environment matter for psychological restoration gained through running? *Psychology of Sport and Exercise, 4*(2), 141–153. doi: 10.1016/s1469-0292(01)00038-3

Bowler, D. E., Buyung-Ali, L. M., Knight, T. M., & Pullin, A. S. (2010). A systematic review of evidence for the added benefits to health of exposure to natural environments. *BMC Public Health, 10*(1), 456. doi: 10.1186/1471-2458-10-456

Brymer, E., & Davids, K. (2013). Ecological dynamics as a theoretical framework for development of sustainable behaviours towards the environment. *Environmental Education Research, 19*(1), 45–63. doi: http://dx.doi.org/10.1080/13504622.2012.677416

Brymer, E., Crabtree, J., & King, R. (2020). Exploring perceptions of how nature recreation benefits mental wellbeing: A qualitative enquiry. https://doi.org/10.1080/11745398.2020.1778494. doi: RANZ-2018-0092.R3

Brymer, E., Davids, K., & Mallabon, L. (2014). Understanding the psychological health and well-being benefits of physical activity in nature: An ecological dynamics analysis. *Ecopsychology, 6*(3), 189–197.

Calogiuri, G., Evensen, K., Weydahl, A., Andersson, K., Patil, G., Ihlebaek, C., & Raanaas, R. K. (2016). Green exercise as a workplace intervention to reduce job stress. Results from a pilot study. *WORK: A Journal of Prevention, Assessment & Rehabilitation, 53*(1), 99–111. doi: 10.3233/wor-152219

Coutts, C., Chapin, T., Horner, M., & Taylor, C. (2013). County-level effects of green space access on physical activity. *Journal of Physical Activity & Health, 10*(2). doi: 10.1123/jpah.10.2.232

De Valck, J., Landuyt, D., Broekx, S., Liekens, I., De Nocker, L., & Vranken, L. (2017). Outdoor recreation in various landscapes: Which site characteristics really matter? *Land Use Policy, 65,* 186–197. doi: 10.1016/j.landusepol.2017.04.009

Dzhambov, A. M., Hartig, T., Tilov, B., Atanasova, V., Makakova, D. R., & Dimitrova, D. D. (2019). Residential greenspace is associated with mental health via intertwined capacity-building and capacity-restoring pathways. *Environmental Research, 178.* doi: 10.1016/j.envres.2019.108708

Focht, B. C. (2009). Brief walks in outdoor and laboratory environments: Effects on affective responses, enjoyment, and intentions to walk for exercise. *Research Quarterly for Exercise and Sport, 80*(3), 611–620.

Gibson, J. (1979). *The ecological approach to visual perception.* Boston, MA, US. In: Houghton, Mifflin and Company.

Hartig, T., Mitchell, R., de Vries, S., & Frumkin, H. (2014). Nature and Health. In J. E. Fielding (Ed.), *Annual Review of Public Health,* a, 207–228).

Kaplan, R., & Kaplan, S. (1989). *The experience of nature: A psychological perspective.* United States of America: Cambridge University Press.

Kuo, M. (2015). How might contact with nature promote human health? Promising mechanisms and a possible central pathway. *Frontiers in Psychology, 6*(1093). doi: 10.3389/fpsyg.2015.01093

Lachowycz, K., & Jones, A. P. (2013). Towards a better understanding of the relationship between greenspace and health: Development of a theoretical framework. *Landscape and Urban Planning, 118,* 62–69.

Lahart, I., Darcy, P., Gidlow, C., & Calogiuri, G. (2019). The effects of green exercise on physical and mental wellbeing: A systematic review. *International Journal of Environmental Research and Public Health, 16*(8). doi: 10.3390/ijerph16081352

Lawrence, R. J., Forbat, J., & Zufferey, J. (2019). Rethinking conceptual frameworks and models of health and natural environments. *Health, 23*(2), 158–179. doi: 10.1177/1363459318785717

Lynch, M., Spencer, L. H., & Tudor Edwards, R. (2020). A systematic review exploring the economic valuation of accessing and using green and blue spaces to improve public health. *International Journal of Environmental Research and Public Health, 17*(11). doi: https://doi.org/10.3390/ijerph17114142

Markevych, I., Schoierer, J., Hartig, T., Chudnovsky, A., Hystad, P., Dzhambov, A. M., … Fuertes, E. (2017). Exploring pathways linking greenspace to health: Theoretical and methodological guidance. *Environmental Research, 158,* 301–317. doi: https://doi.org/10.1016/j.envres.2017.06.028

Masters, R., Anwar, E., Collins, B., Cookson, R., & Capewell, S. (2017). Return on investment of public health interventions: A systematic review. doi: 10.1136/jech-2016-208141

Developing Integrated Conceptual 111

Northridge, M. E., Sclar, E. D., & Biswas, P. (2003). Sorting out the connections between the built environment and health: A conceptual framework for navigating pathways and planning healthy cities. *Journal of Urban Health-Bulletin of the New York Academy of Medicine, 80*(4), 556–568. doi: 10.1093/jurban/jtg064

Rogerson, M., Barton, J., Pretty, J., & Gladwell, V. (2019). The green exercise concept: Two intertwining pathways to health and well-being. In T. E. MacIntyre & A. A. Donnelly (Eds.), *Physical Activity in Natural Settings: Green Exercise and Blue Mind.* Abingdon upon Thames, UK: Routledge.

Rogerson, M., Gladwell, V. F., Gallagher, D. J., & Barton, J. L. (2016). Influences of green outdoors versus indoors environmental settings on psychological and social outcomes of controlled exercise. *International Journal of Environmental Research and Public Health, 13*(4). doi: 10.3390/ijerph13040363

Ryan, R. M., Weinstein, N., Bernstein, J., Brown, K. W., Mistretta, L., & Gagne, M. (2010). Vitalizing effects of being outdoors and in nature. *Journal of Environmental Psychology, 30*(2), 159–168. doi: 10.1016/j.jenvp.2009.10.009

Song, C. R., Ikei, H., Igarashi, M., Takagaki, M., & Miyazaki, Y. (2015). Physiological and psychological effects of a walk in urban parks in fall. *International Journal of Environmental Research and Public Health, 12*(11), 14216–14228. doi: 10.3390/ijerph121114216

Thompson Coon, J., Boddy, K., Stein, K., Whear, R., Barton, J., & Depledge, M. (2011). Does participating in physical activity in outdoor natural environments have a greater effect on physical and mental wellbeing than physical activity indoors? A systematic review. *Environmental Science & Technology, 45*(5). doi: 10.1021/es102947t

Tzoulas, K., Korpela, K., Venn, S., Yli-Pelkonen, V., Kazmierczak, A., Niemela, J., & James, P. (2007). Promoting ecosystem and human health in urban areas using green infrastructure: A literature review. *Landscape and Urban Planning, 81*(3), 167–178. doi: 10.1016/j.landurbplan.2007.02.001

Ulrich, R. S., Simons, R. F., Losito, B. D., Fiorito, E., Miles, M. A., & Zelson, M. (1991). Stress recovery during exposure to natural and urban environments. *Journal of Environmental Psychology, 11*(3), 201–230. doi: 10.1016/s0272-4944(05)80184-7

White, M., Smith, A., Humphryes, K., Pahl, S., Snelling, D., & Depledge, M. (2010). Blue space: The importance of water for preference, affect, and restorativeness ratings of natural and built scenes. *Journal of Environmental Psychology, 30*(4), 482–493.

Wooller, J. J., Rogerson, M., Barton, J., Micklewright, D., & Gladwell, V. (2018). Can simulated green exercise improve recovery from acute mental stress? *Frontiers in Psychology, 9.* doi: 10.3389/fpsyg.2018.02167

Yeh, H.-P., Stone, J., Churchill, S., Wheat, J., Brymer, E., & Davids, K. (2015). Physical, psychological and emotional benefits of green physical activity: An ecological dynamics perspective. *Sports Medicine, 46*(7), 947–953.

9 Physical Activity in Nature: An Ecological Dynamics Perspective

Hsiao-Pu Yeh, Duarte Araújo,
Eric Brymer, and Keith Davids

9.1 The Complex and Coinfluenced Relationship Between Humans, Nature, and Physical Activity

Recalling your last visit to nature, whether it was walking, mountain biking, climbing, horse riding, sailing, kayaking, or any other activity undertaken in the mountains, woodlands, sea, or reservoir, you likely observed and detected differences or changes that existed in the environment. These differences might have encouraged you to change the way you behaved or impacted on how you felt. Such differences were likely associated with the weather, temperature, sunlight, natural views, terrain, or even other organisms. It is also likely personal factors such as physical fatigue, mood, expectations, or purpose, impacted on your physical activity. If you were with companions, it is possible that they contributed to the way you behaved. The physical activity itself (intensity, duration, and type) might have also influenced the experience or outcome of the visit. For these reasons, exploring the impacts of physical activity in nature is complex and requires a comprehensive underpinning theoretical framework to analyze and explain the processes and outcomes involved. The ecological dynamics framework is a robust and comprehensive approach to exploring physical activity in nature (Araújo et al., 2019; Brymer & Davids, 2013; Brymer et al., 2014; Davids, Araújo & Brymer, 2016; Yeh et al., 2016; Yeh, 2017). The ecological dynamics framework integrates ecological psychology and dynamical systems theory, with three features of significance for understanding human behavior: emergence of behaviors from multiple subsystems, interacting constraints, and affordances. This approach emphasizes the interplay between ***individual, environment, task*** categories of constraints, when perceiving, and realizing ***affordances*** (i.e. possibilities for action) offered by the relationship between the exerciser and natural environments.

This chapter aims to elucidate salient points from the ecological dynamics framework for understanding the impact of physical activity in nature and offer research or intervention suggestions. Emphasis is placed on the role of affordances in nature, and how perception–action couplings can be captured and influenced.

DOI: 10.4324/9781003154419-11

9.2 Affordances

Gibson defined affordances as:

> The *affordances* of the environment are what it *offers* the animal, what it *provides* or *furnishes*, either for good or ill. The verb to *afford* is found in the dictionary, but the noun *affordances* is not. I have made it up. I mean by it something that refers to both the environment and the animal in a way that no existing term does. It implies the complementarity of the animal and the environment. (Gibson, 1986 p. 127).

The notion of affordances suggests that the relationship between the individual and the environment invites behaviors. For example, a flat, extended, and rigid grass surface invites various activities such as walking, running, or lying down. But if a flat, extended, and rigid surface is made of ice, the affordances might change depending on the organism. Humans might be too heavy for the surface to support but for light bodyweight animals, such as rats or cats, this ice surface is still walkable, run-over-able or lying-down-able. In this example, humans can still detect the function of support from this ice surface but would refuse to use it because of safety concerns. This example shows that affordances abundantly exist in an environment for individuals with different capacities to perceive or utilize. The existence of objects in the environment might or might not offer affordances, i.e. *meaningful* interactions for a certain function. The ice surface previously noted might not be functional for humans to perform physical activity, but an ice surface might reflect the clear blue sky or moving clouds which can provide humans with an image of natural beauty. Gibson (1986) mentioned that affordances cannot be measured in the same way we might attempt to measure phenomenon in physics as environments might offer more than one affordance for an organism to detect and utilize. For example, a chair can be used as a seat, a table when putting paper on it for writing, a temporary ladder to reach the top of a cupboard, a weapon to attack people when needed, and a tool to perform a dance or stretch your body. The utilization of affordances would vary between organisms and even for the same individual at different times. Similarly, the same environment can be used for different purposes. Duzenli, Bayramoglu, and Ozbilen (2010) analyzed psychosocial affordances provided to adolescents in different urban environments. The youths in this study used the city centre for shopping, recreation, and being with friends and schools for other functions such as trying new activities, obtaining new information, and hanging out. This shows the various functions of affordances offered by the same space to adolescents.

Any object or property of the environment provides affordances related to an animal's capabilities. When we learn to perceive a given affordance, we learn to perceive the *information* about the world conveyed by ambient

114 H.-P. Yeh, D. Araújo, E. Brymer, and K. Davids

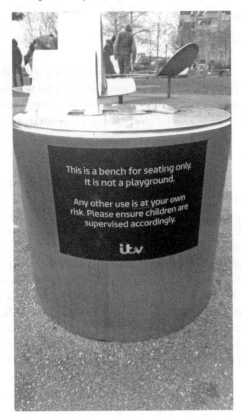

Figure 9.1 A public seat used by children for playing rather than sitting.

light, sound, odour, and so on as ambient patterns of energy (Gibson, 1986). We learn to detect what is offered by the environment which confers *meaning on information* that is detected and related to what can be affected (Gibson & Pick, 2000). Here, instead of simply detecting the object by its physical features, such as color, shape, size, or quality, we are actually detecting the offerings from this object as a whole. For example, a stick can be grasped or wielded. A building block can be grasped or thrown. In Figure 9.1, you can see how a public seat offers additional action possibilities when it is detected for different meanings or functions. Children detected opportunities for playing, climbing, sliding, and walking rather than simply sitting.

Humans learn to perceive and realize affordances from an early age and continue to develop skills in perceiving and acting upon affordances throughout the lifespan (Gibson & Pick, 2000). Infants can only perform limited physical activity and communication, but they actively perceive their surroundings and act on it when possible. Infants start to perform exploratory movements to gain knowledge of environmental possibilities,

Physical Activity in Nature   115

affordances, and capabilities. They also learn to pick up distinctive features to differentiate various types of information via exploratory activity (Gibson & Pick, 2000). During perceptual learning, humans learn how to perceive a selection of affordances such as how far we can reach, how heavy we can carry, or how high we can step over, etc. These body-scaled affordances have been studied for various actions, such as reachability (Huang et al., 2013; Ishak, Adolph & Lin, 2008), barrier-crossing ability (Snapp-Childs & Bingham, 2009), ability to walk under barriers (Wagman & Malek, 2008) or the ability to jump and reach (Ramenzoni et al., 2010).

As we develop, we continuously gain an understanding of our capabilities and experiences of various physical activities and become sensitive to some new affordances. We become experts in perceiving and acting upon certain sets of affordances which we are familiar with. These sets of affordances could be understood as our niche of affordances. Gibson (1986) explained a niche as referring to *how* an animal lives its particular life, from daily activities to specific events. For example, people involved in particular sports display higher accuracy on perceiving sport-related affordances than nonplayers (Weast et al., 2014). When faced with a landscape of affordances, most affordances can be perceived by most people, but some affordances will only be perceived by people with particular capacities and experiences. The skill level required to participate in a particular physical activity plays a role in whether a person perceives and utilises particular affordances, which consequently results in different exercise experiences. For example, expert climbers and beginners were tested on their interlimb coordination patterns when perceiving icefall properties as affordances during performances. Results showed that beginners were less sensitive and lacked perceptual attunement to environmental properties, with lower levels of functional intraindividual variability. Experts, on the other hand, displayed a wide range of upper and lower limb coordination patterns and fewer exploratory movements, suggesting they were more sensitive and effective in using affordances to regulate performance (Seifert et al., 2014). The experience and skill of an individual actor underpin the capacity to attune to some affordances and not to others. In this sense, an affordance is perceived according to the particular skills of the person who exercises in nature. Therefore, affordances refer to the fit between individuals' capabilities and the environmental opportunities that make a given activity possible (Gibson & Pick, 2000).

This unique fit between the organism and environment requires that both adapt to each other when performing behaviors. Humans can adapt more quickly than the environment. For example, walking along a forest trail requires humans to be mobile with the essential ability of posture control, muscle strength, and balance while the trail is flat, solid, and extended, to afford the possibility of walking on it. During the interactive process for the person to walk on the trail, any changing components either from the individual or environment might lead to different behaviors. If it started to rain, the walker might decide to run or do speed walking if she/he was concerned about the possibility of slipping and falling. During the journey, if a rabbit suddenly showed up on the side of the road, the walker might stop and look or if being frightened by its unexpected appearance, the individual might jump and shout. Any changes (the rabbit or the rain) during the process of perceiving or realizing nature affordances might lead to different outcomes (walking, stop walking, jumping, or running) but it is worth noting affordances remained available without being used (the trail can still be used for walking). This indicates that affordances are dynamic, in the individual–environment interplay, constantly changing the perception–action reciprocity.

Although affordances always exist even if they are not perceived or realized, certain sets of affordances invite specific behaviors. For example, the sound of the morning alarm encourages people to quickly react; the dark and cloudy sky prompts people to bring umbrellas with them. In sport, the posture of a defender would have an influence on the direction of an attacker's drive (Esteves, De Oliveira & Araújo, 2011). Information such as this offers functional meanings to the perceiver for corresponding behaviors. On the same note, the objects and layout of the environment encourage or discourage human behaviors accordingly. Withagen and Caljouw (2016) conducted an empirical study which aimed to stop sitting in an office environment by designing workspaces with no tables and chairs. Hence, there are no obvious sit-on-able offerings for humans in this given environment. Results showed 83% of participants worked in different non-sitting postures in multiple locations, thus stimulating movement but interestingly no impact on concentration, satisfaction, or the work produced. When designing environments for particular purposes, it is vital to thoroughly consider all the presented information in the environment, which might offer positive and negative invitations for behaviors.

9.3 The Rich Landscape of Affordances in Nature

Physical environments play a vital role in shaping human behaviors through the coinfluenced relationship between human behaviors and environments in terms of affordances, perceptions, and realizations, and the unique individual niche of affordances. A growing body of research also suggests that natural environments make positive contributions to health promotion (Chawla et al., 2014; Gilchrist, 2009; Gladwell et al., 2013; McCormick, 2017; Twohig-Bennett & Jones, 2018; van den Berg et al., 2016; van den Bosch & Ode Sang, 2017; Wood et al., 2017). Natural environments offer affordances which are more likely to be positive and meaningful to the perceivers and encourage health-enhancing behaviors to emerge. For example, the acoustic, aesthetic, and semantic properties of bird sounds were considered to be vital in perception and experiences of restoration (Ratcliffe, 2015). Woodland areas and trees offer positive effects on stress reduction (Gilchrist, 2009). Walking in forests exposes people to phytoncides (wood essential oils) which offer the chance to enhance human natural killer cell activity and levels of intracellular anticancer proteins (Li et al., 2006; 2008). Even bringing nature (plants) indoors creates a health-promoting environment because of healthier air, and feelings of comfort, calm, and pleasure (Lohr, 2010).

In nature, there are many diverse sets of olfactory, visual, haptic, and acoustic information offered for individuals to perceive and utilize, which consequently provides a rich landscape of affordances for humans, and suggests a greater perceptual and action availability for individuals to draw upon to stay physically, psychologically, or emotionally attuned to information in nature (Araújo et al., 2019). There is value in "engaging" with nature, whether a person performs physical activities or not. The benefits of engaging with nature have been presented in previous chapters. There is now robust evidence and a developing body of research, advocating the abundant benefits from engaging with nature in different formats (the three levels of *green exercise* which was based on the level of engagement with nature; viewing nature indoors, passively and actively interacting with nature) (Barton, Griffin & Pretty, 2012; Gladwell & Rogerson, 2016; Pasanen et al., 2018; Pretty, 2004).

9.4 Three Interactive Constraints: Individual, Environmental, and Task

The previous sections presented an ecological dynamics perspective on how "bird sounds," "trees," "forests," and "plants" might be beneficial for some people, in certain contexts, and at specific times. For example, bird sounds might not be perceived by people with hearing impairment. If bird song is heard, then it might impact on perception differently for different people, perhaps related to knowledge of specific bird calls. This individual difference might facilitate distinct behaviors. Trees and forests might offer little extra meaning for people with low-stress levels. An indoor plant that looks like it is dying might induce negative feelings. These examples indicate that different constraints impact on behaviors, mental status, and related health outcomes. The rich landscape of affordances in nature functions differently, dependent on the particular person–environment relationship. Engagement with nature (perceiving and utilizing affordances in nature) should not be considered a fixed process where the same person consistently exhibits the same behaviors. There may also be differences in observed behavior dependent on many interacting constraints such as the type of natural environment (environmental constraint), type of physical activity (task constraint), and how an individual is feeling at any particular time (individual constraint). Engagement is a dynamic process of ongoing perception–action cycles under different constraints which suggests that the relationship between

118　*H.-P. Yeh, D. Araújo, E. Brymer, and K. Davids*

all constraints is important to consider (individual, environmental, and task constraints).

In this section, individual, environmental, and task constraints are presented with selected research to demonstrate the diversity of each constraint in the context of nature engagement and health promotion.

9.4.1 Individual Constraint

Individuals are different in all aspects, such as physical capabilities, mental states, age, preferences, history, experience, and thoughts on the environments, and so on. These individual differences are classified as individual constraints, which are important to consider when designing specific programmes for different target groups. For example, the generation difference might lead to inconsistent results between adults, adolescents, and children when measuring engagement with nature (Duncan et al., 2014; Wood et al., 2013). Age difference might also be relevant to an individual's experience of nature connectedness (Duncan et al., 2014) but more work is needed to further our understanding. Even within the same age group, individual differences are important. Barton et al. (2014) examined the physical activity level in playground and nature-based interventions among rural and urban children and found a positive relationship between fitness and time spent in physical activity for the playground intervention, while no correlation was found between fitness levels and time spent in physical activity during the nature-based intervention. This study indicated one of the individual differences (fitness level) leads to different outcomes even in the same age group. The study also supported the notion that nature-based activities offer higher availability for a wider range of abilities.

Experiences of engaging with nature in childhood were found to correlate with fewer symptoms of depression in adulthood. Contact with nature has the potential to facilitate a learned coping mechanism that may improve mental health in adulthood (Snell et al., 2017). Contact with nature or engagement with nature brings out multifarious benefits and promotes children's healthy development, wellbeing, and positive environmental attitudes and value (Adams & Savahl, 2017; Tim, 2014). Connectedness with nature is seen as a personal disposition which might be an indicator of wellbeing, particularly meaningfulness (Cervinka, Roderer & Hefler, 2012).

9.4.2 Environmental Constraint

Environmental constraints are both global, physical variables in nature, such as ambient light, temperature, or altitude, and social, such as other people (Davids, Button & Bennett, 2008). In nature, the layout of surfaces, weather, wind, or animals, and so on fall into the category of environmental constraints, which provide action possibilities, or present limitations

Physical Activity in Nature 119

for people when performing physical activity. The richness of information offered from the human–environment relationship, for example, the surface condition for running, provides meaning and different engagement opportunities for the individual perceiver. For example, a runner in a forest trail is likely to pay more attention than on an urban park pathway, if only to avoid injury or falls. The uneven and irregular forest trail surface offers more haptic information for the runner or invites the runner to be more responsive to it. The urban park runner would still receive haptic information from each step as it contacts the park pathway surface, but the lower diversity of uneven and irregular running surfaces requires little extra engagement with the environment.

This level of affordance richness in the natural environment might also be linked to biodiversity (Marselle et al., 2015). As an example, bird sounds (Ratcliffe, 2015) have been associated with perceptions and experiences of restoration for mental wellbeing. The abundance of information in natural environments is also likely to be available as positive influences for a wider range of users and a wider range of outcomes (Araújo et al., 2019). For example, increasing the level of greenness in urban nearby environments improves children's cognitive functions (Wells, 2000). Increased neighborhood greenness was also related to lower risks of poor mental health and cardiovascular disease (Richardson et al., 2013). Gascon and colleagues (2018) suggested that there is a potential protective role of long-term exposure to green spaces on mental health (depression and anxiety) in adults.

9.4.3 Task Constraint

Task constraints are usually more specific to performance contexts and include task goals, rules associated with an activity, and activity-related tools and equipment (Davids, Button & Bennett, 2008). The duration, intensity, and type of physical activity are all task constraints. All these task-related factors would play a role in exercise performances. For example, performing a 5-mile field run would be different from doing a 20-mile field run for the same runner in terms of energy expenditure, and exertion, time, or running strategy, and so on. Certain exercises require essential equipment adjustment/setting when performing in different types of environment, for example, cycling. The styles and width of tyres used on mountain bikes and on-road bikes are different because each requires different types of tyres to maximize contact with surfaces. Different models of footwear and footwear characteristics would have an impact on running economy (Fuller et al., 2015).

While we have listed the three types of constraints as if they are separate, it is important to note that there is a mutual relationship between them all and, in particular, between the individual and the environment. Individuals often develop habitual ways to interact with the environment and sometimes even choose their preferred environments. People tend to perceive and utilize a particular set of affordances for physical activity, which might be strongly associated with previous experiences. Evidence indicates that children learn to perceive nature-based affordances from a young age and associate these with positive effects. In turn, these experiences facilitate a close connection with nature, which brings its own benefits (Montgomery, 2015). Childhood experiences of natural environments can influence adult behaviors and attitudes to natural environments (Thompson, Aspinall & Montarzino, 2008).

The influences of the three interacting constraints can be observed easily in our lives. For example, a simple walk to school for a mother and daughter requires a choice between two routes. One is long but flat and the other is short but a little steeper. To get to school efficiently (the goal), the mother might judge that taking the short route is better than taking the longer route. However, this may not be the case. An adult may not find the steepness of the shorter route influences the task (walking speed/time) in any meaningful way because of her adult body structure and capabilities (e.g. fitness and leg length). However, for the child, the steepness might have a considerable impact on her task performance (slower walking speed/longer time) because the short and steep route challenges her physical abilities (shorter legs and muscular strength). The three constraints interact with each other and form distinct exercise experiences for each performer. This interaction is dynamic and personal. As a researcher or programme designer, it is vital to consider the three categories of constraints as equally important when designing exercise programmes or carefully manipulating one of the constraints to meet research purposes when designing studies.

9.5 Suggestions for Future Research

Investigating how people perform physical activities (tasks) in natural environments facilitates the analysis of the process of how people engage with nature and the outcomes of this engagement. How people engage with nature illuminates how individuals perceive and realize affordances from nature, channeled by individual, task, and environmental constraints. The outcomes of the engagement can be the behaviors or performances we observe. Some tasks require more engagement than others. For example, outdoor climbing requires a deep engagement with the environment when using the whole body to make contact with the rock. Haptic information offered from contact points between the body and the rock, combined with relevant visual information, facilitates decision-making on climbing routes. In comparison, walking in a woodland demands lower engagement with the environment.

Certain tasks might require attunement to a higher level of particular sensory source than others. For instance, birdwatching might mean that the birdwatcher is particularly aware of acoustic and visual information for

Physical Activity in Nature 121

identifying, locating, and watching birds. Even when undertaking the same type of physical activity (task), the intensity or duration of the physical activity changes the engagement characteristics with nature. A 5-km field run within 20 minutes might be different even to one that takes 30 minutes. In the first instance, exercisers might focus on their pace, breathing, running surfaces, or other environmental obstacles to achieve the under-20 minute requirement. In the second instance, more nontask-related perception and action could possibly occur between exercisers and the environment, such as actively observing other organisms or objects during the run. The characteristics of each type of physical activity should be considered when investigating the link between exercise experience and engagement with nature. A mixed methods or qualitative approach would more likely capture these differences. Qualitative data offers the opportunity to gather rich information and descriptions of personal experience of engaging with nature.

Engaging with nature is a complex and dynamic process and understanding how engagement happens from an ecological perspective is about how affordances have been realized and how the three categories of constraints interact with each other. In Duvall's (2011) study, the outdoor walking group was given tasks, such as focusing on sounds or imagining themselves as an artist, to increase their engagement with the environment. Participants in this group experienced significant improvements in multiple dimensions of psychological wellbeing. Moreover, they were more likely to obtain psychological benefits when walking at low-to-moderate levels. This method encouraged participants to actively engage with the environment by using various awareness plans. That is, they were deliberately taught to perceive and utilize a range of affordances while performing physical activity.

Virtual nature might also be worth exploring as possible opportunities for those unable to engage with natural environments, such as those with limited mobility. Current virtual reality technology means that people are more likely to be fully immersed in the environment created by the technology. The impact of engagement with virtual nature can be investigated by manipulating the presented virtual environment. Given the increased interest in using technology in health care, the use of virtual nature-based programmes for patients could be a useful tool for health promotion. Studies are urgently required to examine feasibility and outcomes.

Given the influences of affordance perception and utilization on performance, outcomes, and personal experience, it is critical for researchers and program designers to consider how and what information is presented. Presentation of essential information is not only about displaying key information for participants to perceive, but also about removing distracting information. When designing nature-based exercise programmes for health promotion, it is important to carefully consider what aspects of an environment might be vital to accrue expected benefits or outcomes. This process needs to take into account the various attributes impacting the effectiveness of exercise, such as the presentation of essential information, available physical activities, exercise intensity, duration, and the target group. Group differences and individual differences are equally important and designers need to be flexible while allowing for individual-specific exercise behaviors. Flexibility within a programme can have a crucial influence on the impact of designed programmes. This point is also important when designing interventions, especially for people with special needs. Research on how best to design interventions and programmes designed to impact health and performance is needed.

9.6 Conclusion

In this chapter, we broadly outlined the main principles of an ecological dynamics framework. We showed how behavior is related to three interactive categories of constraints (individual, environmental, and task) and the reciprocal individual–environment interplay. We argued that an effective understanding of how nature-based physical activity impacts health and wellbeing needs an ecological approach. Further, design of interventions and programmes is based on a completed understanding of these key ecological principles. Researchers and intervention designers need to thoroughly consider the implications and purpose of the research question or intervention and the impact of both interactive constraints and the mutual person–environment system. Consideration should be given to individual characteristics such as age, fitness levels, childhood experience with nature, or medical conditions. Different types of environments, including greenness, and biodiversity (urban parks or forests) need to be taken into account. Greenness can impact individuals differently and individuals might also perceive greenness differently (e.g. an urban park might be green for some people and urban for others). Type and intensity of physical activity, jogging, or sprint training in a park can also lead to distinct nature engagement differences.

References

Adams, S., & Savahl, S. (2017). Nature as children's space: A systematic review. *Journal of Environmental Education, 48*(5), 291–321. https://doi.org/10.1080/00 958964.2017.1366160

Araújo, D., Brymer, E., Brito, H., Withagen, R., & Davids, K. (2019). The empowering variability of affordances of nature: Why do exercisers feel better after performing the same exercise in natural environments than in indoor environments? *Psychology of Sport and Exercise, 42*, 138–1455. https://doi.org/10.1016/j.psychsport.2018.12.020

Barton, J. Griffin, M., & Pretty, J. N. (2012). Exercise-, nature- and socially interactive-based initiatives improve mood and self-esteem in the clinical population. *Perspectives in Public Health, 132*(2), 89–96. https://doi.org/10.1177/1757913910393862

Barton J, Sandercock G, Pretty J, & Wood C. (2015). The effect of playground- and nature-based playtime interventions on physical activity and self-esteem in UK school children. *International Journal of Environmental Health Research*. 25(2), 196–206. doi: 10.1080/09603123.2014.915020. Epub 2014 May 12. PMID: 24814948.

Brymer, E., & Davids, K. (2013). Ecological dynamics as a theoretical framework for development of sustainable behaviours towards the environment. *Environmental Education Research*, 19(1), 45–63. https://doi.org/10.1080/13504622.2012.677416

Brymer, E., Davids, K., & Mallabon, L. (2014). Understanding the psychological health and well-being benefits of physical activity in nature: An ecological dynamics analysis. *Ecopsychology*, 6(3), 189–197. https://doi.org/10.1089/eco.2013.0110

Cervinka, R., Roderer, K., & Hefler, E. (2012). Are nature lovers happy? On various indicators of wellbeing and connectedness with nature. *Journal of Health Psychology*, 17(3), 379–388.

Chawla, L., Keena, K., Pevec, I., & Stanley, E. (2014). Green schoolyards as havens from stress and resources for resilience in childhood and adolescence. *Health and Place*, 28, 1–13. https://doi.org/10.1016/j.healthplace.2014.03.001

Davids, K., Araújo, D., & Brymer, E. (2016). Designing affordances for health-enhancing physical activity and exercise in sedentary individuals. *Sports Medicine*, 46(7), 933–8. https://doi.org/10.1007/s40279-016-0511-3

Davids, K., Button, C., & Bennett, S. (2008). *Dynamics of skill acquisition: A constraints-led approach*. IL: Human Kinetics.

Duncan, M. J., Clarke, N. D., Birch, S. L., Tallis, J., Hankey, J., Bryant, E., & Eyre, E. L. J. (2014). The effect of green exercise on blood pressure, heart rate and mood state in primary school children. *International Journal of Environmental Research and Public Health*, 11, 3678–3688. https://doi.org/10.3390/ijerph110403678

Duvall, J. (2011). Enhancing the benefits of outdoor walking with cognitive engagement strategies. *Journal of Environmental Psychology*, 31(1), 27–35. https://doi.org/10.1016/j.jenvp.2010.09.003

Duzenli, T., Bayramoglu, E., & Ozbilen, A. (2010). Needs and preferences of adolescents in open urban spaces. *Scientific Research and Essays*, 5(2), 201–216.

Esteves, P. T., De Oliveira, R. F., & Araújo, D. (2011). Posture-related affordances guide attacks in basketball. *Psychology of Sport and Exercise*, 12(6), 639–644. https://doi.org/10.1016/j.psychsport.2011.06.007

Fuller, J. T., Bellenger, C. R., Thewlis, D., Tsiros, M. D., & Buckley, J. D. (2015). The effect of footwear on running performance and running economy in distance runners. *Sports Medicine*, 45(3), 411–22. https://doi.org/10.1007/s40279-014-0283-6

Gascon, M., Sánchez-Benavides, G., Dadvand, P., Martínez, D., Gramunt, N., Gotsens, X., ... Nieuwenhuijsen, M. (2018). Long-term exposure to residential green and blue spaces and anxiety and depression in adults: A cross-sectional study. *Environmental Research*, 162, 231–239. https://doi.org/10.1016/j.envres.2018.01.012

Gibson, E. J., & Pick, A. D. (2000). *An ecological approach to perceptual learning and development*. New York: Oxford University Press.

Gibson, J. J. (1986). *The ecological approach to visual perception*. New Jersey: Lawrence Erlbaum Associates, Inc.

Gilchrist, K. (2011, April 13-14). Promoting wellbeing through environment: The role of urban forestry. Trees, people and the built environment. Edinburigh. Scotland. United Kingdom. http://www.forestry.gov.uk/PDF/FCRP01...

124 *H.-P. Yeh, D. Araújo, E. Brymer, and K. Davids*

Gladwell, V., & Rogerson, M. (2016). A lunchtime walk in nature enhances restoration of autonomic control during night-time sleep results from a preliminary study. *International Journal of Environmental Research and Public Health*, 13(3), 280.. https://doi.org/10.3390/ijerph13030280

Gladwell, V. F., Brown, D. K., Wood, C., Sandercock, G. R., & Barton, J. L. (2013). The great outdoors: How a green exercise environment can benefit all. *Extreme Physiology & Medicine*, 2(1), 3. https://doi.org/10.1186/2046-7648-2-3

Huang, H. -H., Ellis, T. D., Wagenaar, R. C., & Fetters, L. (2013). The impact of body-scaled information on reaching. *Physical Therapy*, 93(1), 41–49. https://doi.org/10.2522/ptj.20110467

Ishak, S., Adolph, K. E., & Lin, G. C. (2008). Perceiving affordances for fitting through apertures. *Journal of Experimental Psychology: Human Perception and Performance*, 43(6), 1501–1514. https://doi.org/10.1037/a0011393

Li, Q., Morimoto, K. I., Kobayashi, M., Inagaki, H., Katsumata, M., Hirata, Y., … Products, F. (2008). Visiting a forest, but not a city, increases human natural killer activity and expression of anti-cancer proteins. *International Journal of Immunopathology and Pharmacology*, 21(I), 117–127.

Li, Q., Nakadai, A., Matsushima, H., Miyazaki, Y., Krensky, A. M., Kawada, T., & Morimoto, K. (2006). Phytoncides (wood essential oils) induce human natural killer cell activity. *Immunopharmacol Immunotoxicol*, 28(2), 319–333. https://doi.org/10.1080/08923970600809439

Lohr, V. I. (2010). What are the benefits of plants indoors and why do we respond positively to them? *Acta Horticulturae*, 881(2), 675–682.

Marselle, M. R., Irvine, K. N., Lorenzo-Arribas, A., & Warber, S. L. (2015). Moving beyond green: Exploring the relationship of environment type and indicators of perceived environmental quality on emotional well-being following group walks. *International Journal of Environmental Research and Public Health*, 12(1), 106–130. https://doi.org/10.3390/ijerph120100106

McCormick, R. (2017). Does access to green space impact the mental well-being of children: A systematic review. *Journal of Pediatric Nursing*, 37, 3–7. https://doi.org/10.1016/j.pedn.2017.08.027

Montgomery, J. M. (2015). *Nature as healer and teacher: The importance of reconnecting children to the earth for physical and emotional wellbeing (master thesis)*. Vancouver, Canada: City University of Seattle. Retrieved from http://repository.cityu.edu/handle/20.500.11803/45

Pasanen, T., Johnson, K., Lee, K., & Korpela, K. (2018). Can nature walks with psychological tasks improve mood, self-reported restoration, and sustained attention? Results from two experimental field studies. *Frontiers in Psychology*, 9, 2057. https://doi.org/10.3389/fpsyg.2018.02057

Pretty, J. (2004). How nature contributes to mental and physical health. *Spirituality and Health International*, 5(2), 68–78. https://doi.org/10.1002/shi.220

Ramenzoni, V. C., Davis, T. J., Riley, M. A., & Shockley, K. (2010). Perceiving action boundaries: Learning effects in perceiving maximum jumping-reach affordances. *Attention, Perception, and Psychophysics*, 72, 1110–1119. https://doi.org/10.3758/APP.72.4.1110

Ratcliffe, E. (2015). *Restorative perceptions and outcomes associated with listening to birds (doctoral thesis)*. Surrey, United Kingdom: University of Surrey. Retrieved from http://epubs.surrey.ac.uk/808249/

Richardson, E. A., Pearce, J., Mitchell, R., & Kingham, S. (2013). Role of physical activity in the relationship between urban green space and health. *Public Health, 127*(4), 318–324. https://doi.org/10.1016/j.puhe.2013.01.004

Seifert, L., Wattebled, L., Herault, R., Poizat, G., Adé, D., Gal-Petitfaux, N., & Davids, K. (2014). Neurobiological degeneracy and affordance perception support functional intra-individual variability of inter-limb coordination during ice climbing. *PLOS ONE, 9*(2). https://doi.org/10.1371/journal.pone.0089865

Snapp-Childs, W., & Bingham, G. P. (2009). The affordance of barrier crossing in young children exhibits dynamic, not geometric, similarity. *Experimental Brain Research, 198*(4), 527–533. https://doi.org/10.1007/s00221-009-1944-9

Snell, T. L., Lam, J. C. S., Lau, W. W., Lee, I., Eleanor, M., Mulholland, N., ... Mulholland, N. (2017). Contact with nature in childhood and adult depression, *26*(1), 111–124. https://doi.org/10.7721/chilyoutenvi.26.1.0111

Thompson, C. W., Aspinall, P., & Montarzino, A. (2008). The childhood factor: Adult visits to green places and the significance of childhood experience. *Environment and Behavior, 40*(1), 111–143. https://doi.org/10.1177/0013916507300119

Tim, G. (2014). The benefits of children's engagement with nature: A systematic literature review. *Children, Youth and Environments, 24*(2), 10–34. https://doi.org/10.7721/chilyoutenvi.24.2.0010

Twohig-Bennett, C., & Jones, A. (2018). The health benefits of the great outdoors: A systematic review and meta-analysis of greenspace exposure and health outcomes. *Environmental Research, 166,* 628–637. https://doi.org/10.1016/j.envres.2018.06.030

van den Berg, M., van Poppel, M., van Kamp, I., Andrusaityte, S., Balseviciene, B., Cirach, M., ... Maas, J. (2016). Visiting green space is associated with mental health and vitality: A cross-sectional study in four European cities. *Health and Place, 38,* 8–15. https://doi.org/10.1016/j.healthplace.2016.01.003

van den Bosch, M., & Ode Sang. (2017). Urban natural environments as nature-based solutions for improved public health: A systematic review of reviews. *Environmental Research, 158,* 373–384. https://doi.org/10.1016/j.envres.2017.05.040

Wagman, J. B., & Malek, E. A. (2008). Perception of affordances for walking under a barrier from proximal and distal points of observation. *Ecological Psychology, 20*(1), 65–83. https://doi.org/10.1080/10407410701766650

Weast, J. A., Walton, A., Chandler, B. C., Shockley, K., & Riley, M. a. (2014). Essential kinematic information, athletic experience, and affordance perception for others. *Psychonomic Bulletin & Review, 21*(3), 823–829. https://doi.org/10.3758/s13423-013-0539-4

Wells, N. M. (2000). At home with nature: Effects of greenness on children's cognitive functioning. *Environment and Behavior, 32,* 775–795. https://doi.org/10.1177/00139160021972793

Withagen, R., & Caljouw, S. R. (2016). "The end of sitting": An empirical study on working in an office of the future. *Sports Medicine, 46*(7), 1019–1027. https://doi.org/10.1007/s40279-015-0448-y

Wood, C., Angus, C., Pretty, J., Sandercock, G. R. H., & Barton, J. L. (2013). A randomised control trial of physical activity in a perceived environment on self-esteem and mood in UK adolescents. *International Journal of Environmental Research, 23*(4), 311–320.

Wood, L., Hooper, P., Foster, S., & Bull, F. (2017). Public green spaces and positive mental health: Investigating the relationship between access, quantity and types of parks and mental wellbeing. *Health and Place, 48*, 63–71. https://doi.org/10.1016/j.healthplace.2017.09.002

Yeh, H.-P. (2017). Physical, psychological and emotional effects of nature-based affordances of green physical activity (doctoral thesis). Sheffield, United Kingdom: Sheffield Hallam University.

Yeh, H.-P., Stone, J. A., Churchill, S. M., Wheat, J. S., Brymer, E., & Davids, K. (2016). Physical, psychological and emotional benefits of green physical activity: An ecological dynamics perspective. *Sports Medicine, 46*(7), 947–53. https://doi.org/10.1007/s40279-015-0374-z

10 Physical Activity and Virtual Nature: Perspectives on the Health and Behavioral Benefits of *Virtual* Green Exercise

Giovanna Calogiuri, Sigbjørn Litleskare, and Fred Fröhlich

10.1 Introduction

Some believe that virtual reality (VR) will have, on people's lives, the same impact as the advent of smartphones (and cell phones before them). VR might change the way we search and assimilate information, as well as the way we communicate long distance or organize our travels. For example, we can already virtually visit any place on the globe, using platforms such as Google Earth VR, which may facilitate our decision-making process about what places to visit or not visit as well as plan how to move within those places. Facebook's acquisition of Oculus was a milestone in the development of VR-based communication and social-media use, allowing people to interact through virtual avatars in virtual spaces. The continuous development of commercial (relatively affordable and user-friendly) VR technology is indicative of an increasing presence of VR in people's homes. With respect to the human-nature interaction, gaming platforms (see e.g. *Nature Treks VR* in Steam) and mobile applications (see e.g. *VR Video 360 Nature*) already exist to access virtual nature that can be experienced using different types of VR-headsets. This suggests that the "VR revolution" has begun and is already shaping our way of interacting with nature, and we are left to wonder what we are going to lose and what we are going to gain along the way. At the same time, we may still be on time to take action to reduce potential negative effects, as well as take advantage of the technological advances.

In 1999, when the commercial availability of virtual nature technology was seen as imminent, Levi and Kocher (1999) investigated the impact that this technology might have on society. They found that although virtual nature may have the advantage of bringing nature to people, as well as to increase people's support for remote natural environments, this may come at the cost of devaluating local natural areas. These findings are emblematic of a change in people's perceptions of the natural world, from seeing nature as a fundamental part of the world in which we live to seeing nature as a consumer good, a change that may be (if not prompted) at least accelerated by the commercialization and increased use of VR technology. As

DOI: 10.4324/9781003154419-12

128   G. Calogiuri, S. Litleskare, and F. Fröhlich

Levi and Kocher warn, "the problem with virtual nature – like the problem with plastic trees – is that the value of nature is more than the experiential and recreational benefits it provides to people. Nature provides a variety of benefits beyond human's immediate experience; nature exists and has value separate from human beings" (1999; p. 224). Although we share the concerns expressed herewith, and acknowledge both the challenges and potential unintended negative consequences associated with the promotion of virtual nature, we also believe that, used with caution, virtual nature might be part of a strategy to tackle different health and environmental challenges.

The present chapter will explore ways in which virtual nature can not only act as a tool to supplement nature experiences for people for whom access to real nature is limited (or impossible), but also how it may be used as a strategy to enhance the health benefits of physical activity. Focusing on so-called *immersive virtual nature* (IVN), the chapter will provide an overview of VR technology, how this tool emerged in the broader landscape of *technological nature*, and how it can be combined with physical activity (*virtual green exercise*). Then, the "green exercise concept" will be applied as a conceptual model to explain in what way (and to what extent) IVN can augment the health benefits of physical activity. Eventually, a series of recommendations will be provided regarding how to design interventions and research that involve IVN.

10.2 Immersive Virtual Nature: An Overview

10.2.1 Technological Nature, Virtual Reality, and Immersive Virtual Nature

Technological nature is quite a broad concept, which encompasses any technology that in various ways mediates, augments, and/or simulates our experience of the natural world (Kahn et al., 2009). Abiding by the very definition of technology, i.e. the application of scientific knowledge for practical purposes, this term comprises artefacts such as pictures, stuffed animals, or plastic plants. Further technological development has instituted the rise of robot-pets, ranging from simpler robot-toys for children to more sophisticated robot-pets showing life-like interactions with humans, e.g. using facial recognition technology to make the robot-pet stare in a person's eyes and respond to petting with affectionate motions (see, for example, PARO Therapeutic Robot, www.parorobots.com). Arguably, the most recent development in the field of technological nature is the advancement of VR.

Sherman and Craig (2003) defined VR as "a medium composed of interactive computer simulation that senses the participant's position and actions and replaces or augments the feedback to one or more senses, giving the feeling of being mentally immersed or present in the simulation (a virtual world)" (p. 13). Different types of VR technology exist, although, in later years, the type based on so-called *immersive-virtual environment* technology arguably became most popular. This technology consists of synthetic sensory information that provide a surrounding and continuous stream of stimuli, creating the illusory perception of being enclosed within and interacting with a real environment (Smith, 2015). Immersive-virtual environment technology is made possible by the development of so-called head-mounted devices (HMDs), more commonly known as "VR masks" or "VR goggles." The relatively recent launch of affordable HMDs on the consumer market allow people to immerse themselves in a virtual environment by plugging their smartphones to these devices, which allowed VR to take off and become a phenomenon of mass consumption (for example, Google Cardboard™ can cost less than 20$). Relatively inexpensive cameras are also available that take 360° pictures and film 360° videos, i.e. omnidirectional cameras that can capture 360° images that can be viewed using HMDs (a technique made famous by Google Street View).

Immersive virtual nature (IVN) consists in immersive-virtual environments representing *natural* environments, thus providing the illusory perception of being enclosed within a natural environment. Different types of IVNs exist, which differ in their degree of resemblance with real nature as well as in the level of interactivity they provide, and such differences are often dictated by the techniques used to create IVN (see Section 10.4.1). Note, the definition of IVN primarily refers to *visual* stimulation (i.e. images or videos of nature). Such visual stimulations however can be augmented by auditory stimuli (soundscapes) or other sensory stimuli. For example, devices have been developed that can reproduce scents (see e.g. *FEELREAL Multisensory VR Mask*™).

10.2.2 Virtual Green Exercise

As green exercise is generally defined as any physical activity taking place in contact with nature (Pretty et al., 2003), we specifically define virtual green exercise as any physical activity taking place while being exposed to virtual nature. While this definition may apply also to nonimmersive forms of virtual nature (e.g. images or videos of nature projected on screens), this chapter will focus on the combination of physical activity (e.g. pedalling on a stationary bike or walking on a treadmill) and exposure to IVN. Technology that allows this combination already exists. For example, different consoles for VR gaming can be connected to special stationary bikes that replace the function of the controller so that the gamer must pedal to make the in-game avatar move in the virtual space, and the faster one pedals, the faster the avatar moves. These bikes are not only made for gaming as they also offer training sessions simulating outdoor bike tours in beautiful landscapes. This technology is quite expensive, but more affordable solutions also exist to engage in virtual green exercise. For instance, people

130   *G. Calogiuri, S. Litleskare, and F. Fröhlich*

can use different indoor endurance apparatus (e.g. stationary bikes, manually driven treadmills, rowing machines, etc.) while wearing a low-cost HMD displaying a 360° video of a tour in a natural environment. Bluetooth speed monitors can also be used so that the pace in the video corresponds to the treadmill speed or the watt levels of a stationary bike. Furthermore, mobile applications exist to connect VR systems to Google Street View to allow virtual navigation through different itineraries.

10.3 How can Virtual Nature Augment the Benefits of Physical Activity: An Application of the "Green Exercise Concept"

10.3.1 *Two Intertwining Pathways to Health and Wellbeing*

Through an extensive review of the literature on green exercise, Rogerson et al. (2019) have previously explained the underlying mechanisms that link green exercise and health by describing two intertwining pathways: i) physical activity facilitates exposure to nature, and thus enables people to benefit from nature's salutogenic properties; and ii) natural environments shape people's physical activity behaviors, promoting participation in health-enhancing exercise. According to this conceptual framework, these two pathways intertwine and support each other: not only do natural environments provide a venue for exercise, their psycho-physio-social benefits can lead to increased exercise duration and/or intensity (thus leading to greater health outcomes) as well as long-term exercise adherence. The conceptual framework proposed by Rogerson et al. could be applied to explain how VR, and especially *virtual green exercise*, can augment the benefits of physical activity.

Indoor exercise is widely prevalent. For example, figures from England show that indoor activities such as swimming (performed by 11% of the population)[1] and gym-based exercise (e.g. fitness classes [14%], general gym sessions [12%], exercise machines [9%], and weights sessions [5%]) are *cumulatively* more common than outdoor activities such as running (15%), climbing/mountaineering (5%), and golf (2%) (The House of Commons, 2017). Furthermore, the fact that an activity is performed outdoors does not necessarily imply that it is performed in contact with nature. In fact, while walking and cycling for leisure or transport are highly prevalent, with figures indicating that about 50% of the English population perform these activities for at least 150 minutes/week (The House of Commons, 2017), a 2016 study indicates that only about 20% of the population in England perform "active visits" in natural environments of a duration of at least 30 minutes during a regular week (White et al., 2016).

Even in Norway, where, compared to England, green exercise is more popular (51% of the adult population reported to engage in this activity for at least 1 hour/week), exercise in the gym still remains a largely popular mode of exercise (26%) (Calogiuri, Patil & Aamodt, 2016). Moreover, there is a dose-response pattern in the prevalence of exercising in the gym with respect to centrality (i.e. whether one lives in the countryside, a town/village, small city or large city), with a greater prevalence (about 35%) among people living in major cities as compared with those living in rural areas (about 20%) (Calogiuri, Patil & Aamodt, 2016). With increasing urbanization, it can be expected that an increasing number of people will make the shift to exercising indoors, especially if the growing cities will leave little space to exercise-supportive green spaces. Thus, virtual green exercise might represent a way for people who mainly exercise indoors to integrate nature into their exercise routines. This might augment the health benefits of exercise and encourage people to sustain regular exercise as well as help them exercise at higher intensities and/or for longer durations.

It should be noted that the applicability of the "green exercise concept" to *virtual green exercise* contexts is strictly limited by the extent to which virtual nature can provide psychological, physiological, and behavioral benefits equivalent to those provided by real nature. The evidence in this field is still relatively scarce, especially with respect to *IVN-based* green exercise, while more studies exist on virtual green exercise based on nonimmersive technology (for an overview, see Lahart et al., 2019). In recent years, however, studies examining the extent to which IVN can provide psychological, physiological, and behavioral benefits equivalent to those provided by real natural environments have been published, including some studies in which exposure to IVN was combined with physical activity (e.g. walking on a treadmill or cycling on a stationary bike). In the following sections, we will provide a brief, narrative, summary of such studies in relation to the two pathways described in the conceptual framework by Rogerson et al. (2019).

10.3.2 Pathway 1: Psycho-physio-social Benefits of Virtual Green Exercise (Is Virtual Nature as Good as the Real Thing?)

10.3.2.1 Psychological Benefits

There is accumulating evidence demonstrating that IVN can provide restorative and mood-enhancing experiences, at least when administered in sedentary conditions (i.e. participants not engaging in physical activity). Studies have shown that sedentary exposure to IVN can elicit quicker psychological restoration (reduction of anxiety/stress and increasing positive affect) as compared to control conditions (Valtchanov & Ellard, 2010; Valtchanov, Barton & Ellard, 2010) and to a greater extent than simply watching images of nature on a screen (Liszio et al., 2018). Moreover, some studies that have compared IVN with either virtual urban environments (Yu et al., 2018) or real natural environments (Chirico & Gaggioli, 2019;

132   G. Calogiuri, S. Litleskare, and F. Fröhlich

Nukarinen et al., 2020) indicate that IVN can elicit affective responses similar to those observed or expected in real nature-exposure contexts (e.g. increase in vigour and decrease in negative emotions). However, a recent meta-analysis indicates that the improvements of mood elicited by exposure to real nature are greater than those elicited by exposure to IVN (Browning et al., 2020). Interestingly, a study comparing exposure to a real natural environment to two types of IVN that were developed using different techniques showed that the affective responses to the IVN may differ depending on the type of IVN used. In particular, the study found that as compared with an IVN based on a 360° video (see Chapter 10.4.1), an IVN based on a 3-dimensional model elicited affective responses that were more similar to those elicited by a real natural environment (Nukarinen et al., 2020).

Unlike the studies based on sedentary exposure to IVN, studies that have combined IVN with physical activity have produced less consistent results. Studies comparing a real nature-walk to a walk on a treadmill combined with a virtual reproduction of the same nature walk (i.e. a 360° video filmed in the same natural environment) show that the real and virtual green exercise elicit equivalent ratings of perceived environmental restorativeness (Calogiuri et al., 2018), but also that the virtual green exercise was perceived as less enjoyable (Calogiuri et al., 2018; Plante et al., 2006) and elicited lower levels of positive affect/energy (Calogiuri et al., 2018; Plante at al., 2003b; Plante et al., 2006). Some evidence exists on virtual green exercise eliciting a reduction of negative emotions (e.g. negative affect/tension, fatigue, and calmness) that is equivalent to real green exercise (Plante at al., 2003b; Plante et al., 2006). However, some evidence also suggests that IVN can, to the contrary, trigger negative emotions, especially if participants experience discomforts such as cyber sickness (Calogiuri et al., 2018). On the other hand, studies comparing virtual green exercise with indoor exercise suggest that the former only provide limited (Plante et al., 2003a; 2003b) or no (Alkahtani et al., 2019) additional psychological benefits as compared to the latter.

10.3.2.2 Physiological Benefits

The currently available literature indicates that IVN can elicit physiological benefits that are only to a limited extent similar to those elicited by contact with real nature. On the one hand, exposure to an IVN (a photorealistic forest) was found to provide quicker reduction of physiological stress (assessed through heart rate and skin conductance levels) as compared with a control condition (Valtchanov, Barton & Ellard, 2010), outcomes that are in line with studies in real natural environments (see e.g. Park et al., 2010). Studies in the health-care field have reported the effectiveness of IVN as a palliative treatment in patients, especially in reducing perceived pain during treatment (Chirico et al., 2016, White et al., 2018),

Physical Activity and Virtual Nature 133

outcomes that resample classic studies on how exposure to nature benefits hospitalized patients (Raanaas, Patil & Haritg, 2012; Ulrich, 1984). On the other hand, unlike what has been described when comparing exposure to real natural vs. urban environments (Hartig et al., 2003; Park et al., 2010), no differences in physiological stress indicators (blood pressure, salivary α amylase, and heart-rate variability) were found when comparing an IVN with a virtual urban environment (Yu et al., 2018). This finding could be explained by the fact that VR technology does not provide the full range of stimuli (sounds, smells, temperature, etc.) that a person would experience in a real environment. In particular, real urban environments are likely to *trigger* a stress response because of noises, traffic, and crowds, while such responses would be much less pronounced in virtual settings. Moreover, a study comparing IVN with a matching real natural environment showed that while the IVN elicited a "fight and flight" response (measured as electrodermal activity) equivalent to that elicited the real natural environment, the IVN was associated with an increased "rest and digest" response (measured as heart rate and heart rate variability) (Nukarinen et al., 2020).

The studies described herewith refer to sedentary exposure to IVN. Fewer studies have examined users' physiological parameters when exposed to IVN in combination with physical activity. These studies have mainly focused on heart rate during exercise and found no differences in mean heart rate when comparing virtual green exercise with exercise alone (Plante et al., 2003a; Alkahtani et al., 2019), or with real green exercise (Calogiuri et al., 2018). This suggests that IVN might be effective in providing opportunities for health-enhancing physical activity.

10.3.3 Pathway 2: Virtual Green Exercise to Shape People's Exercise Behaviors (Can IVN Enhance Indoor or Green Exercise Behavior?)

10.3.3.1 Acute Impacts on Exercise Behavior

Since the 1990s, using different types of VR technology, researchers have studied how VR can influence people's locomotion patterns, such as gate behavior (see e.g. Jaffe et al., 2004; Peruzzi et al., 2016; Sheik-Nainar & Kaber, 2007), or how physical activity can influence the VR experience (see e.g. Slater, Usoh & Steed, 1995). However, to the best of our knowledge, few of these studies have attempted to combine physical activity with *immersive* VR technology (i.e. HMDs allowing a 360° range of vision) or focused on examining the impact of the specific virtual environment on health indicators or exercise behavior (e.g. exercise output, future exercise intention, etc.).

One of the ways in which natural environments impact people's physical activity behaviors is that exercising in natural environments is often associated with a lower perception of effort, stimulating people to exercise for a longer time or at higher intensities than they would do if they exercised

134 *G. Calogiuri, S. Litleskare, and F. Fröhlich*

indoors (Gladwell et al., 2013; Lahart et al., 2019). This phenomenon has been explained by the fact that the natural setting provides a distraction from internal feelings of fatigue (Harte & Eifert, 1995). When comparing virtual green exercise with indoor exercise, it seems that VR could provide behavioral benefits somewhat similar to those provided by natural environments, at least in the extent to which it can provide greater engagement and, thus, leading to greater exercise output. On the other hand, it would appear that virtual green exercise is not associated with the lower *perceived* exertion that is often associated with real green exercise. For example, when comparing an exercise condition (cycling on a stationary bike) with a combined exercise-VR condition (interactive VR bicycle experience), Plante et al. (2003a) found that in the latter condition, the participants cycled faster (more revolutions per minute). The greater exercise output appeared to be explained by a greater engagement (e.g. greater enjoyment), but it was at the same time associated with a corresponding increase in perceived exertion. Accordingly, in a study by Calogiuri et al. (2018), participants underwent a walk in a real natural environment and then walked (for an equivalent amount of time) on a self-paced manually driven treadmill whilst watching a first-person 360° video showing the same nature walk. No differences were found between the real vs. virtual nature walk for objective exercise indicators (heart rate and walking speed), indicating that the participants spontaneously generated the same exercise output in the two conditions. The virtual walk, however, was associated with greater ratings of perceived exertion as compared with the real nature walk.

10.3.3.2 Long-term Impacts on Exercise Behavior

A big promise of VR technology in the exercise domain is that through gamification and engaging virtual exercise contexts, VR can help people sustain regular exercise over time. The findings of a recent scoping review found, indeed, that highly immersive VR had, generally, more positive effects on motivation, affect, enjoyment, and engagement during exercise, as compared with less immersive VR (Mouatt et al, 2020). VR can also transform leisure activities that are traditionally associated with sedentary behavior (e.g. playing videogames), into opportunities for being physically active. The potential of VR as an integrative tool in physical education and lifestyle change interventions has been acknowledged (see e.g. Miller et al., 2013; Pasco, 2013; Thomas & Bond, 2014). Because of its benefits, IVN might, in particular, play an important role in this scenario. However, to the best of our knowledge, to date, there is no scientific evidence on the extent to which IVN can help people sustain physical activity and exercise behaviors in the long term. On the other hand, IVN and virtual green exercise may have the potential to promote participation in real green exercise. It has been previously suggested that the positive experiences associated with green exercise can result in more stable exercise behaviors (Calogiuri and Chroni, 2014; Calogiuri, Nordtug & Weydahl, 2015). Similar mechanism may be elicited by virtual green exercise. These authors have reported some promising (though preliminary) findings indicating that a single bout of virtual green exercise can elicit increased future green exercise intention (Calogiuri, Litleskare & MacIntyre, 2019). This particular field of research, however, is still at its infancy.

10.3.4 Strengths and Limitations of the Evidence

To date, there is inconclusive evidence supporting the assumption that virtual green exercise can provide equivalent (or at least similar) health benefits as outlined for real green exercise. It should be, however, considered that the research in this field is still at its infancy. Differences might exist depending on the type of VR technology used, whether or not the IVN exposure is combined with physical activity, and whether the IVN consists in either static images or dynamic videos. However, VR technology is advancing rapidly and future developments might lead to more effective ways to produce virtual experiences of nature.

10.4 Design IVN Interventions for Research and Health Promotion: Some Recommendations

10.4.1 Creating Immersive Virtual Natural Environments

One way to create IVN is to use video game development techniques and game engines to create artistic representations of natural elements and landscapes with which the viewers can interact, for example, by moving relatively freely within the virtual space. Advancements in this field allow creating 3-dimensional models containing *photorealistic representations of nature* that can achieve high levels of realism. Another way to create IVN is by means of 360° cameras, which allow creation of 360° pictures and videos that can be displayed in HMD (Figure 10.1). It is important to note that the commercialization and the continuous development of relatively affordable and user-friendly 360° cameras, along with programs that allow the manipulation of 360° images and videos post-production, makes it possible for most people to create IVN even if they don't have advanced skills in programming. Although 360° images and videos may be perceived as more realistic compared to IVN created using 3-dimensional modeling, they usually allow a smaller degree of interaction with the virtual environment. The viewer does not have, for example, the possibility to move freely within the virtual space. This is especially apparent in the case of *static* 360° images or videos (i.e. images or videos that allow 360° vision from a single fixed viewer-perspective). Commercial 360° cameras often don't allow high degrees of image resolution. Moreover, dynamic 360° videos (i.e. 360° videos in which the viewer perspective moves in the space, following movements of the camera operator at the moment of filming) may, on the other hand, provide some, although still limited, illusory agency in "exploring" a

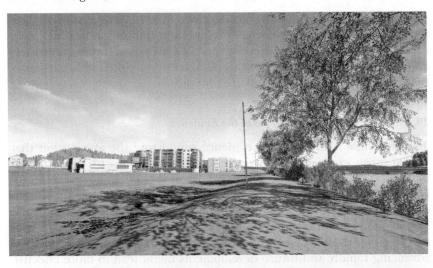

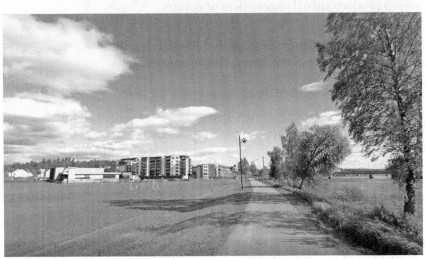

Figure 10.1 A snapshot of two different IVNs reproducing the same environment, which were created using different techniques: 3-dimensional modeling (top image) and commercial 360° camera (bottom image). Images developed by the research team of the project "Green VR: Nature experiences in IVE 2.0: developing virtual settings for green-exercise and health promotion research." Credits to Fred Fröhlich, Ole Einar Flaten, Sigbjørn Litleskare, and Giovanna Calogiuri.

natural environment (Calogiuri et al., 2018). To date, very little published evidence exists on the effectiveness of the different techniques in eliciting life-like experiences of nature (Litleskare, MacIntyre and Calogiuri, 2020). To the best of the authors' knowledge, two published studies have compared static 360° video with a matching 3-dimensional model (Nukarinen et al., 2020; Yeo et al., 2020), and one has compared different techniques in producing dynamic 360° videos (Litleskare and Calogiuri, 2019).

10.4.2 Combining Physical Activity and IVN

Physical activity is often a component of nature experiences (e.g. when walking in a natural environment) and this needs to be taken into account as the physical activity alone not only can influence peoples' physiology (e.g. increased heart and body temperature), it can also produce positive or negative emotional responses that contribute to the overall experience in nature. Combining physical activity and exposure to IVN, however, is not a simple task. Because IVN impedes visual contact with the external (real) world, users' balance is likely to be challenged; so, it is important to take precautions to avoid injuries. It is also impossible for the users to manoeuvre apparatuses, such as set the speed on the display of a treadmill. For these reasons, it is therefore recommended to use manually driven treadmills or stationary bikes (see e.g. in Figure 10.2). Furthermore, it is

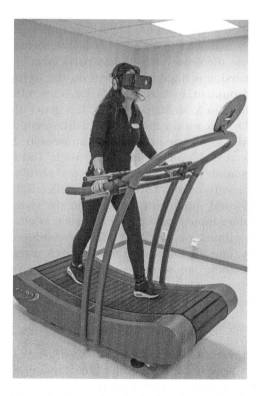

Figure 10.2 A participant in the study Calogiuri et al. (2018) walking on a manually driven treadmill while viewing a first-person 360° video showing a walk by a river. Picture by Tore L. Rydgren.

138   G. Calogiuri, S. Litleskare, and F. Fröhlich

considered important that the participants' movements matches the movements of their virtual avatars in the IVN to avoid cyber sickness while, at the same time, increase the sense of presence (Weech, Kenny & Barnett-Cowman, 2019); more details in the next section). This can be accomplished through special sensors that can connect the VR system with the treadmill or stationary bike.

10.4.3 Central Issues to Consider for Effective Experiences in Virtual Reality

Experiences in virtual reality are influenced by a multitude of factors, including technological, personal, and content-related factors. To give an exhaustive overview of all known (and potentially unknown) factors is beyond the scope of this book chapter. Instead, an insight into three key factors is presented herewith. It should be noted that although the three key factors: i) immersion, ii) presence, and iii) cyber sickness are presented separately, they are highly intertwined.

10.4.3.1 Immersion

Immersion is defined as the extent to which a computer-generated environment is "capable of delivering an inclusive, extensive, surrounding, and vivid illusion of reality to the senses of a human participant" (Slater & Wilbur, 1997). Thus, immersion is highly dependent on the technological aspects of the virtual environment, such as field of view, frame rate, and resolution of the display (Bowman & McMahan, 2007). It is generally deemed necessary to enclose the user within the virtual environment and shut out the "real world" in order to achieve high levels of immersion. This feat is partly achieved by modern HMDs by occupying the users' full field of view and also by replacing sounds from the surrounding real world with soundscapes from the virtual environment. This procedure effectively replaces visual and auditive real-world input with inputs from the virtual environment, but does not consider input from other senses such as olfactory and tactile inputs. Despite this limitation, modern HMDs are considered highly immersive. Theoretically, one should be able to objectively assess a systems level of immersion, but there are no universally agreed upon criteria for such assessments, which complicate comparisons between different technologies. Nevertheless, immersion is considered a key component of a successful IVE.

10.4.3.2 Presence

While immersion refers to the ability of the technology to deliver a vivid illusion of reality, presence, on the other hand, relates to the users' perception of the virtual environment. Presence describes the subjective feeling of "being in the virtual environment" (Slater and Wilbur, 1997). This concept describes the psychological feeling of being transported from the

Physical Activity and Virtual Nature 139

physical location and to the virtual location. This feat is considered pivotal to the effectiveness of an IVE and relates to the ability of the virtual environment to fulfil the purposes set by the virtual environment (Botella et al., 2017; Steuer, 1992; Triberti, Repetto & Riva, 2014). The likelihood of achieving a high degree of presence is believed to depend on the level of immersion. However, as presence is a subjective psychological feeling, it logically also depends on personality traits, which complicates the relationship between immersion and presence.

10.4.3.3 Cyber Sickness

The effectiveness of virtual environments does not only rely on increasing positive aspects such as immersion and presence, but also on reducing the impact of negative aspects. Cyber sickness is a malaise that can occur in users of virtual environments presented through a visual medium, including cell phones, computer screens, and head-mounted displays. Cyber sickness is considered a specific type of visually induced motion sickness (Kennedy, Drexler & Kennedy, 2010) and is known to induce dizziness, nausea, and general discomfort (Smith, 2015). Cyber sickness is reported to occur in as much as 100% of viewers depending on the technology used, the duration of immersion, and the content of the virtual environment (Allen et al., 2016; Merhi et al., 2007; Murata, 2004). The discomfort caused by cyber sickness will naturally influence the user's experience of a virtual environment. Calogiuri et al. (2018) demonstrated the impact on user experience and showed that the potential psychophysiological benefit from virtual green exercise was masked by the occurrence of cyber sickness. Furthermore, a review by Weech, Kenny and Barnett-Cowman (2019) suggests that cyber sickness also reduces the sense of presence in virtual environments. The discomfort caused by cyber sickness and the impact on positive aspects of VR exposure has made it a top priority for manufacturers and researchers. This work has enabled researchers to identify several factors that contribute to or limit the susceptibility to cyber sickness, such as habituation, exposure time, scene oscillation, movement lag, and type of display (Calogiuri et al., 2018; Duzmanska, Strojny & Strojny, 2018; Gavgani et al., 2017; Litleskare & Calogiuri, 2019; Sharples et al., 2008). However, research has also revealed that visual displays that are considered more advanced and immersive, such as head-mounted displays, generally induce higher levels of cyber sickness (LaViola, 2000; Sharples et al., 2008). This creates a paradox as the most advanced displays may provide higher degrees of immersion and presence, but these displays may at the same time be more prone to induce cyber sickness. Thus, the complicated procedure of creating effective virtual environments relies on the ability to make use of highly immersive technology to create content that invokes a high degree of presence, while avoiding the occurrence of cyber sickness.

140   *G. Calogiuri, S. Litleskare, and F. Fröhlich*

10.4.4 Recommendations for Future Research on Virtual Green Exercise

IVN technology has great potential as a tool in green exercise research (as well as other research fields) as it allows researchers to investigate the way people respond to and behave in different environments while, at the same time, controlling for possible confounders. In particular, IVN can allow for more rigour in green exercise experiments through standardization of key environmental conditions (temperature, humidity, less variability in the virtual environments due to weather changes, etc.) and concealment of treatment allocation (both for assessors and, to a certain extent, research subjects). However, this would assume that IVN validly and reliably reproduces the same emotional and behavioral responses people experience in real environments. Unfortunately, evidence supporting such assumption is still scarce and inconclusive as previously noted.

Research combining dynamic IVNs (especially IVN based on HMDs with 360° range of vision) with physical activity is especially scarce. Although the research in this field is likely to be hindered by known limitations of the currently available technology (see e.g. the challenge given by cyber sickness), more studies are needed in order to better understand if and to what extent IVN could represent a valid instrument for green exercise research, and if it could be part of the solution in integrating more nature into people's everyday life.

When planning research on virtual green exercise, it is also important to carefully consider specific aspects that might influence the outputs (Litleskare, MacIntyre and Calogiuri, 2020). In particular, we recommend that four aspects, briefly summarized herewith, are carefully considered: i) Duration of IVN exposure; ii) Type of technology; iii) Combining physical activity and IVN; and iv) Possible confounders.

10.4.4.1 Duration of IVN Exposure

Cyber sickness symptoms generally increase with time, at least until a certain threshold (~75 minutes) (Duzmanska, Strojny & Strojny, 2018). Previous studies that combine IVN and physical activity have used exposure durations ranging from 10 to 30 minutes (Calogiuri et al., 2018; Plante et al., 2003a; Plante et al., 2003b; Plante et al., 2006). However, shorter bouts (e.g. 5 minutes) of nature experiences have previously been associated with the largest effect sizes on self-esteem and total mood, while benefits on biological indicators of stress (e.g. blood pressure) would peak at 10-minutes duration (Barton & Pretty, 2010). Thus, an exposure duration of 5–10 minutes is recommended.

10.4.4.2 Type of IVN Technology

Different ways of producing IVN have been described herewith; each method has associated advantages and disadvantages. Different techniques are also employed for creating sounds in IVN, resulting in different levels of realism (for an overview on this issue, see Hong et al., 2019). Moreover, the VR systems and equipment used can have a big impact on the users' experiences, especially in relation to comfort, image-resolution, and risk of inducing cyber sickness. Rebenitsch and Owen (2016) provided an exhaustive list of display characteristics that may influence the users' experiences. The type of technology used should be carefully considered to suit the needs of the specific experimental design.

10.4.4.3 Possible Confounders

Studies have shown that VR experiences can be influenced by individual characteristics. For example, it has been demonstrated that the incidence and severity of cyber sickness can depend on the users' sex (Weech, Kenny & Barnett-Cowman, 2019), genetic predisposition (Hromatka et al., 2015), habituation, due to repeated VR exposure, (Duzmanska, Strojny & Strojny, 2018), visual acuity (Allen et al., 2016), and postural control (Munafo, Diedrick & Stoffregen, 2017). Previous physical activity habits were found to influence the extent to which a person is able to correctly estimate the visual speed of their virtual avatar (Caramenti et al., 2019). Individuals' personality has also been found to influence the way users perceive and respond to IVNs (Senese et al., 2020). The influence of individual characteristics on experiences in VR is not fully understood and it is to be expected that further characteristics will be identified in future studies.

10.5 Conclusion

VR technology has been developing remarkably in the past few decades, demonstrating great potential for people's health, especially in the field of rehabilitation and palliative health care. Moreover, VR may bare great potential also in relation to exercise promotion. In particular, in view of the progressive urbanization process, IVN technology can make nature more accessible and exercise more enjoyable, thus contributing to two major societal challenges of modern times: pervasive mental health issues and insufficient physical activity levels. This technology, however, yet holds a number of limitations and possible undesirable consequences, including among others, social isolation and further detachment from the real natural world. The scientific research in this field is still limited; more studies investigating the extent to which IVN and virtual green exercise can provide benefits similar to those provided by real green exercise experiences are especially warranted, as well as studies that focus on possible undesirable consequence of long-term exposure to VR devices. In other words, although more work still needs to be done, if the research community succeeds in creating lifelike virtual experiences of nature, this may become part of the solution to tackle some of the major health challenges of our modern society.

142 *G. Calogiuri, S. Litleskare, and F. Fröhlich*

Note

1. The percentages presented refer to individuals who reported having performed the specific activity at least twice in the 28 days previous the survey.

References

Allen, B., Hanley, T., Rokers, B., & Green, C. S. (2016). Visual 3D motion acuity predicts discomfort in 3D stereoscopic environments. *Entertainment Computing, 13*, 1–9. doi: 10.1016/j.entcom.2016.01.001

Alkahtani, S., Eisa, A., Kannas, J., & Shamlan, G. (2019). Effect of acute high-intensity interval cycling while viewing a virtual natural scene on mood and eating behavior in men: A randomized pilot trial. *Clinical Nutrition Experimental, 28*, 92–101. doi: 10.1016/j.yclnex.2019.10.003

Barton, J., & Pretty, J. (2010). What is the best dose of nature and green exercise for improving mental health? A multi-study analysis. *Environmental science & technology, 44*(10), 3947–3955. doi: 10.1021/es903183r

Botella, C., Fernandez-Alvarez, J., Guillen, V., Garcia-Palacios, A., & Banos, R. (2017). Recent progress in virtual reality exposure therapy for phobias: A systematic review. *Current Psychiatry Reports, 19*(7), 42. Retrieved from https://www.ncbi.nlm.nih.gov/pubmed/28540594. doi: 10.1007/s11920-017-0788-4

Bowman, D. A., & McMahan, R. P. (2007). Virtual reality: How much immersion is enough? *Computer, 40*(7), 36. doi: 10.1109/Mc.2007.257

Browning, M. H., Shipley, N., McAnirlin, O., Becker, D., Yu, C. P., Hartig, T., & Dzhambov, A. M. (2020). An actual natural setting improves mood better than its virtual counterpart: a meta-analysis of experimental data. *Frontiers in psychology, 11*, 2200. doi: 10.3389/fpsyg.2020.02200

Calogiuri, G., & Chroni, S. (2014). The impact of the natural environment on the promotion of active living: An integrative systematic review. *BMC Public Health, 14*, 873. doi: 10.1186/1471-2458-14-873

Calogiuri, G., Litleskare, S., Fagerheim, K. A., Rydgren, T. L., Brambilla, E., & Thurston, M. (2018). Experiencing Nature through Immersive Virtual Environments: Environmental Perceptions, Physical Engagement, and Affective Responses during a Simulated Nature Walk. *Frontiers in Psychology, 8*(2321). doi: 10.3389/fpsyg.2017.02321

Calogiuri G., Litleskare, S., & MacIntyre, T. E. (2019). (From) virtual (to) reality: Can virtual experiences help people reconnect with nature? *Conference on Environmental Psychology 2019, Lillehammer, Norway.*

Calogiuri, G., Nordtug, H., & Weydahl, A. (2015). The potential of using exercise in nature as an intervention to enhance exercise behavior: Results from a pilot study. *Percept Mot Skills, 121*(2), 350–370. doi: 10.2466/06.PMS.121c17x0

Calogiuri, G., Patil, G. G., & Aamodt, G. (2016). Is green exercise for all? A descriptive study of green exercise habits and promoting factors in adult Norwegians. *International Journal of Environmental Research and Public Health, 13*(11), 1165. doi: 10.3390/ijerph13111165

Caramenti, M., Lafortuna, C. L., Mugellini, E., Khaled, O. A., Bresciani, J. P., & Dubois, A. (2019). Regular physical activity modulates perceived visual speed when running in treadmill-mediated virtual environments. *PLOS ONE, 14*(6), e0219017. doi: 10.1371/journal.pone.0219017

Chirico, A., & Gaggioli, A. (2019). When virtual feels real: Comparing emotional responses and presence in virtual and natural environments. *Cyberpsychology, Behavior, and Social Networking, 22*(3), 220–226. doi: 10.1089/cyber.2018.0393

Chirico, A., Lucidi, F., De Laurentiis, M., Milanese, C., Napoli, A., & Giordano, A. (2016). Virtual reality in health system: Beyond entertainment. A mini-review on the efficacy of VR during cancer treatment. *Journal of Cellular Physiology, 231*(2), 275–287. doi: 10.1002/jcp.25117

Duzmanska, N., Strojny, P., & Strojny, A. (2018). Can simulator sickness be avoided? A review on temporal aspects of simulator sickness. *Frontiers in Psychology, 9*(2132). doi: 10.3389/fpsyg.2018.02132

Gavgani, A. M., Nesbitt, K. V., Blackmore, K. L., & Nalivaiko, E. (2017). Profiling subjective symptoms and autonomic changes associated with cybersickness. *Autonomic Neuroscience, 203*, 41–50. doi: 10.1016/j.autneu.2016.12.004

Gladwell, V. F., Brown, D. K., Wood, C., Sandercock, G. R., & Barton, J. L. (2013). The great outdoors: How a green exercise environment can benefit all. *Extreme Physiology & Medicine, 2*(1), 3. doi: 10.1186/2046-7648-2-3

Harte, J. L., & Eifert, G. H. (1995). The effects of running, environment, and attentional focus on athletes' catecholamine and cortisol levels and mood. *Psychophysiology, 32*(1), 49–54. doi: 10.1111/j.1469-8986.1995.tb03405.x

Hartig, T., Evans, G. W., Jamner, L. D., Davis, D. S., & Garling, T. (2003). Tracking restoration in natural and urban field settings. *Journal of Environmental Psychology, 23*(2), 109–123. doi: 10.1016/s0272-4944(02)00109-3

Hong, J. Y., Lam, B., Ong, Z. T., Ooi, K., Gan, W. S., Kang, J., ... Tan, S. T. (2019). Quality assessment of acoustic environment reproduction methods for cinematic virtual reality in soundscape applications. *Building and Environment, 149*, 1–14. doi: 10.1016/j.buildenv.2018.12.004

Hromatka, B. S., Tung, J. Y., Kiefer, A. K., Do, C. B., Hinds, D. A., & Eriksson, N. (2015). Genetic variants associated with motion sickness point to roles for inner ear development, neurological processes and glucose homeostasis. *Human Molecular Genetics, 24*(9), 2700–2708. doi: 10.1093/hmg/ddv028

Jaffe, D. L., Brown, D. A., Pierson-Carey, C. D., Buckley, E. L., & Lew, H. L. (2004). Stepping over obstacles to improve walking in individuals with poststroke hemiplegia. *Journal of Rehabilitation Research and Development. 41*, 283–292. doi: 10.1682/JRRD. 2004.03.0283

Kahn, P. H., Severson, R. L., & Ruckert, J. H. (2009). The human relation with nature and technological nature. *Current Directions in Psychological Science, 18*(1), 37–42.

Kennedy, R. S., Drexler, J., & Kennedy, R. C. (2010). Research in visually induced motion sickness. *Applied Ergonomics, 41*(4), 494–503. doi: 10.1016/j.apergo.2009.11.006

Lahart, I., Darcy, P., Gidlow, C., & Calogiuri, G. (2019). The effects of green exercise on physical and mental wellbeing: A systematic review. *International Journal of Environmental Research and Public Health, 16*(8), 1352. doi: 10.3390/ijerph16081352

LaViola, J. J. Jr. (2000). A discussion of cybersickness in virtual environments. *Newsletter ACM SIGCHI Bulletin, 32*, 47–56. doi: 10.1145/333329.333344

Levi, D., & Kocher, S. (1999). Virtual nature: The future effects of information technology on our relationship to nature. *Environment and Behavior, 31*(2), 203–226.

Liszio, S., Graf, L., & Masuch, M. (2018). The relaxing effect of virtual nature: Immersive technology provides relief in acute stress situations. *Annual Review of Cybertherapy and Telemedicine, 16*, 87–93.

Litleskare, S., & Calogiuri, G. (2019). Camera stabilization in 360° videos and its impact on cyber sickness, environmental perceptions and psychophysiological responses to a simulated nature walk – A single-blinded randomized trial. *Frontiers in Psychology, 10*(2436). doi: 10.3389/fpsyg.2019.02436

Litleskare, S., MacIntyre, T. E., & Calogiuri, G. (2020). Enable, reconnect and augment: A new era of virtual nature research and application. *International Journal of Environmental Research and Public Health, 17*(5). doi: 10.3390/ijerph17051738

Merhi, O., Faugloire, E., Flanagan, M., & Stoffregen, T. A. (2007). Motion sickness, console video games, and head-mounted displays. *Human Factors, 49*(5), 920–934. doi: 10.1518/001872007X230262

Miller, K. J., Adair, B. S., Pearce, A. J., Said, C. M., Ozanne, E., & Morris, M. M. (2013). Effectiveness and feasibility of virtual reality and gaming system use at home by older adults for enabling physical activity to improve health-related domains: A systematic review. *Age and Ageing, 43*(2), 188–195. doi: 10.1093/ageing/aft194

Mouatt, B., Smith, A. E., Mellow, M. L., Parfitt, G., Smith, R. T., & Stanton, T. R. (2020). The Use of Virtual Reality to Influence Motivation, Affect, Enjoyment, and Engagement During Exercise: A Scoping Review. *Frontiers in Virtual Reality, 1*, 39. doi: 10.3389/frvir.2020.564664

Munafo, J., Diedrick, M., & Stoffregen, T. A. (2017). The virtual reality head-mounted display Oculus Rift induces motion sickness and is sexist in its effects. *Experimental Brain Research, 235*(3), 889–901. doi: 10.1007/s00221-016-4846-7

Murata, A. (2004). Effects of duration of immersion in a virtual reality environment on postural stability. *International Journal of Human-Computer Interaction, 17*(4), 463–477. doi: 10.1207/s15327590ijhc1704_2

Nukarinen, T., Istance, H. O., Rantala, J., Mäkelä, J., Korpela, K., Ronkainen, K., Surakka, V., & Raisamo, R. (2020). Physiological and psychological restoration in matched real and virtual natural environments. Extended Abstracts of the 2020 CHI Conference on Human Factors in Computing Systems Extended Abstracts, 1–18. doi: http://dx.doi.org/10.1145/3334480.3382956

Park, B. J., Tsunetsugu, Y., Kasetani, T., Kagawa, T., & Miyazaki, Y. (2010). The physiological effects of Shinrin-yoku (taking in the forest atmosphere or forest bathing): Evidence from field experiments in 24 forests across Japan. *Environmental Health and Preventive Medicine, 15*(1), 18–26.

Pasco, D. (2013). The potential of using virtual reality technology in physical activity settings. *Quest, 65*(4), 429–441.

Peruzzi, A., Cereatti, A., Della Croce, U., & Mirelman, A. (2016). Effects of a virtual reality and treadmill training on gait of subjects with multiple sclerosis: A pilot study. *Multiple Sclerosis and Related Disorders. 5*, 91–96. doi: 10.1016/j.msard.2015.11.002

Plante, T. G., Aldridge, A., Bogden, R., & Hanelin, C. (2003a). Might virtual reality promote the mood benefits of exercise?. *Computers in Human Behavior, 19*(4), 495–509.

Plante, T. G., Aldridge, A., Su, D., Bogdan, R., Belo, M., & Kahn, K. (2003b). Does virtual reality enhance the management of stress when paired with exercise? An exploratory study. *International Journal of Stress Management, 10*, 203–216.

Physical Activity and Virtual Nature 145

Plante, T. G., Cage, C., Clements, S., & Stover, A. (2006). Psychological benefits of exercise paired with virtual reality: Outdoor exercise energizes whereas indoor virtual exercise relaxes. *International Journal of Stress Management, 13*, 108–117.

Pretty, J., Griffin, M., Sellens, M., & Pretty, C. (2003). Green Exercise: Complementary Roles of Nature, Exercise and Diet in Physical and Emotional Well-Being and Implications for Public Health Policy. Retrieved from Colchester: http://www.outdoorfoundation.org/pdf/GreenExercise.pdf

Raanaas, R. K., Patil, G. G., & Hartig, T. (2012). Health benefits of a view of nature through the window: A quasi-experimental study of patients in a residential rehabilitation center. *Clinical Rehabilitation, 26*(1), 21–32. doi: 10.1177/0269215511412800

Rebenitsch, L., & Owen, C. (2016). Review on cyber sickness in applications and visual displays. *Virtual Reality, 20*(2), 101–125. doi: 10.1007/s10055-016-0285-9

Rogerson, M., Barton, J., Pretty, J., & Gladwell, V. (2019). The green exercise concept: Two intertwining pathways to health and well-being. In Aoife A. Donnelly, A. A., & MacIntyre, T. E. (Ed.), *Physical Activity in Natural Settings: Green Exercise and Blue Mind.* Routledge.

Senese, V. P., Pascale, A., Maffei, L., Cioffi, F., Sergi, I., Gnisci, A., & Masullo, M. (2020). The influence of personality traits on the measure of restorativeness in an urban park: A multisensory immersive virtual reality study. In *Neural Approaches to Dynamics of Signal Exchanges*, 347–357. Singapore: Springer.

Sharples, S., Cobb, S., Moody, A., & Wilson, J. R. (2008). Virtual reality induced symptoms and effects (VRISE): Comparison of head mounted display (HMD), desktop and projection display systems. *Displays, 29*(2), 58–69. doi: 10.1016/j.displa.2007.09.005

Sheik-Nainar, M. A., & Kaber, D. B. (2007). The utility of a virtual reality locomotion interface for studying gait behavior. *Human Factors, 49*, 696–709. doi: 10.1518/001872007X215773

Sherman, W. R., & Craig, A. B. (2003). *Understanding Virtual Reality. Interface, Application and Design.* Boston, MA: Morgan-Kaufmann Publishers.

Slater, M., & Wilbur, S. (1997). A framework for immersive virtual environments (FIVE): Speculations on the role of presence in virtual environments. *Presence-Teleoperators and Virtual Environments, 6*(6), 603–616. doi: 10.1162/pres.1997.6.6.603

Slater, M., Usoh, M., & Steed, A. (1995). Taking steps: The influence of a walking technique on presence in virtual reality. *ACM Transactions on Computer-Human Interaction. 2*, 201–219. doi: 10.1145/210079.210084

Smith, J. W. (2015). Immersive virtual environment technology to supplement environmental perception, preference and behavior research: A review with applications. *International Journal of Environmental Research and Public Health, 12*(9), 11486–11505. doi: 10.3390/ijerph120911486

Steuer, J. (1992). Defining virtual reality: Dimensions determining telepresence. *Journal of Communication, 42*(4), 73–93. doi: 10.1111/j.1460-2466.1992.tb00812.x

The House of Commons (2017). *Sports Participation in England (8181).* Retrieved from https://researchbriefings.files.parliament.uk/documents/CBP-8181/CBP-8181.pdf

Thomas, J. G., & Bond, D. S. (2014). Review of innovations in digital health technology to promote weight control. *Current Diabetes Reports, 14*(5), 485. doi: 10.1007/s11892-014-0485-1

146   G. Calogiuri, S. Litleskare, and F. Fröhlich

Triberti, S., Repetto, C., & Riva, G. (2014). Psychological factors influencing the effectiveness of virtual reality-based analgesia: A systematic review. *Cyberpsychology, Behavior, and Social Networking, 17*(6), 335–345. doi: 10.1089/cyber.2014.0054

Ulrich, R. S. (1984). View through a window may influence recovery from surgery. *Science, 224*(4647), 420–421.

Valtchanov, D., & Ellard, C. (2010). *Physiological and Affective Responses to Immersion in Virtual Reality: Effects of Nature and Urban Settings. Journal of Cyber Therapy & Rehabilitation.* 3(4), 359–373.

Valtchanov, D., Barton, K. R., & Ellard, C. (2010). Restorative effects of virtual nature settings. *Cyberpsychology, Behavior, and Social Networking. 13*, 503–512. doi: 10.1089/cyber. 2009.0308

Weech, S., Kenny, S., & Barnett-Cowan, M. (2019). Presence and cybersickness in virtual reality are negatively related: A review. *Frontiers in Psychology, 10*. doi: ARTN 158

White, M. P., Elliott, L. R., Taylor, T., Wheeler, B. W., Spencer, A., Bone, A., ... Fleming, L. E. (2016). Recreational physical activity in natural environments and implications for health: A population based cross-sectional study in England. *Preventive Medicine, 91*, 383–388. doi: 10.1016/j.ypmed.2016.08.023

White, M. P., Yeo, N. L., Vassiljev, P., Lundstedt, R., Wallergard, M., Albin, M., & Lohmus, M. (2018). A prescription for "nature": The potential of using virtual nature in therapeutics. *Neuropsychiatric Disease and Treatment, 14*, 3001–3013. doi: 10.2147/Ndt.S179038

Yeo, N., White, M., Alcock, I., Garside, R., Dean, S., Smalley, A., & Gatersleben, B. (2020). What is the best way of delivering virtual nature for improving mood? An experimental comparison of high definition TV, 360° video, and computer generated virtual reality. *Journal of Environmental Psychology, 72*, 101500. doi: 10.1016/j.jenvp.2020.101500

Yu, C. P., Lee, H. Y., & Luo, X. Y. (2018). The effect of virtual reality forest and urban environments on physiological and psychological responses. *Urban Forestry & Urban Greening, 35*, 106–114. doi: 10.1016/j.ufug.2018.08.013

11 Emerging Psychological Wellbeing Frameworks for Adventure Recreation, Education, and Tourism

Susan Houge Mackenzie

11.1 Introduction

While participation rates across many traditional organized sports and exercise activities are declining or stagnating, the popularity of outdoor adventure pursuits, such as skydiving, rock climbing, whitewater kayaking, and snowboarding, has steadily increased (e.g. Brymer & Schweitzer, 2017; Outdoor Industry Foundation, 2018). This trend in recreation was reflected in the growth of adventure tourism globally prior to the COVID-19 pandemic, which expanded by 195% from 2010–2014 (UNWTO, 2014). Even in the face of unprecedented mobility restrictions adopted to slow the spread of COVID-19, people continued to seek adventure benefits, either through creative "microadventures" close to home or by violating government mandates and thereby endangering public health (Houge Mackenzie & Goodnow, 2020). These trends, both before and during a global pandemic, highlight the value many individuals place on adventure. Puchan (2004, p. 177) argued that increasing interest and engagement in adventure is "not… just a 'flash in the pan' but a sign of the times in which people are looking for a new way to define their lives and to escape from an increasingly regulated and sanitized way of living." This conjecture is supported by findings across recreation, education, and tourism domains. Outdoor adventure experiences across these domains have been shown to facilitate a range of positive affective and cognitive outcomes, such as increased self-confidence, self-esteem, resilience, intrinsic motivation, enjoyment, educational engagement, competence, relatedness, and autonomy, in addition to personal transformations and the development of ecocentric perspectives (e.g. Brymer & Houge Mackenzie, 2017; Brymer & Schweitzer, 2013; Ewert & Yoshino, 2011; Hattie et al., 1997; Houge Mackenzie, Son & Eitel, 2018; Scarf et al., 2018; Sibthorp et al., 2008).

Outdoor adventure has been defined in a number of ways over the past three decades. The terms extreme, action, high-risk, alternative, or lifestyle sports have often been used interchangeably to describe adventure across bodies of literature, including medical and legal (e.g. Pain & Kerr, 2004), marketing (e.g. Shoham, Rose & Kahle, 2000), and psychological (Clough

DOI: 10.4324/9781003154419-13

148 *S.H. Mackenzie*

et al., 2016). While defining adventure remains an ongoing challenge for the field, the following definition encapsulates core components of modern outdoor adventure pursuits: *self-initiated nature-based physical activities that generate heightened bodily sensations (e.g. vestibular sensations arising from quick acceleration in varying dimensions of space) and require skill development to manage unique perceived and objective risks* (Boudreau, Houge Mackenzie & Hodge, 2020). This definition offers two important perspectives that may be overlooked in the literature defining adventure. First, this definition highlights the bodily sensations arising from adventure as heightened relative to typical bodily sensations experienced in everyday life. Second, in contrast to traditional, risk-focused adventure definitions, this perspective characterizes the perceived and objective risks encountered in adventure as unique, rather than inherently or purposefully higher, compared to the risks encountered in everyday experiences (e.g. driving a car).

Framing the risks encountered in adventure as *unique* rather than *inherently or purposefully higher* than those in everyday life challenges traditional models of outdoor adventure participation that have characterized adventure as being primarily focused on risk, danger, hedonism, and thrill or sensation-seeking. Not only have these traditional frameworks demonstrated limited predictive power and depth, but they have also precluded and restricted considerations of how outdoor adventure may benefit broader populations in terms of general public health and wellbeing (e.g. Clough et al., 2016; Houge Mackenzie & Brymer, 2020). Moreover, traditional adventure definitions and perspectives have largely disconnected adventure studies from rapidly developing research on links between nature and health. This chapter aims to identify fruitful avenues of theoretical development and further study that may help bridge these disparate lines of research. To this end, the chapter will explore emerging frameworks that focus on psychological wellbeing outcomes of outdoor adventure and suggest key mechanisms through which these outcomes may be facilitated.

11.1.1 Psychological Wellbeing Benefits of Adventure

Research suggests that adventure activities enhance physical health and psychological wellbeing in a variety of unexpected ways and that these experiences of wellbeing encourage further participation (Brymer & Schweitzer, 2017). Adventure participants report a range of hedonic and eudaimonic wellbeing outcomes, including positive life transformations, emotional regulation, improved quality of life, goal achievement, social connections, overcoming fears and challenges, nature connection, and transcendence (e.g. Brymer & Gray, 2010; Willig, 2008; Woodman, Cazenave & Le Scanff, 2008; Woodman et al., 2010). Large meta-analyses demonstrate efficacy of adventure programmes, particularly for longer programs and younger participants, with outcomes that include improved

Emerging Psychological Wellbeing 149

self-concept, self-awareness, and acceptance, and reduced behavioral and emotional symptoms (e.g. Gass, Gillis & Russell, 2012; Hattie et al., 1997). While the evidence base is smaller, the tourism domain also suggests how adventure may foster psychological wellbeing for clients and guides (e.g. Houge Mackenzie & Kerr, 2012, 2013, 2014, 2017).

A variety of mechanisms may explain links between psychological wellbeing and outdoor adventure. For instance, the aesthetic, spiritual, and novel qualities of natural environments have been found to promote personal development, self-awareness, and environmental consciousness (e.g. D'Amato & Krasny, 2011). Adventure is posited to restore attentional resources, improve cognitive function, and foster healthy behavioral changes and ecocentric perspectives (e.g. Berman, Jonides & Kaplan, 2008; Pryor, Carpenter & Townsend, 2012), which in turn support psychological wellbeing. In adventure education, Sibthorp and colleagues (e.g. Ramsing & Sibthorp, 2008; Sibthorp & Arthur-Banning, 2004) have repeatedly identified how enhanced autonomy and personal relevance may account for the positive psychological outcomes of adventure programmes. These findings challenge traditional risk-focused theories of adventure and suggest that (i) underlying psychological processes; and (ii) natural settings may be critical mechanisms through which adventure fosters psychological wellbeing. Thus, these concepts are further explored in the following sections.

11.1.2 Nature, Physical Activity, and Psychological Wellbeing in Adventure

As outdoor adventure involves physical activity in nature, this may be an important, but overlooked, mechanism through which adventure supports psychological wellbeing. Physical activity in outdoor contexts has been shown to benefit both psychological function and psychological wellbeing (e.g. Frumkin et al., 2017; Kamijo, Takeda & Hillman, 2011; Maller et al., 2002). For example, "green exercise" studies have identified synergistic benefits of physical activity in nature (e.g. Pretty et al., 2005). Evidence suggests that even viewing pictures of pleasant natural scenes during physical activity results in enhanced physical and psychological benefits compared with non-natural scenes (e.g. Pretty et al., 2007). While physical activity may account for some of the psychological benefits of adventure, the natural context also plays a significant role in wellbeing outcomes. For instance, both vigorous and less active outdoor leisure afford important wellbeing benefits, and nature exposure alone is linked to mental recovery, resilience, and general wellbeing (e.g. Frumkin et al., 2017; Mutz & Müller, 2016). In an experimental design across indoor, urban, and natural settings, Ryan et al. (2010) found that nature significantly enhanced subjective vitality beyond the influence of physical activity alone. These findings suggest that the nature contact inherent in adventure may independently contribute to wellbeing outcomes, beyond other aspects of the experience.

150 *S.H. Mackenzie*

The importance of nature to psychological wellbeing has been attributed to the role of nature in attention restoration (Kaplan, 1995). This hypothesis is supported by research showing brain wave patterns associated with meditative calm documented during nature exposure (Aspinall, Mavros, Coyne & Roe, 2013). Drawing on Fredrickson's (2001) "broaden and build" theory of positive emotions, Aspinall et al. (2013) examined cortical correlates of emotional states in green and urban spaces. Consistent with attention restoration theories, these authors found cortical evidence of lower frustration, engagement, arousal, and higher meditation in natural settings, and concluded that creating access to nature may enhance emotional responses and mood among the general public. Chawla et al. (2014) found similar psychological wellbeing benefits for children who were exposed to nature, such as enhanced relatedness, autonomy, competence, vitality, creativity, and positive emotions. As nature appears to play a vital role in psychological wellbeing, and adventure activities are inherently conducted in nature, it is likely that nature both directly and indirectly facilitates a number of psychological wellbeing outcomes associated with adventure. Thus, future adventure research should utilize models that (i) directly examine the relationship between nature contact or nature connection and psychological wellbeing outcomes; and (ii) incorporate nature contact or nature connection as a key mediator or moderator of psychological wellbeing outcomes.

11.1.3 Hedonia, Eudaimonia, Basic Psychological Needs, and Adventure

In addition to the role of nature, recent conceptual developments suggest that adventure may foster both hedonic and eudaimonic psychological wellbeing outcomes via basic psychological need fulfilment (Houge Mackenzie & Hodge, 2020). This approach is informed by the two long-standing traditions in wellbeing research: hedonia and eudaimonia. Hedonic wellbeing consists of pleasure, positive emotions, and avoidance of pain (e.g. Waterman, Schwartz & Conti, 2008), whereas eudaimonic wellbeing encompasses meaning, purpose, optimal functioning, self-realization, and flourishing (e.g. Huppert & So, 2013). Although these perspectives define wellbeing in distinct ways, scholars increasingly support holistic approaches that incorporate both hedonic and eudaimonic elements (e.g. Henderson & Knight, 2012; Lomas & Ivtzan, 2016). For instance, Huta and Ryan (2010) argue that pursuing eudaimonic wellbeing results in a meaningful life, which fosters stable and enduring hedonic happiness. Importantly, this literature has robustly demonstrated how eudaimonic benefits stem directly from the immediate satisfaction of basic psychological needs for autonomy (e.g. exercising volition, freedom from external control), competence (e.g. feeling capable of achieving personally meaningful goals), and relatedness (e.g. feeling deeply connected to important others) (Ryan, Huta & Deci,

2013). The degree to which basic psychological needs for autonomy, competence, and relatedness are supported (or frustrated) has been shown to significantly impact wellbeing in many life domains, such as business, education, health, and leisure (e.g. Ryan & Deci, 2017), and basic psychological need fulfillment predicts both daily wellbeing (Reis et al., 2000) and life satisfaction (Ryan & Huta, 2009). While some adventure literature has demonstrated support for these constructs (e.g. Houge Mackenzie & Raymond, 2020; Houge Mackenzie, Boudreau & Raymond, 2020; Houge Mackenzie, Son & Eitel, 2018; Scarf et al., 2018; Sibthorp et al., 2008), frameworks based around basic psychological need fulfillment have not been widely applied to adventure research.

Using basic psychological needs frameworks, and indicators of hedonia and eudaimonia, can improve our understanding of adventure experiences and psychological wellbeing outcomes. Adventure activities provide unique physical and psychological challenges resulting from the person–environment relationship, rather than other people or sporting situations that are "contrived." Successfully creating and mastering these challenges can fulfil the basic psychological need for competence and thereby increase outcomes such as positive affect, self-efficacy and resilience. In psychological wellbeing models, these outcomes are recognized as essential components of wellbeing. The concept of resilience, generally defined as a range of capacities that mitigate factors which threaten an individual's health (e.g. Kaplan, 1999), has been increasingly examined as an important outcome of adventure that can buffer the impact of stressful life events (e.g. D'Amato & Krasny, 2011; Ewert & Yoshino, 2011; Neill & Dias, 2001). Identifying mechanisms beyond those related to risk that may underlie the development of resilience, such as fulfilling the need for competence, can improve adventure models and practices.

In addition to fulfilling the psychological need for competence and associated wellbeing outcomes, adventure appears to support autonomy, both in the immediate adventure context and in participants' everyday lives (Houge Mackenzie, Boudreau & Raymond, 2020; Houge Mackenzie & Raymond, 2020; MacGregor, Woodman & Hardy, 2014; Sibthorp et al., 2008; Wurdinger & Paxton, 2003). This is logical considering that adventure participants arguably have greater opportunities for volitional choice about potential courses of action than they would in traditional sporting activities with more formalized "rules." These opportunities can support eudaimonic wellbeing by potentially increasing the salience of autonomous decision-making processes and personal meaning. Adventure frameworks incorporating the role of autonomy may more fully account for the psychological wellbeing outcomes identified in adventure contexts, and inform the development of more positive adventure experiences across recreation, education, and tourism settings.

Adventure also appears to support the psychological need for relatedness in various ways, such as working cooperatively with small groups in

152   *S.H. Mackenzie*

natural environments. Nature has been shown to enhance interpersonal connections (e.g. Maas et al., 2009), and adventure participants often work with others to reach common goals. The majority of adventure activities require high levels of trust and cooperation as both the activity and natural environment activity pose unique challenges, ranging from physical discomfort or serious injury to psychological distress that participants must overcome together. Participants may also have prolonged contact on adventures such as multiday mountaineering or river trips, which can promote a strong sense of relatedness. Recent studies have further suggested that beyond opportunities to connect deeply to others, adventure guiding, in particular, may promote wellbeing outcomes by facilitating a sense of "beneficence" (having a positive impact on others) (Houge Mackenzie & Raymond, 2020; Houge Mackenzie, Boudreau & Raymond, 2020). However, this is an emergent proposition requiring further research across larger samples and a broader range of adventure contexts. As adventure activities often foster intimate relationships that may be more meaningful than everyday social interactions, it is important to consider the role of relatedness, and the potential role of beneficence, in fostering psychological wellbeing outcomes of adventure.

While "relatedness" is defined in terms of relationships with other people in Self-Determination Theory (Ryan & Deci, 2017), this need may be met in other ways. Adventure could potentially foster psychological wellbeing by promoting feelings of connection with nature, in addition to other people. Evidence to support this conjecture is provided by BASE jumpers who report the central importance of nature connection in this adventure activity (Brymer & Gray, 2010; Kerr & Houge Mackenzie, 2020). This form of nature connection is reflected in the emerging concept of Nature Relatedness, which describes the affective, cognitive, and experiential aspects of human–nature relationships (Nisbet, Zelenski & Murphy, 2009). Studies by Nisbet and colleagues suggest that nature relatedness may uniquely contribute to human wellbeing and happiness, as well as promoting environmental sustainability (Nisbet, Zelenski & Murphy, 2011; Zelenski & Nisbet, 2014). Repeated positive adventure experiences (e.g. positive emotions; hedonia) may, over time, facilitate place attachment and eudaimonic psychological wellbeing outcomes, such as identity formation and sense of purpose (Morgan, 2010; Twigger-Ross & Uzzell, 1996). Future models should consider how adventure may support wellbeing by fostering relationships with nature, as well as other people.

Research supports these potential links between adventure experiences, connection to nature, and psychological wellbeing. Relationships with nature have been linked to high self-esteem, life satisfaction, and subjective wellbeing (Cervinka, Röderer & Hefler, 2012; Zhang, Howell & Iyer, 2014). Feeling connected to nature is also significantly correlated with lower anxiety and higher wellbeing (Martyn & Brymer, 2016). This relationship also appeared to be moderated to a degree by autonomy (Martyn

& Brymer, 2016), which further suggests that (i) nature contact and connection, autonomy, competence, and relatedness each play an important role in adventure outcomes; and (ii) these constructs may influence each other in adventure contexts.

The following section examines a recent example to illustrate how these diverse concepts may be developed into a coherent framework that can be used to examine psychological processes and outcomes involved in adventure experiences. Houge Mackenzie and Hodge (2020) proposed a potential framework for examining the psychological wellbeing processes and outcomes of adventure recreation (see Figure 11.1). This conceptual framework synthesized recent advances in psychological wellbeing literature and linked these to many of the adventure processes and outcomes discussed in this chapter. While it is important to note that this is a working model requiring testing and refinement, it highlights many of the key mechanisms that may underpin psychological wellbeing outcomes of adventure by integrating basic psychological need constructs (e.g. basic psychological need satisfaction; autonomous motivation; autonomy-supportive social environments; Ryan & Deci, 2017) and nature contact. This framework offers one example of how gaps in the literature can be addressed by modeling how adventure may foster eudaimonic subjective wellbeing (e.g. meaning, life satisfaction) by fulfilling basic psychological needs for autonomy, competence, and relatedness, as well as the recently proposed fourth basic need for beneficence (e.g. Martela, Ryan & Steger, 2018). In this model, autonomy is defined as having an authentic sense of

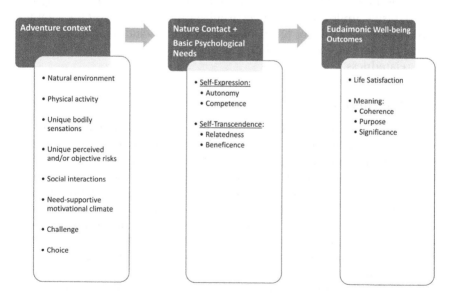

Figure 11.1 Proposed conceptual framework of adventure and psychological wellbeing (adapted from Houge Mackenzie & Hodge, 2020).

154   S.H. Mackenzie

self-direction and volition, and being the perceived origin of one's own behavior (Ryan & Deci, 2017). Competence refers to individuals feeling effective in their ongoing interactions with their environment and experiencing opportunities to exercise and express their capacities. Relatedness refers to feeling connected to others, caring about and being cared for by others, and having a sense of belonging both with other individuals and with one's community. Beneficence is characterized by feeling that one has a positive impact on the lives of other people and engaging in prosocial behavior (Martela, Ryan, & Steger, 2018). This model is rooted in evidence showing how people experience positive psychological development and optimal psychological wellbeing across diverse contexts when psychological needs are satisfied (Ryan & Deci, 2017).

While this framework is limited in that it focuses on eudaimonic outcomes, it highlights the importance of (i) identifying underlying mechanisms that may result in positive wellbeing outcomes, and (ii) identifying various components of psychological wellbeing (e.g. coherence, purpose, significance; Martela & Steger, 2016) in order to effectively differentiate amongst specific psychological wellbeing outcomes. To enhance this framework and increase its predictive value, a broader range of both hedonic (e.g. positive affect, subjective vitality), eudaimonic (e.g. life satisfaction), and psychological wellbeing outcomes could be added and examined. While there are many ways to conceptualize adventure and psychological wellbeing, adventure researchers should strive to advance theory in this field by elucidating *how* and *why* adventure fosters psychological wellbeing. This can be achieved by proposing and evaluating key mechanisms underpinning diverse adventure outcomes. This chapter has identified a range of promising constructs, including nature contact or connection and basic psychological needs for autonomy, competence, and relatedness.

11.2 Conclusion

Reframing adventure requires a movement away from models focused on risk, danger, hedonism, and thrill-seeking. Risk-focused models not only lack predictive value in terms of being able to account for the wide range of psychological wellbeing outcomes, they also lack robust psychological explanations of how positive outcomes are achieved. This chapter identified a number of promising constructs that can inform future adventure frameworks and models. At a theoretical level, expanding adventure models to include links to literature and measurement tools across psychology, health, and nature literature will improve our understanding of how and when adventure may support psychological wellbeing. In order to successfully develop adventure theory in this vein, researchers will also need to evaluate models across more heterogeneous participants and adventure experiences.

Advancing theoretical models of adventure have a range of potential practical benefits. These advancements can inform how we practice adventure and hopefully lead to safer, more inclusive adventure opportunities that provide a wide range of much-needed mental health benefits for diverse populations. Reframing how we understand adventure experiences can provide valuable means of enhancing individual and social wellbeing. These shifts have the potential to benefit community groups, educational institutions, tourism operators, and public health agencies. For example, adventure could be considered as a preventative health strategy for promoting mental health and wellbeing (Clough at al., 2016). Examining adventure through psychological wellbeing lenses may also advance the recent movement toward "green prescriptions" (e.g. Buckley & Brough, 2017). While the current chapter illustrated some of the ways that adventure may be reframed in terms of psychological wellbeing, this is simply a starting point. Future researchers should continue to critically examine traditional and emerging adventure frameworks by considering complementary disciplines and findings. Adopting broader, more holistic perspectives of adventure can help expand the vision of what adventure is and how adventure may impact wellbeing.

References

Aspinall, P., Mavros, P., Coyne, R., & Roe, J. (2013). The urban brain: Analysing outdoor physical activity with mobile EEG. *British Journal of Sports Medicine, 49,* 272–276. doi: 10.1136/bjsports-2012-091877

Berman, M. G., Jonides, J., & Kaplan, S. (2008). The cognitive benefits of interacting with nature. *Psychological Science, 19*(12), 1207–1212.

Boudreau, P., Houge Mackenzie, S., & Hodge, K. (2020). Flow states in adventure recreation: A systematic review and critical thematic synthesis. *Psychology of Sport and Exercise, 46,* 101611. https://doi.org/10.1016/j.psychsport.2019.

Brymer, E., & Houge Mackenzie, S. (2017). Psychology and the extreme sport experience. In F. Feletti (Ed.), *Science and extreme sport medicine* (pp. 3–13). Cham, Switzerland: Springer International Publishing.

Brymer, E., & Schweitzer, R. D. (2013). Extreme sports are good for your health: A phenomenological understanding of fear and anxiety in extreme sport. *Journal of Health Psychology, 18*(4), 477–487.

Brymer, E., & Schweitzer, R. D. (2017). Evoking the ineffable: The phenomenology of extreme sports. *Psychology of Consciousness: Theory, Research, and Practice, 4*(1), 63–74. http://dx.doi.org/10.1037/cns0000111

Buckley, R. C., & Brough, P. (2017). Nature, eco, and adventure therapies for mental health and chronic disease. *Frontiers in Public Health, 5,* 220.

Cervinka, R., Röderer, K., & Hefler, E. (2012). Are nature lovers happy? On various indicators of well-being and connectedness with nature. *Journal of Health Psychology, 17*(3), 379–388.

Chawla, L., Keena, K., Pevec, I., & Stanley, E. (2014). Green schoolyards as havens from stress and resources for resilience in childhood and adolescence. *Health & Place, 28,* 1–13. doi: 10.1016/j.healthplace.2014.03.001

Clough, P., Houge Mackenzie, S., Mallabon, L., & Brymer, E. (2016). Adventurous physical activity environments: A mainstream intervention for mental health. *Sports Medicine, 46*, 963–968.

D'Amato, L. G., & Krasny, M. E. (2011). Outdoor adventure education: Applying transformative learning theory to understanding instrumental learning and personal growth in environmental education. *The Journal of Environmental Education, 42*(4), 237–254.

Ewert, A., & Yoshino, A. (2011). The influence of short-term adventure-based experiences on levels of resilience. *Journal of Adventure Education & Outdoor Learning, 11*, 35–50.

Fredrickson, B. L. (2001). The role of positive emotions in positive psychology: The broaden-and-build theory of positive emotions. *American Psychologist, 56*, 218–226.

Frumkin, H., Bratman, G. N., Breslow, S. J., Cochran, B., Kahn Jr, P. H., Lawler, J. J., … & Wood, S. A. (2017). Nature contact and human health: A research agenda. *Environmental Health Perspectives*, 125(7). doi: 10.1289/EHP1663

Gass, M. A., Gillis, H. L., & Russell, K. C. (2012). *Adventure therapy: Theory, research, and practice.* New York: Routledge.

Hattie, J., Marsh, H. W., Neill, J. T., & Richards, G. E. (1997). Adventure education and outward bound: Out-of-class experiences that make a lasting difference. *Review of Educational Research, 67*, 43–87.

Henderson, L. W., & Knight, T. (2012). Integrating the hedonic and eudaimonic perspectives to more comprehensively understand wellbeing and pathways to wellbeing. *International Journal of Wellbeing, 2*(3), 196–221. doi: 10.5502/ijw.v2i3.3

Houge Mackenzie, S., & Brymer, E. (2020). Conceptualizing adventurous nature sport: A positive psychology perspective. *Annals of Leisure Research, 23*(1), 79–91.

Houge Mackenzie, S., & Goodnow, J. (2020). Adventure in the age of COVID-19: Embracing microadventures and locavism in a post-pandemic world. *Leisure Sciences*, 1–8. https://doi.org/10.1080/01490400.2020.1773984

Houge Mackenzie, S., & Hodge, K. (2020). Adventure recreation and subjective well-being: A conceptual framework. *Leisure Studies, 39*(1) 26–40.

Houge Mackenzie, S., & Kerr, J. H. (2012). A (mis)guided adventure tourism experience: An autoethnographic analysis of mountaineering in Bolivia. *Journal of Sport & Tourism, 17*(2), 125–144.

Houge Mackenzie, S., & Kerr, J. H. (2013). Can't we all just get along? Emotions and the team guiding experience in adventure tourism. *Special edition of Journal of Destination Marketing and Management, 2*(2), 85–93.

Houge Mackenzie, S., & Kerr, J. H. (2014). The psychological experience of river guiding: Exploring the protective frame and implications for guide well-being. *Journal of Sport & Tourism, 19*(1), 5–27.

Houge Mackenzie, S., & Kerr, J. H. (2017). Co-creation and experience brokering in guided adventure tours. In S. Filep, J. Laing and M. Csikszentmihalyi (Eds.), *Positive tourism.* New York, NY: Routledge.

Houge Mackenzie, S., & Raymond, E. (2020). A conceptual model of adventure tour guide well- being. *Annals of Tourism Research, 84*, 102977. https://doi.org/10.1016/j.annals.2020.102977

Houge Mackenzie, S., Boudreau, P., & Raymond, E. (2020). Well-being and adventure: The experiences of women tour guides in New Zealand. *Journal of Tourism and Hospitality Management, 45*, 410–418.

Houge Mackenzie, S., Son, J. S., & Eitel, K. (2018). Using outdoor adventure to enhance intrinsic motivation and engagement in science and physical activity: An exploratory study. *Journal of Outdoor Recreation and Tourism, 21*, 76–86.

Huppert, F. A., & So, T. T. (2013). Flourishing across Europe: Application of a new conceptual framework for defining well-being. *Social Indicators Research, 110*(3), 837–861.

Huta, V., & Ryan, R. M. (2010). Pursuing pleasure or virtue: The differential and overlapping well-being benefits of hedonic and eudaimonic motives. *Journal of Happiness Studies, 11*(6), 735–762.

Kamijo, K., Takeda, Y., & Hillman, C. H. (2011). The relation of physical activity to functional connectivity between brain regions. *Clinical Neurophysiology, 122*, 81–89.

Kaplan, H. B. (1999). Toward an understanding of resilience: A critical review of definitions and models. In M. D. Glantz and J. L. Johnson (Eds.), *Resilience and development* (pp. 17–83). New York: Kluwer Academic.

Kaplan, S. (1995). The restorative benefits of nature: Toward an integrative framework. *Journal of Environmental Psychology, 15*, 169–182.

Kerr, J. H., & Houge Mackenzie, S. (2020). "I don't want to die. That's not why I do it at all": Multifaceted motivation, psychological health, and personal development in BASE jumping. *Annals of Leisure Research, 23*, 223–242. https://doi.org/10.108 0/11745398.2018.1483732

Lomas, T., & Ivtzan, I. (2016). Second wave positive psychology: Exploring the positive-negative dialectics of wellbeing. *Journal of Happiness Studies, 17*(4), 1753–1768.

Maas, J., van Dillen, S. M. E., Verheij, R. A., & Groenewegen, P. P. (2009). Social contacts as a possible mechanism behind the relation between green space and health. *Health Place, 15*(2), 586–595.

MacGregor, A., Woodman, T., & Hardy, L. (2014). Risk is good for you: An investigation of the processes and outcomes associated with high-risk sport. *Journal of Exercise, Movement, and Sport, 46*(1), 175.

Maller, C., Townsend, M., Brown, P., & St. Leger, L. (2002). *Healthy parks, healthy people: The health benefits of contact with nature in a park context.* Report to Parks Victoria and the International Park Strategic Partners Group. Melbourne: Deakin University.

Martela, F., & Steger, M.F. (2016). The three meanings of meaning in life: Distinguishing coherence, purpose and significance. *Journal of Positive Psychology, 11*, 531–545.

Martela, F., Ryan, R., & Steger, M. (2018). Meaningfulness as satisfaction of autonomy, competence, relatedness, and beneficence: Comparing the four satisfactions and positive affect as predictors of meaning in life. *Journal of Happiness Studies, 19*, 1261–1282.

Martyn P., & Brymer E. (2016). The relationship between nature relatedness and anxiety. *Journal of Health Psychology, 21*(7), 1436–1445.

Morgan, P. (2010). Towards a developmental theory of place attachment. *Journal of Environmental Psychology, 30*(1), 11–22.

Mutz, M., & Müller, J. (2016). Mental health benefits of outdoor adventures: Results from two pilot studies. *Journal of Adolescence, 49*, 105–114.

Neill, J. T., & Dias, K. L. (2001). Adventure education and resilience: The double-edged sword. *Journal of Adventure Education & Outdoor Learning, 1*(2), 35–42.

158   S.H. Mackenzie

Nisbet, E. K., Zelenski, J. M., & Murphy, S. A. (2009). The nature relatedness scale: Linking individuals' connection with nature to environmental concern and behavior. *Environment and Behavior, 41*(5), 715–740.

Nisbet, E. K., Zelenski, J. M., & Murphy, S. A. (2011). Happiness is in our nature: Exploring nature relatedness as a contributor to subjective well-being. *Journal of Happiness Studies, 12*(2), 303–322.

Outdoor Industry Foundation. (2018). Outdoor Industry Foundation report. Retrieved from: https://outdoorindustry.org/resource/2018-outdoor-participation-report/ on 25 October 2019.

Pain, M., & Kerr, J. H. (2004). Extreme risk taker who wants to continue taking part in high risk sports after serious injury. *British Journal of Sports Medicine, 38*(3), 337–339.

Pretty, J., Peacock, J., Hine, R., Sellens, M., South, N., & Griffin, M. (2007). Green exercise in the UK countryside: Effects on health and psychological well-being, and implications for policy. *Journal of Environmental Planning and Management, 50*(2), 211–231.

Pretty, J., Peacock, J., Sellens, M., & Griffin, M. (2005). The mental and physical health outcomes of green exercise. *International Journal of Environmental Health Research, 15*, 319–337.

Pryor, A., Carpenter, C., & Townsend, M. (2012). Outdoor education and bush adventure therapy: A social-ecological approach to health and wellbeing. *Australian Journal of Outdoor Education, 9*(1), 3–13.

Puchan, H. (2004). Living 'extreme': Adventure sports, media and commercialisation. *Journal of Communication Management, 9*(2), 171–178.

Ramsing, R., & Sibthorp, J. (2008). The role of autonomy support in summer camp programs: Preparing youth for productive behaviors. *Journal of Park and Recreation Administration, 26*(2), 61–77.

Reis, H. T., Sheldon, K. M., Gable, S. L., Roscoe, R., & Ryan, R. (2000). Daily well-being: The role of autonomy, competence, and relatedness. *Personality & Social Psychology Bulletin, 26*, 419–435.

Ryan, R. M., & Deci, E. L. (2017). *Self-determination theory: Basic psychological needs in motivation, development, and wellness.* New York, NY: Guilford Press.

Ryan, R. M., & Huta, V. (2009). Wellness as healthy functioning or wellness as happiness: The importance of eudaimonic thinking (response to the Kashdan et al. and Waterman discussion). *Journal of Positive Psychology, 4*, 202–204.

Ryan R. M., Huta V., & Deci E. L. (2013). Living well: A self-determination theory perspective on eudaimonia. In A. Delle Fave (Ed.), *The exploration of happiness* (pp. 117–139). Dordrech: Springer.

Ryan, R. M., Weinstein, N., Bernstein, J., Brown, K.W., Mistretta, L., & Gagné, M. (2010). Vitalizing effects of being outdoors and in nature. *Journal of Environmental Psychology, 30*, 159–169.

Scarf, D., Kafka, S., Hayhurst, J., Jang, K., Boyes, M., Thomson, R., & Hunter, J. A. (2018). Satisfying psychological needs on the high seas: Explaining increases self-esteem following an adventure education programme. *Journal of Adventure Education & Outdoor Learning, 18*, 165–175.

Shoham, A., Rose, G. M., & Kahle, L. R. (2000). Practitioners of risky sports: A quantitative examination. *Journal of Business Research, 47*(3), 237–251.

Sibthorp, J., & Arthur-Banning, S. (2004). Developing life effectiveness through adventure education: The roles of participant expectations, perceptions of empowerment, and learning relevance. *Journal of Experiential Education, 27*(1), 32–50.

Emerging Psychological Wellbeing 159

Sibthorp, J., Paisley, K., Gookin, J., & Furman, N. (2008). The pedagogic value of student autonomy in adventure education. *Journal of Experiential Education, 31*, 136–151.

Twigger-Ross, C. L., & Uzzell, D. L. (1996). Place and identity processes. *Journal of Environmental Psychology, 16*(3), 205–220.

UNWTO World Tourism Organisation (2014). Global Report on Adventure Tourism, 2014. Retrieved from: http://cf.cdn.unwto.org/sites/all/files/pdf/final_1global_report_on_adventure_tourism.pdf

Waterman, A. S., Schwartz, S. J., & Conti, R. (2008). The implications of two conceptions of happiness (hedonic enjoyment and eudaimonia) for the understanding of intrinsic motivation. *Journal of Happiness Studies, 9*(1), 41–79.

Willig, C. (2008). A phenomenological investigation of the experience of taking part in extreme sport. *Journal of Health Psychology, 13*, 690–702.

Woodman, T., Cazenave, N., & Le Scanff, C. (2008). Skydiving as emotion regulation: The rise and fall of anxiety is moderated by alexithymia. *Journal of Sport & Exercise Psychology, 30*, 424–433.

Woodman, T., Hardy, L., Barlow, M., & Le Scanff, C. (2010). Motives for prolonged engagement high-risk sports: An agentic emotion regulation perspective. *Psychology of Sport and Exercise, 11*, 345–352.

Wurdinger, S., & Paxton, T. (2003). Using multiple levels of experience to promote autonomy in adventure education students. *Journal of Adventure Education & Outdoor Learning, 3*(1), 41–48.

Zelenski, J. M., & Nisbet, E. K. (2014). Happiness and feeling connected: The distinct role of nature relatedness. *Environment and Behavior, 46*(1), 3–23.

Zhang, J. W., Howell, R. T., & Iyer, R. (2014). Engagement with natural beauty moderates the positive relation between connectedness with nature and psychological well-being. *Journal of Environmental Psychology, 38*, 55–63.

12 *In Vivo* Nature Exposure as a Positive Psychological Intervention: A Review of the Impact of Nature Interventions on Wellbeing

Jillian T. Hunt, Andrew J. Howell, and Holli-Anne Passmore

12.1 Introduction

Appreciating the beauty of a blossom, the loveliness of a lilac, or the grace of a gazelle are all ways in which people can, in some small measure, fill their daily lives with evolutionarily inspired epiphanies of pleasure. (Buss, 2000, p. 22)

In this eloquent description of the effect of spending time in nature on human wellbeing, Buss (2000) suggests that exposure to nature may be an important source of both hedonic and eudaimonic wellbeing in the form of pleasure and moments of epiphany, respectively. He emphasizes the ready accessibility of nature, with daily exposure possible for many people, and further suggests that the impact of nature is likely to be modest in magnitude, presumably reflecting the fact that well-being has many determinants. Finally, Buss emphasizes the evolutionary basis of the relationship between affiliating with nature and well-being among humans, suggesting that this relationship is relatively hard-wired within our species. This chapter narratively reviews current quantitative research examining the impact of nature interventions on well-being. Our aim is to explore the relationship between human wellness and the experience of nature.

We have chosen the framework of positive psychology to examine current research findings regarding nature experiences and well-being. Positive psychology's primary goal is to understand and support the good life, and then to apply this knowledge toward the betterment of the human collective (Pawelski, 2016). One method by which positive psychology aims to achieve this goal is via the development and empirical validation of positive psychological interventions – activities designed specifically to promote feeling good (hedonic well-being) and functioning well (eudaimonic well-being) (Keyes & Annas, 2009).

12.2 Hedonic and Eudaimonic Aspects of Wellbeing

Hedonia and eudaimonia represent two overlapping aspects of well-being, both of which are integral to human flourishing (Ryan & Deci, 2001). Hedonistic wellness, centering around the presence of positive affect and the absence of negative affect, is often contrasted against eudaimonia, conceptualized as "living a complete human life, or the realization of

DOI: 10.4324/9781003154419-14

In Vivo *Nature Exposure* 161

valued human potentials" (Ryan et al., 2008, p. 140). In accordance with this, Proctor and Tweed (2016) offered suggestions for researchers seeking to differentiate measures of eudaimonia from hedonia. They propose that hedonic well-being be measured by positive affect, negative affect and life satisfaction, and that main categories of eudaimonia (i.e. motivation, behavior, or outcome) be measured by such constructs as awe, meaning, intrinsic motivation, transcendence, and spirituality. Additionally, vitality overlaps with both eudaimonic and hedonic aspects of well-being (see Ryan & Frederick, 1997); in the current review, we chose to place vitality into the hedonic category of wellbeing, along with energy, and its opposite, tiredness.

12.3 The Current Review of Nature Intervention Studies

Research has consistently demonstrated that experiences with real nature provide greater boosts to mood than does technologically mediated or virtual exposure to nature (e.g. videos, photos; Kahn et al., 2009; Kjellgren & Buhrkall, 2010; Mayer et al., 2009; McMahan & Estes, 2015). Moreover, Baxter and Pelletier (2019) argue that the need to affiliate with nature is not only a basic human need (see also Hurly & Walker, 2019), but that this need for nature is inherently experiential and thus can only be satisfied fully through *in vivo* experiences in natural environments. In light of this, we included only studies with *in vivo* nature conditions in this review. Other inclusion criteria for selected studies necessitated them: (1) to be randomized controlled trials with at least one non-nature condition; (2) to include a nature intervention of a minimum duration of 10 minutes; and (3) to employ a measure at post-treatment that assesses an aspect of hedonic or eudaimonic well-being according to Proctor and Tweed's (2016) classification. Figure 12.1 presents a detailed process of the search for and selection of articles for review. Table 12.1 summarizes the well-being measures used in articles reviewed herein.

The narrative review of studies meeting our selection criteria focuses upon the main content of relevance to our inquiry: differences (or the lack thereof) in wellbeing outcomes between nature immersion and control conditions. Studies are reviewed in chronological order so as to reflect progression of the field; however, articles are listed alphabetically in Table 12.2 for ease of reference.

12.3.1 Review of Studies

Mayer et al., 2009. Introductory psychology students were randomly assigned to a 10-minute walk in either a nature preserve or a concrete urban area. Before their respective walk, participants were asked to silently reflect on a "loose end" in their life (an easily resolvable problem that needed tending to). Well-being (positive/negative emotions) was measured with the PANAS. Results showed that, relative to those in the urban condition, those in the nature condition reported significantly more positive affect but not significantly less negative affect.

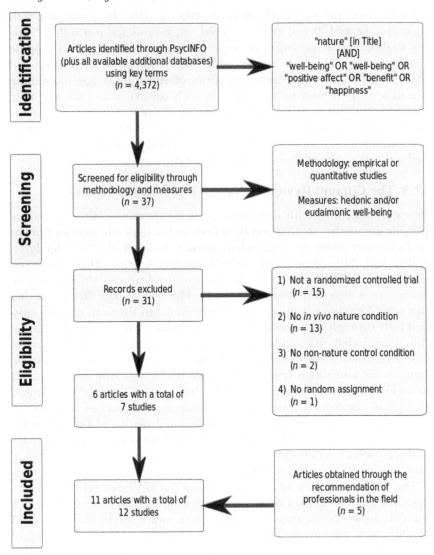

Figure 12.1 Process of the search for and selection of articles for review.

Ryan et al., 2010. Ryan and colleagues randomly assigned undergraduates to a 15-minute walk through either an indoor series of underground tunnels or outdoors along a tree-lined footpath alongside a river. Well-being (vitality) was measured using the SVS. Results revealed a significantly greater increase in vitality for those in the outdoor condition than for those in the indoor condition.

Nisbet & Zelenski, 2011. These two studies also involved participants walking either indoors in outdoors.

Table 12.1 Summary of well-being measures used in articles reviewed

Aspect of Wellbeing	Acronym	Full Name of Measure	Citation
Hedonia			
• energy and tiredness	A–DAC	Activation–Deactivation Adjective Checklist	Thayer, 1986
• positive/negative emotions	PANAS	Positive and Negative Affect Scale	Watson et al., 1988
• vitality	SVS	Subjective Vitality Scale	Ryan & Frederick, 1997
• life satisfaction	SWL	Satisfaction with Life Scale	Diener et al., 1985
• general well-being	WEMWBS	Warwick-Edinburgh Mental Well-Being Scale	Tennant et al., 2007
Eudaimonia			
• elevation	EES	Elevating Experiences Scale	Huta & Ryan, 2010
• meaning in life	MLQ	Meaning in Life Questionnaire	Steger et al., 2006
• transcendent connectedness	MSS	Metapersonal Self Scale	DeCicco & Stroink, 2007
• meaning in life	SMS	Sense of Meaning Scale	Huta & Ryan, 2010
• spiritual transcendence	STS	Spiritual Transcendence Scale	Piedmont, 1999

Study 1. In Study 1, participants were randomly assigned to a 17-minute walk through indoor tunnels between buildings or along a bike pathway following a canal to an arboretum. Well-being (positive/ negative emotions) was measured with a version of the PANAS that was modified to include low-arousal pleasant states such as relaxation and fascination. Those in the nature condition reported significantly higher levels of positive affect, along with significantly lower levels of negative affect, compared to those in the indoor condition.

Study 2. University students again took walks on either indoor or outdoor routes (comparable to the routes in Study 1). As in Study 1, well-being (positive/negative emotions) was measured with the PANAS. Findings demonstrated a significant increase in positive affect and a significant decrease in negative affect for those in the nature condition relative to the control condition.

Passmore & Howell, 2014. Moving beyond one-time nature-experience manipulations, Passmore and Howell conducted a two-week nature-intervention study involving undergraduate students randomly assigned to either a nature or a control condition. In the nature condition, participants were instructed to engage in a nature activity as often as possible for the next two weeks; participants in the control condition were instructed to engage in solving anagram puzzles as often as possible over the next two weeks. Well-being aspects assessed were positive/negative emotions (PANAS), elevation (EES), and meaning in life (SMS). Results indicated that netPA (i.e. positive affect minus negative affect) and elevation were significantly

Table 12.2 Summary of randomized controlled trials of in vivo nature interventions: Effects on well-being

Study	Size and Type of Sample	Manipulation of the Nature Variable	Well-Being Measures	Cohen's d Effect Size, for Each Well-Being Measure	p
Ballew & Omoto, 2018	*N* = 100 American university students	Nature Condition: 15-minute solitary immersion in a local arboretum reflecting on feelings. Built Condition: 15-minute solitary immersion in a stadium reflecting on feelings.	~ Question items developed by researchers for study	Awe: 0.43 Positive emotions: 0.58	p = .036 p = .005
Fuegen & Breitenbecher, 2018	*N* = 181 American university students	*Comparison 1:* Outdoor Exercise: 15-minute outdoor walk on campus circling a lake with nature elements and built elements. Indoor Exercise: 15-minute walk on treadmill watching slideshow/video of images of sights seen by outdoor group. *Comparison 2:* Outdoor Rest: 15-minute rest sitting on a bench adjacent to lake. Indoor Rest: sat at computer desk watching slideshow/video of images of sights seen from bench of outdoor group rested.	~ PANAS ~ A-DAC	*Comparison 1:* Positive affect: 0.09 Negative affect: 0.08 Energy: 0.09 Tiredness: 0.00 *Comparison 2:* Positive affect: 0.80 Negative affect: 0.28 Energy: 0.79 Tiredness: 1.09	p = .682 p = .701 p = .650 p = 1.00 p < .001 p = .207 p < .001 p < .001
Hamann & Ivtzan, 2016	*N* = 62 members of nature and positive psychology Facebook groups, U.S.A., Canada, UK, other	Nature: 30 minutes or more in nature daily for 30 days. Control: Waitlist.	~ PANAS ~ WEMWBS ~ MLQ ~ STS	Positive affect: 0.73 Negative affect: 0.77 General wb: 0.56 Meaning: 0.20 Spirit. Transc.: 0.33	p = .006 p = .004 p = .034 p = .439 p = .200

Study	Sample (N)	Intervention	Measure	Results
Mayer et al., 2009, Study 1	$N = 76$ American introductory psychology students	Nature: 10-minute walk in nature preserve; Control: 10-minute walk in concrete urban area	~ PANAS	Positive affect: 0.65 ($p = .008$); Negative affect: 0.15 ($p = .545$)
Nisbet & Zelenski, 2011, Study 1	$N = 150$ Canadian university students	Nature: 17-minute walk on campus bike path; Control: 17-minute walk through campus indoor tunnels	~ PANAS	Positive affect: 1.15 ($p < .001$); Negative affect: 0.50 ($p = .035$)
Nisbet & Zelenski, 2011, Study 2	$N = 80$ Canadian university students	Nature: 17-minute walk campus bike path; Control: 17-minute walk through campus indoor tunnels	~ PANAS	Positive affect: 1.45 ($p < .001$); Negative affect: 0.49 ($p = .030$)
Nisbet et al., 2019	$N = 100$ Canadian university students	Nature: 20-minute walk outdoors; Control: 20-minute walk indoors	~ PANAS; ~ SVS	Positive affect: 0.98 ($p < .001$); Negative affect: 0.24 ($p = .343$); Vitality: 1.20 ($p < .001$); Nature positive affect: 1.14 ($p < .001$)
Passmore, 2019	$N = 784$ Canadian (518) and Chinese (198), university students, American (73) graduate students and professionals	Nature: for 2-weeks, note daily what emotions evoked by nature encountered in everyday routine, write description of emotions and nature that evoked emotions; Control: for 2 weeks, note daily description of details of the day	~ PANAS; ~ SWLS; ~ MLQ; ~ EES; ~ MSS	NetPA: 0.25 ($p = .004$); Life Satisfaction: 0.16 ($p = .062$); Elevation: 0.62 ($p < .001$); Meaning in life: 0.08 ($p = .364$); Transc. Connect.: 0.24 ($p = .007$)

(Continued)

Table 12.2 *(Continued)*

Study	Size and Type of Sample	Manipulation of the Nature Variable	Well-Being Measures	Cohen's d Effect Size, for Each Well-Being Measure	p
Passmore & Holder, 2017	$N = 364$ Canadian undergraduate students	Nature: for 2 weeks, note daily what emotions evoked by nature encountered in everyday routine, write description of emotions, take photo of nature that evoked them Control: business-as-usual waitlist	~ PANAS ~ EES ~ SMS ~ Composite Transcendent Connectedness	NetPA: 0.46 Elevation: 0.38 Meaning: 0.11 Transc. Connect.: 0.43	$p < .001$ $p = .003$ $p = .370$ $p < .001$
Passmore & Howell, 2014	$N = 84$ Canadian undergraduate students	Nature: as much time immersed in nature activity as can for 2 weeks, recording of daily engagement in nature activities Control: as much solving anagram puzzles as can for 2 weeks, record if completed or not	~ PANAS ~ EES ~ SMS	NetPA: 0.47 Elevation: 0.63 Meaning in Life: 0.36	$p = .036$ $p = .005$ $p = .098$
Passmore, Yang & Sabine, 2019	$N = 173$ Chinese undergraduate students	Nature: for 2 weeks, note daily what emotions evoked by nature encountered in everyday routine, write description of emotions and nature that evoked emotions Control: for 2 weeks, note daily description of details of the day	~ PANAS ~ SWL ~ modified EES ~ MLQ ~ MSS	NetPA: 0.99 PA: 0.63 NA: 0.69 Life satisfaction: 0.48 Elevation: 0.29 Meaning in Life: 0.48 Transc. Connect.: 0.38	$p < .001$ $p = .001$ $p < .001$ $p = .011$ $p = .128$ $p = .012$ $p = .044$
Ryan et al., 2010, Study 2	$N = 80$ American undergraduate students	Nature: 15-minute outdoor walk through tree-lined footpath along a river Control: 15-minute indoor walk through underground tunnels	~ SVS	Not calculable (standard deviations not published)	

higher in the nature condition relative to the control condition; meaning in life was marginally significantly higher in the nature group.

Hamann & Ivtzan, 2016. Using the online Rewild Your Life programme, Hamann and Ivtzan challenged participants to spend at least 30 minutes in nature daily for 30 days. A wait list control group was also employed. Several aspects of well-being were measured: positive/negative emotions (PANAS), general well-being (WEMWBS), meaning in life (MLQ), and spiritual transcendence (STS). Results showed that the nature intervention, relative to the wait list control, significantly increased positive affect and general well-being while significantly decreasing negative affect. No significant difference between conditions emerged for meaning in life or spiritual transcendence (although effect sizes are somewhat notable).

Passmore & Holder, 2017. This study tested the effectiveness of a two-week "Noticing Nature" well-being intervention wherein undergraduate students were randomly assigned to one of three conditions: nature, built, or business-as-usual control. Our focus is on the nature condition relative to the business-as-usual control. In the nature condition, participants were directed to simply notice the nature they encountered in their daily routines and how it made them feel. They were then to snap a photo of the nature that evoked emotions, and to provide a brief written description of their nature-inspired emotions. The control group was instructed to continue with their regular routine. Four aspects of well-being were measured: positive/negative emotions (PANAS), elevation (EES), meaning in life (SMS), and transcendent connectedness (composite measure created for the study). Participants were also assessed for time in nature. Results at postintervention revealed significantly higher scores on netPA, elevation, and transcendent connectedness for those in the nature condition relative to the control condition. Meaning in life was not significantly different between conditions. No significant difference emerged across conditions for time spent in nature.

Ballew & Omoto, 2018. Brief, solitary nature experience was the focus of this study, in which university students were randomly assigned to either a 15-minute solitary natural or built environment condition. Within each condition, participants were instructed to pay attention to and write down their feelings, the features of their surroundings, and to make use of all their senses. Items were developed for the study to measure the well-being aspects of awe and positive emotions. Absorption was also assessed using items developed for the study. Participants in the nature condition reported significantly greater states of awe and positive emotions than those in the built condition; those in the nature condition also experienced greater absorption.

Fuegen & Breitenbecher, 2018. Seeking to explore the effects of exposure to nature during both rest and exercise, Fuegen and Breitenbecher randomly assigned university students to one of four 15-minute experimental conditions: outdoor/nature exercise, indoor exercise, outdoor/nature rest, or indoor rest. We viewed these as providing two experimental comparison groups of nature versus control conditions. The first comparison

168 J.T. Hunt, A.J. Howell, and H.-A.Passmore

was indoor exercise relative to outdoor/nature exercise. Here, the indoor condition involved participants walking on a treadmill while watching a video or slideshow of images of the outdoor nature path that the outdoor exercise groups walked along. The second comparison compared resting indoors versus resting outdoors, wherein the indoor condition involved participants viewing a video or slideshow of images seen from the bench upon which the outdoor participants in the nature condition rested. Well-being aspects assessed were positive and negative emotions (PANAS), along with energy and tiredness (A-DAC). Results showed that, compared to those who rested indoors, those who rested outdoors in nature showed significantly increased positive affect and energy. Negative affect was lower in the nature group, but not significantly so. Interestingly, affect, energy, and tiredness were not significantly different in the two exercise groups.

Nisbet et al., 2019. Building on their previous work (Nisbet & Zelesnki, 2011), Nisbet and colleagues randomly assigned university students to one of three 20-minute walks: indoors/nature, outdoors/nature, or outdoors/nature with mindfulness instruction. We focus only upon the contrast between the first two conditions. Well-being measures were a modified PANAS to measure positive/negative emotions as well as "nature positive affect" (i.e. fascinated, curious, relaxed, in awe, and joyful), and the SVS to assess vitality. Outdoor/nature participants reported significantly greater positive affect, vitality, and "nature positive affect" than did the indoor participants. The groups did not differ significantly on negative affect or mindfulness.

Passmore et al., 2019. Expanding on the first "Noticing Nature" intervention study (Passmore & Holder, 2017), Passmore and colleagues randomly assigned undergraduates from a university in China to one of three conditions: nature, built, and active placebo control. Again, here we focus on emergent differences between the nature and the control group. Instructions for participants in the nature and built conditions were the same as in the original 2017 study described above except that participants jotted down a description of the objects/scenes rather than snapping a photo. As in the 2017 study, participants noted a brief description of what emotions were evoked. Aspects of well-being assessed in this study were: positive/negative emotions and netPA (PANAS), life satisfaction (SWLS), elevation (EES), meaning in life (MLQ), and transcendent connectedness (MSS). Ill-being (depression, anxiety, and stress) and time in nature were also measured. Results indicated that participants who noticed nature (compared to the control condition) reported significantly higher levels of positive emotions, netPA, life satisfaction, meaning in life, and transcendent connectedness, along with significantly lower levels of negative emotions. Elevation was not significantly different between the two groups. Ill-being was significantly lower in the nature group. No significant difference emerged across conditions for time spent in nature.

Passmore, 2019. In this study, Passmore randomly assigned participants (Canada, United States, and China) to one of three conditions: the noticing nature condition described directly above, the Three Good Things positive psychology intervention condition, and an active placebo control condition

In Vivo *Nature Exposure*   169

also described above. For this review, we focus on outcomes of the noticing nature condition compared to the active placebo control. Well-being was assessed via netPA (PANAS), life satisfaction (SWLS), elevation (EES), meaning in life (MLQ), and transcendent connectedness (MSS). Ill-being (depression, anxiety, and stress) and time spent in nature were also assessed. Results indicated that, compared to people in the control condition, people who noticed nature had significantly higher levels of netPA, elevation, and transcendent connectedness. Life satisfaction was marginally significantly higher in the nature group. Meaning in life was not significantly different between the two groups. Stress was significantly lower in the nature group, but no significant differences in depression and anxiety were evidenced. No significant difference emerged across conditions for time spent in nature.

12.4 Discussion

Across the 12 studies reviewed, there were 45 assessments of well-being covering an array of markers of hedonic and eudaimonic well-being. Overall, participants in the nature groups reported significantly higher levels of well-being on 68% (30 of 44) of these assessments relative to the reported well-being of participants in the control conditions. A significant increase emerged for 73% (22 of 30) of the hedonic well-being assessments (22 of 30) and 57% (8 of 14) of the eudaimonic well-being assessments, with the nature conditions emerging as more beneficial to well-being compared to the control conditions.

Effect sizes for these studies ranged from $d = 0.25$ to 1.48.[1] To put this into perspective, across four meta-analyses examining the effectiveness of PPIs, reported meta-analytic effect sizes for well-being interventions have been estimated to range from $d = 0.20$ to $d = 0.61$ (Bolier et al., 2013; Sin & Lyubomirsky, 2009; Weiss et al. 2016; White et al., 2019). All 30 (significant) effect sizes found in our review for nature-based well-being interventions fell within this range, with the majority falling above $d = 0.40$; the 14 non-significant effect sizes ranged from $d = 0.00$ to 0.36.

With regard to hedonic markers of well-being, a significant increase in positive affect was found in eight (of nine) studies measuring positive affect. In contrast, a significant decrease in negative affect was found in only half of the studies which measured negative affect. Net positive affect emerged as significantly enhanced in all four studies which reported netPA. "Nature positive affect" emerged as significantly higher in the one study reporting on this, as did general well-being. Vitality was shown to increase significantly in two studies; however, we were only able to compute the effect size for one of these. Energy and tiredness were revealed to be significantly higher in one of the two studies examining this. Similarly, life satisfaction was found to be significantly higher in the nature condition in only one of the two studies assessing it.

With regard to eudaimonic markers of well-being, awe emerged as significantly higher in the nature group in the study which assessed it. Meaning in life was found to be significantly higher in only one of the five studies measuring meaning. Spiritual transcendence was not found to be significantly impacted by the nature condition in the study which examined this; however, transcendent connectedness (that is, a general sense of connectedness to others, to nature, and to all of life) did emerge as significantly higher in the nature groups compared to the control conditions in all three studies which assessed this construct. Lastly, elevation (a complex mix of emotions including awe, inspiration, and feeling deeply appreciative) emerged as significantly higher in three of the four studies in which it was measured.

Overall, hedonic aspects of well-being (nonweighted average $d = 0.77$) had larger effect sizes relative to eudaimonic aspects (nonweighed average $d = 0.45$). However, more studies are needed to strengthen the validity of this finding, due to the limited number of studies examined in this review ($N = 12$), and the even more limited number of studies that included indices of eudaimonic well-being ($n = 6$). A quantitative meta-analysis is also needed to further assess the average impact of these nature-based well-being interventions.

Nonetheless, the studies reviewed herein lend support for nature-based positive psychology interventions and their ability to enhance both eudaimonic and hedonic forms of well-being. Connecting individuals with nature could have far-reaching implications, perhaps especially if such interventions are designed to also enhance individual's sense of nature connectedness – feeling that one is part of, rather than separate from, the greater-than-human natural world. A large body of research evidences a positive association between nature connectedness and well-being (see meta-analyses by Capaldi et al., 2014; Pritchard et al., 2019).

One framework with which to examine the effectiveness of a positive psychology intervention is provided by Lyubomirsky and Layous' (2013) positive-activity model. This model proposes four variables that might mediate the relationship between a positive psychological activity and a well-being outcome: positive emotions, positive thoughts, positive behaviors, and need satisfaction. Positive emotions are supported by the results of the studies reviewed and, as such, suggest that positive affect may serve both as a process and an outcome variable. The remaining mediators require direct testing in future research on nature interventions. The positive-activity model also posits that features of an activity and characteristics of the person engaging in that activity interact to produce an activity that is optimally effective. Specific features of activities that influence the activity's ability to increase happiness include its sequence, variety, dosage, and built-in social support. For example, dosage in our case would apply to the duration of nature exposure per day throughout the intervention, and to the number of total days that the exposure involves. In the above reviewed studies, single exposure duration ranged from 10 to 20 minutes daily, and total number of exposures ranged from 1 to 30 or more.

However, it is important to consider existing evidence which suggests that it is not time in nature per se that leads to benefits, but rather how one spends that time. For example, in all three of Passmore and colleagues' "Noticing Nature" studies (Passmore, 2019; Passmore & Holder, 2017;

In Vivo *Nature Exposure*   171

Passmore et al., 2019), participants in the nature conditions did not spend significantly more time in nature than did participants in control conditions, yet these participants reported higher levels of well-being. In Nisbet and colleagues' (2019) study, providing mindfulness instructions to participants before they headed into nature resulted in significantly less negative affect (compared to those walking in nature with no mindfulness instructions) and stronger connections with nature. Moreover, Richardson et al. (2021) reported that time in nature did not emerge as a significant predictor of well-being in their large-scale survey analyses involving over 2,000 United Kingdom adults; rather it was nature connectedness and momentary attentive engagement with nature that were prominent in predicting mental health and well-being. Thus, it appears that paying attention to nature – connecting with nature – is a key active ingredient.

Finally, for an individual to benefit most from an activity, they need to "effortfully engage in it, be motivated to become happier, and believe that their efforts will pay off" (Lyubomirsky & Layous, 2013, p. 59). As a result, an instrument to measure effortful engagement in a nature intervention may be an important aspect to consider in future research as a way to explore the extent to which individuals are reaping the full benefits that are able to be gleaned from each therapeutic nature exposure.

12.5 Future Research

Our literature search revealed that presently there are few randomized controlled trials involving *in vivo* nature interventions. Moreover, only two of the twelve studies we reviewed had sample sizes composed of more than 60 participants per condition. As noted by Goulet-Pelletier and Cousineau (2018), the tendency for Cohen's *d* to overestimate the effect size in a population is increased with smaller samples. Most of the studies came from two research labs – three studies from Nisbet and colleagues and four studies from Passmore and colleagues. Moreover, the vast bulk (85%) of participant samples involved Western university students, limiting generalizability to other populations. To add weight to the current conclusions, more studies (utilizing larger sample sizes and conducted by more researchers) examining nature-based positive psychology interventions' impact on well-being using *in vivo* conditions are needed.

Efforts to distinguish hedonic and eudaimonic measures of well-being more clearly in studies on this topic would aid in providing a more nuanced separation between these constructs, as they relate to well-being in different, and important, ways. For example, hedonia, according to Aristotle, is completed in the time it occurs, whereas eudaimonia is described as an ongoing process of pleasures and pains related to the actions of a passionate life (Proctor & Tweed, 2016). Thus, it may be the case that hedonic forms of well-being in relation to nature experiences are more immediate but shorter-lived, whereas eudaimonic aspects may be slow to accumulate, yet prove to be longer lasting and potentially self-reinforcing. For this reason, it may be

172 _J.T. Hunt, A.J. Howell, and H.-A.Passmore_

useful for future studies to observe the impact of the duration of the intervention on long-term eudaimonic well-being specifically. More studies are needed also that use active control conditions in order to control for effects such as expectancy and demand characteristics. Such research would aid in providing clarity regarding nature's unique benefits on our wellness.

Finally, it is worth considering the potential role of physical mobility and exercise in the effects demonstrated in the current body of studies. Among the nature-related experimental conditions, five directly involved participants walking in nature, two requested participants to engage in "nature activity," four led participants to attend to nature, and one involved participants resting in nature. While it is difficult to discern the extent to which physical activity was a significant contributor to the benefits associated with nature involvement, the majority of nature experiences did involve walking or other activity while in nature. Additionally, one study (Fuegen & Breitenbecher, 2018) included two additional nature and control conditions in which people engaged in physical exercise in both locations; interestingly, they showed no difference across these conditions on well-being outcomes, suggesting the possibility of a ceiling effect wherein physical exercise "trumped" the extra benefits that typically accrue with nature involvement. Future research could seek to disentangle the beneficial and possible combined effects of nature involvement, on the one hand, and the engagement in physical activity, on the other.

In sum, the current review demonstrated that positive psychology interventions that involve affiliating with nature increase both hedonic and eudaimonic aspects of well-being. These findings are limited in number and scope, but taken together they contribute to important research that aims to foster greater understanding of humans' connection and ongoing relationship to nature.

Note

1. It is important to note that we provide these general statistics to provide context to this narrative review; these statistics should not be interpreted as meta-analytic averages.

References

Bakker, A., Cai, J., English, L., Kaiser, G., Mesa, V., & Van Dooren, W. (2019). Beyond small, medium, or large: Points of consideration when interpreting effect sizes. _Educational Studies in Mathematics, 102,_ 1–8. doi:10.1007/s10649-019-09908-4

Ballew, M. T., & Omoto, A. M. (2018). Absorption: How nature experiences promote awe and other positive emotions. _Ecopsychology, 10,_ 26–35. doi:10.1089/eco.2017.0044

Baxter, D. F., & Pelletier L. G. (2019). Is nature relatedness a basic human psychological need? A critical examination of the extant literature. _Canadian Psychology, 60,_ 21–34.

Bolier, L., Haverman, M., Westerhof, G. J., Riper, H., Smit, F., & Bohlmeijer, E. (2013). Positive psychology interventions: A meta-analysis of randomized controlled studies. _BMC Public Health, 13,_ 119–138.

In Vivo *Nature Exposure*   173

Buss, D. M. (2000). The evolution of happiness. *American Psychologist, 55,* 15–23.

Capaldi, C. A., Dopko, R. L., & Zelenski, J. M. (2014). The relationship between nature connectedness and happiness: A meta-analysis. *Frontiers in Psychology.* doi:10.3389/fpsyg.2014.00976

DeCicco, T. L., & Stroink, M. L. (2007). A third model of self-construal: The meta-personal self. *International Journal of Transpersonal Studies, 26,* 82–104.

Diener, E., Emmons, R. A., Larsen, R. J., & Griffin, S. (1985). The satisfaction with life scale. *Journal of Personality Assessment, 49,* 71–75.

Fuegen, K., & Breitenbecher, K. H. (2018). Walking and being outdoors in nature increase positive affect and energy. *Ecopsychology, 10,* 14–25.

Goulet-Pelletier, J.-C., & Cousineau, D. (2018). A review of effect sizes and their confidence intervals, Part I: The Cohen's d family. *Tutorials in Quantitative Methods for Psychology, 14,* 242–265.

Hamann, G. A., & Ivtzan, I. (2016). 30 minutes in nature a day can increase mood, well-being, meaning in life and mindfulness: Effects of a pilot programme. *Social Inquiry into Well-Being, 2,* 34–46.

Hurly, J., & Walker, G. J. (2019). Nature in our lives: Examining the human need for nature relatedness as a basic psychological need. *Journal of Leisure Research, 50,* 290–310. doi:10.1080/00222216.2019.1578939

Huta, V., & Ryan, R. (2010). Pursuing pleasure or virtue: The differential and overlapping well-being benefits of hedonic and eudaimonic motives. *Journal of Happiness Studies, 11,* 735–762.

Kahn, P. H. Jr., Severson, R. L., & Ruckert, J. H. (2009). The human relation with nature and technological nature. *Current Directions in Psychological Science, 18,* 37–42. doi:10.1111/j.1467-8721.2009.01602.x

Keyes, C. L. M., & Annas, J. (2009). Feeling good and functioning well: Distinctive concepts in ancient philosophy and contemporary science. *The Journal of Positive Psychology, 4,* 197–201.

Kjellgren, A., & Buhrkall, H. (2010). A comparison of the restorative effect of a natural environment with that of a simulated natural environment. *Journal of Environmental Psychology, 30,* 464–472.

Lyubomirsky, S., & Layous, K. (2013). How do simple positive activities increase well-being? *Current Directions in Psychological Science, 22,* 57–62.

Mayer, F. S., Frantz, C. M., Bruehlman-Senecal, E., & Dolliver, K. (2009). Why is nature beneficial? The role of connectedness to nature. *Environment and Behavior, 41,* 607–643.

McMahan, E., & Estes, D. (2015). The effect of contact with natural environments on positive and negative affect: A meta-analysis. *The Journal of Positive Psychology, 10,* 507–519.

Nisbet, E. K., & Zelenski, J. M. (2011). Underestimating nearby nature: Affective forecasting errors obscure the happy path to sustainability. *Psychological Science, 22,* 1101–1106.

Nisbet, E. K., Zelenski, J. M., & Grandpierre, Z. (2019). Mindfulness in nature enhances connectedness and mood. *Ecopsychology, 11,* 81–91.

Passmore, H.-A. (2019). *Comparing hedonic, eudaimonic, and social well-being benefits of engaging in noticing nature to benefits of engaging in a common positive psychology intervention* (T). University of British Columbia. Retrieved from https://open.library.ubc.ca/collections/ubctheses/24/items/1.0380859

Passmore, H.-A., & Holder, M. D. (2017). Individual and social benefits of a two-week intervention. *Journal of Positive Psychology, 12,* 537–546.

Passmore, H.-A., & Howell, A. J. (2014). Nature involvement increases hedonic and eudaimonic well-being: A two-week experimental study. *Ecopsychology, 6*, 148–154.

Passmore, H.-A., Yang, Y., & Sabine, S. (2019, in preparation). *Noticing nature as a well-being intervention: Replication and expansion in a Chinese sample.*

Pawelski, J. O. (2016). Defining the 'positive' in positive psychology: Part II. A normative analysis. *The Journal of Positive Psychology, 11*, 1–9.

Piedmont, R. L. (1999). Does spirituality represent the sixth factor of personality? Spiritual transcendence and the five-factor model. *Journal of Personality, 67*, 985–1013.

Pritchard, A., Richardson, M., Sheffield, D., & McEwan, K. (2019). The relationship between nature connectedness and eudaimonic well-being: A meta-analysis. *Journal of Happiness Studies*, 1–23.

Proctor, C., & Tweed, R. (2016). Measuring eudaimonic well-being. In J. Vitterso (Ed.), *Handbook of eudaimonic well-being* (pp. 277–294). Cham, Switzerland: Springer International Publishing.

Richardson, M., Passmore, H-A., Lumber, R., Thomas, R., & Hunt, A. (2021). Moments, not minutes: The nature-wellbeing relationship. *International Journal of Wellbeing, 11*(1), 8–33. doi:10.5502/ijw.v11i1.1267.

Ryan, R M.., & Deci, E. L. (2001). On happiness and human potentials: A review of research on hedonic and eudaimonic well-being. *Annual Review of Psychology, 52*, 141–166.

Ryan, R. M., & Frederick, C. (1997). On energy, personality, and health: Subjective vitality as a dynamic reflection of well-being. *Journal of Personality, 65*, 529–565.

Ryan, R., Huta, V., & Deci, E. (2008). Living well: A self-determination theory perspective on eudaimonia. *Journal of Happiness Studies, 9*, 139–170.

Ryan, R. M., Weinstein, N., Bernstein, J., Brown, K. W., Mistretta, L., & Gagné, M. (2010). Vitalizing effects of being outdoors and in nature. *Environmental Psychology, 30*, 159–168.

Sin, N. L., & Lyubomirsky, S. (2009). Enhancing well-being and alleviating depressive symptoms with positive psychology interventions: A practice-friendly meta-analysis. *Journal of Clinical Psychology, 65*, 467–487.

Steger, M. F., Frazier, P., Oishi, S., & Kaler, M. (2006). The meaning in life questionnaire: Assessing the presence of and search for meaning in life. *Journal of Counseling Psychology, 53*, 80–93.

Tennant, R., Hiller, L., Fishwick, R., Platt, S., Joseph, S., Weich, S, ... Stewart-Brown, S. (2007). The Warwick-Edinburgh Mental Well-being Scale (WEMWBS): Development and UK validation. *Health and Quality of Life Outcomes 5*, 63. doi:10.1186/1477-7525-5-63

Thayer, R. E. (1986). Activation-deactivation check list: Current overview and structural analysis. *Psychological Reports, 58*, 607–614.

Watson, D., Clark, L. A., & Tellegen, A. (1988). Development and validation of brief measures of positive and negative affect: The PANAS scales. *Journal of Personality and Social Psychology, 54*, 1063–1070.

Weiss, L. A., Westerhof, G. J., & Bohlmeijer, E. T. (2016). Can we increase psychological well-being? The effects of interventions on psychological well-being: A meta-analysis of randomized controlled trials. *PLOSONE, 11*, doi: e0158092. doi:10.1371/journal.pone.0158092

White, C. A., Uttl, B., & Holder, M. D. (2019). Meta-analyses of positive psychology interventions: The effects are much smaller than previously reported. *PLOS ONE, 14*, e0216588.

Part III

Real-World Application

13 Care Farms: A Health-Promoting Context for a Wide Range of Client Groups

Simone de Bruin, Jan Hassink, Lenneke Vaandrager, Bram de Boer, Hilde Verbeek, Ingeborg Pedersen, Grete Grindal Patil, Lina H. Ellingsen-Dalskau, and Siren Eriksen

13.1 Introduction

13.1.1 What is a Care Farm?

This chapter synthesizes the knowledge that has been generated in recent years on care farming.

Care farming is a form of intervention for promoting human health and wellbeing through the use of a farm environment as the central element (Hassink, Elings et al., 2010; Hassink, Hulsink & Grin, 2014). Care farms serve a wide range of client groups, including people with learning disabilities, people with mental health problems, youngsters with social problems, people who are long-term unemployed, and people with dementia (Hassink et al., 2007; Prestvik, Nebell & Pettersen, 2013). In care farming, a series of activities and interactions with nature take place with the aim to provide health, social, or educational care services, employment skills, and support through the provision of a supervised, structured program in a supportive social community, rather than occasional one-off visits (Garcia-Llorente et al., 2018; Murray et al., 2019). Many farmers and staff members have an education in agriculture, health care and/or social care (e.g. social workers, registered nurses, nurse assistants, nurse aides, occupational therapists, and educational staff). There are often volunteers assisting in the services. Care farms often collaborate with and/or hire staff of regular care institutions (de Boer et al., 2019; Hassink et al., 2019; Ibsen, Eriksen & Patil, 2018).

Care farming has different representations and varies both between and within countries. They generally have some degree of commercial farming (i.e. crops, livestock, and woodland) combined with health, social, and/or educational care services. There is great variation among care farms regarding the ratio between farming and these services and the types of farming activities (e.g. dairy farm, industrial livestock farm, mixed farm, and forestry). Many farms have conventional agricultural production, while others are primarily care providers (Hassink et al., 2012; Ibsen, Eriksen & Patil, 2018; Murray et al., 2019). The majority of the care farms

DOI: 10.4324/9781003154419-16

178 S. de Bruin, J. Hassink, and L.Vaandrager et al.

offer day services, meaning that the client groups live in their own homes and come to the farm one day or several days a week, depending on their needs and home situations. Other farms offer 24-hour services, such as care farms providing 24-hour nursing home care to people with dementia or care farms offering living and working programs for youngsters with severe social and mental health problems. Additionally, there are a small number of care farms providing evening or weekend services as respite services to family caregivers (de Boer et al., 2015; de Bruin, Oosting, van der Zijpp et al., 2010; Ibsen, Eriksen & Patil, 2018).

13.1.2 How Many Care Farms are There Around the World?

Care farming is a growing field in Europe and other parts of the world. It remains, however, difficult to estimate the exact number of care farms for each country. Outcomes of national surveys, national registries (e.g. registries with the number of care farms signed up for a national quality approval scheme), and funding schemes (e.g. number of care farms financially supported by the national government) provide some insight. The Netherlands and Norway are often seen as frontrunners in providing care at care farms with 1250 in the Netherlands and 400 registered and an unknown number of unregistered care farms in Norway. Gradually, the concept of care farming is being implemented in other countries, including Austria (n = 600), Belgium (n = 670), France (n = 900), Ireland (n = 100), Italy (n = 675), Japan (*no estimations available*), Poland (*no estimations available*), South Korea (n = 30), Switzerland (n = 1000), United Kingdom (n = 230), and the USA (*no estimations available*) (de Bruin et al., 2020; Garcia-Llorente et al., 2018; Hassink et al., 2020; Haubenhofer, 2015; Murray et al., 2019; Yewon Cho, 2020).

13.1.3 What will You Find in This Chapter?

Over the last couple of years, several research projects have been carried out addressing the potential of care farms to promote health and wellbeing. In this chapter, we will specifically focus on what the care farm environment looks like, the programs and activities that are offered to different types of client groups, and the benefits of care farms in terms of health and wellbeing of different types of client groups. We additionally propose recommendations for policy and practice to further advance the field.

13.2 Activities at a Care Farm

Care farms have a wide range of health-promoting environmental characteristics, including the presence of outdoor spaces (e.g. farmyard, vegetable garden, and paddocks), farm and companion animals, plants, daily life stimuli, and a familiar, homelike and social supportive environment (de Boer et al., 2018; de Bruin et al., 2017; Garcia-Llorente et al., 2018; Ibsen, Eriksen & Patil, 2018; Myren et al., 2017; Pedersen & Patil, 2018). The different health-promoting characteristics are naturally present in the farm environment and are therefore extensively used in the wide range of activities care farms offer to their clients (Ellingsen-Dalskau, Pedersen & de Boer, 2019; Ibsen & Eriksen, 2020; Pedersen & Patil, 2018). These activities, which are regarded as stimulating and meaningful, include walking outside, indoor horticulture activities, meal preparation, feeding and viewing the animals, picking eggs, gardening, sweeping the yard, crafts, woodworking, and playing games (de Bruin et al., 2009; Ibsen, Eriksen & Patil, 2018; Myren, Enmarker & Hellzen, 2013; Myren et al., 2017; Pedersen & Patil, 2018; Strandli et al., 2016). Activities can be adjusted to fit the needs of individuals with functional disabilities.

In this section, we more specifically focus on care farms for three types of client groups that are frequent users of care farming services. To demonstrate the variety of care farms and illustrate their activities, some case descriptions are provided below.

13.2.1 Care Farms for People with Dementia

Care farms for people with dementia generally have a small-scale and homelike character. The majority of care farms for people with dementia provide adult day care services, aimed at providing clients with a structured and meaningful day program and providing relief and support to family caregivers (de Bruin et al., 2015). In the Netherlands, in particular, care farms providing 24-hour nursing home care have recently been established as an alternative to regular nursing homes (de Boer et al., 2015).

Care farms provide people with a wide range of stimuli and daily activities such as domestic, work-related, social, nutritional, and leisure/recreational activities, which are incorporated into standard daily life. Examples include folding laundry, preparing meals, weeding the soil, sweeping the lawn, fixing broken furniture/tools, taking care of the animals, and getting wood for the fireplace.

Care farm environments are radically different from those of regular care institutions for people with dementia. The physical environment contains elements which invite people with dementia to perform common daily tasks such as watering the plants, walking the dog, feeding the animals, woodwork, raking, or shoveling snow (also see Figures 13.1, 13.2 and 13.3). Furthermore, people have more freedom of movement, go outside more often, and can choose themselves how and where they want to spend their days (de Boer et al., 2018; de Bruin et al., 2009; Ellingsen-Dalskau, Pedersen & de Boer, 2019; Ibsen, Eriksen & Patil, 2018). This can facilitate feelings of autonomy and meaning in life, as people with dementia still have the opportunity to contribute to the life at the farm (de Bruin et al., 2017; Ibsen & Eriksen, 2020). The social context resembles a family-like structure

Case 1: Buiten Gewoon – People with Dementia

"And here I am, in my boots, doing outdoor work, like a kind of farmer, or well, whatever...With a shovel and a spade. And at the end of the day, when I am going home, I'm feeling really great" (client).

Arjo and Marinel Buijs are managers of two care farms in the western part of the Netherlands. Before they started to work on a care farm, both of them worked in other types of care institutions (e.g. nursing home, home care organization, and mental health institution). At one of the farms, they provide adult day services to 10–12 people with dementia or acquired brain injury. These participants still live in their own homes, but attend adult day services one to five days a week, depending on their needs and their home situations. The other farm provides 24-hour nursing home care to fourteen people with dementia. This farm additionally provides respite services to family caregivers. The daily program starts at 10:00 h with a cup of coffee, during which tasks for the day are assigned. People participate in familiar daily activities such as preparing meals, caring for the animals, and gardening. Other activities include going for a walk and cycling at the "duo bike". At lunchtime, participants together share a hot meal which is prepared by themselves. After lunch, participants either take a nap or participate in activities. The day ends at 16:00 h. In total, care farm Buiten Gewoon is taking care of 50 people attending adult day services, 14 residents, and 1 carer that uses the respite service. They are cared for by 60 qualified staff members and volunteers.

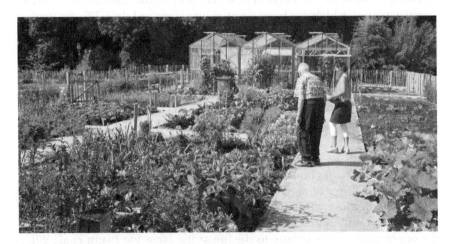

Figure 13.1 Photo by Arjo Buijs, the Netherlands.

Care Farms 181

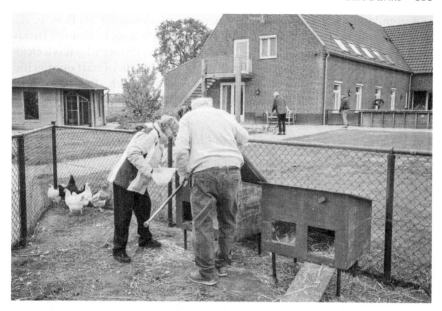

Figure 13.2 Photo by Anita Janssen, the Netherlands.

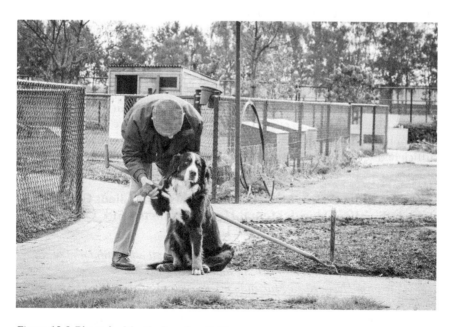

Figure 13.3 Photo by Martin Lundsvoll, Norway.

182 S. de Bruin, J. Hassink, and L.Vaandrager et al.

and stimulates social participation of people with dementia (de Boer et al., 2017; de Bruin et al., 2015), which is important for their social health (Dröes et al., 2016). Finally, there is strong leadership by the farmer who has a clear vision on care delivery, training of staff, and recruitment of staff on specific competencies (e.g. creativity, person-centered approach, flexibility, and progressive mindset) (de Bruin et al., 2017; de Bruin et al., 2020).

13.2.2 Care Farms for People with Mental Health Problems

Care farming services/vocational rehabilitation on farms for people with mental health problems commonly include a diverse range of meaningful activities and work tasks. These vary from taking care of the animals (cleaning stable, feeding, and petting), working on the field and growing vegetables, herbs and flowers, green maintenance, and creative activities like painting, pottery, wood carving, writing, or music. Some care farms run a restaurant, café, or tea garden in which the people with mental problems can participate (Ellingsen-Dalskau, Berget et al., 2016; Granerud & Eriksson, 2014; Pedersen et al., 2012; Pedersen, Ihlebæk & Kirkevold, 2012). Since there is such a wide range of possibilities, activities can be easily tailored to the users' aspirations and interests (Pedersen et al., 2016), an adaptation that is highly important at the individual user level (Kogstad, Agdal & Hopfenbeck, 2014; Pedersen, Ihlebæk & Kirkevold, 2012). Participating in farm activities is considered meaningful by users. They feel valued as an employee and feel they have a meaningful contribution (Granerud & Eriksson, 2014; Hassink, Zweekhorst et al., 2010). This leads to feelings of mastery and competence. Moreover, people gain self-confidence, become more independent and learn new skills (Berget, Ekeberg & Braastad, 2008; Elings & Hassink, 2008; Ellingsen-Dalskau, Morken et al., 2016; Kogstad, Agdal & Hopfenbeck, 2014; Pedersen, et al., 2012).

People with mental health problems appreciate the safe environment of the farm, the possibilities to participate in society, being part of a community (Iancu et al., 2014). They perceive the care farm as an informal setting between illness, labor market, and society. It is a place where they can develop new contacts and practice working skills by performing useful activities with sufficient attention for their health problems (Elings & Hassink, 2008).

Case 2: Hoeve Klein Mariendaal – Diversity of Client Groups, Including People with Mental Health Problems and People with Dementia

"I really appreciate the work in the flower garden. In this beautiful and peaceful and calm environment, I feel safe and relaxed." (client).

Care farm Hoeve Klein Mariendaal is located in Arnhem. The farm provides adult day care services for a diversity of clients and integrates them in society by establishing a close connection with citizens from the nearby city and surrounding villages. The 12 employees of the care farm have diverse backgrounds like agriculture, arts, and hospitality. They are all educated in social care. They are supported by more than 30 volunteers. More than 100 clients make use of the care farm for day activities. The care farm offers services to a range of client groups: adults with severe mental health problems and intellectual disabilities, youngsters that drop out from school temporarily and people with dementia living at home. On Saturdays, the care farm offers a program for children with autism spectrum disorder or ADHD to unburden the parents. The participants can choose from a range of activities like working in the field and growing vegetables, herbs, and flowers, taking care of the animals, working in the tea garden, green maintenance in the city of Arnhem and creative activities. The care farm has a contract with the municipality of Arnhem and surrounding municipalities for the provision of care services. Other sources of income are the selling of boxes with vegetables grown at the farm to families in the neighborhood, the rent of a meeting room for organizations and companies, lunches and drinks of the tea garden, and selling of firewood. The participants appreciate the practical, useful, and diverse activities in the green environment. A daily activity that is valued by a range of participants is the daily walk with the donkeys after lunch time in the beautiful estate where the care farm is located.

13.2.3 Care Farms for Youngsters with Behavioral and Social Problems

Care farms for youngsters with severe behavioral and social problems are offering programs in which youngsters are individually placed on a farm for a period of six months. The farms are private productive dairy and pig farms run by a farmers' family. The youngsters have their own living unit on the farm. They have lunch and dinner with the farmers' family and participate in all farming activities. Activities include feeding the animals and cleaning the stables. Most youngsters live in a city and have never experienced farm life. The farm environment and participating in a farming family life is a completely new experience for them (Hassink et al., 2011; Schreuder et al., 2014).

Case 3: Care Farm Topaze – Youngsters with Behavioral and Social Problems

"Taking good care of the cows motivated me to continue the work and do it properly." (client)

The "living and working programme" is developed for youngsters aged between 16 and 23 with severe social and mental health problems, varying

184 S. de Bruin, J. Hassink, and L.Vaandrager et al.

*from externalizing (acting out, e.g. aggression) to more internalizing prob-
lems (inward, e.g. anxiety and mood disorders, and social withdrawal). The
young people concerned face problems in the following domains: a) family
(they cannot stay at home due to aggression and running away), b) school
or work (they do not attend school or have no job) and c) friends and free
time (they do not spend their free time in a constructive way). The youngsters
live and work on the farm for 6 months on an individual base. 15 farms in
the province of Noord Brabant, the southern part of the Netherlands, participate in this program. They are all productive dairy or pig farms where
the youngsters can participate in all farming activities like milking the cows
and feeding the pigs. The first period focusses on adjusting to living and
working on the farm. Objectives focus on learning to listen to the farmer and
maintaining their own living unit. Contacts with family and friends are
restricted. In the second period, youngsters compare their actual situation
with past experiences. Weekly telephone contact with parents is allowed. In
the third period, the focus is on reflection of changes in behavior over this
time. More contact with parents is allowed. In the last period, the focus is on
making plans for the future. Youngsters stay with their parents during two
weekends. Parents are required to participate in classes to enhance parenting
skills. Both the individual living and working on the farm and the training
for clients and parents are the basis for the aftercare program. In most cases,
clients return to live with their parents. A counselor of the youth care organization visits the youngster and the family on a weekly basis. Learning goals
related to improved functioning in school, work, and free-time are discussed
and agreed between youngster, parents, and counsellor. The farmers and
youngsters indicate that the physical demanding work with the animals is an
important element of the program on the farm. The youngsters are generally
not used to working hard. Their physical condition improves considerably,
they learn to appreciate to work with their hands, to take care of the animals,
and it gives them structure and meaningfulness in their lives. (Schreuder
et al., 2014)*

13.3 Evidence for Impact of Care Farms on Health and Wellbeing

13.3.1 People with Dementia

In several Dutch and Norwegian studies, the potential benefits of care
farms for people with dementia in terms of health and wellbeing have been
evaluated. These studies show that care farms support contact with nature
and animals, time spent outdoors, activity engagement, physical activity,
structure, social interactions, healthy eating, and a sense of meaning in life

Care Farms 185

(de Boer et al., 2017; de Bruin et al., 2009; de Bruin et al., 2019; de Bruin, Oosting, Tobi, et al., 2010; Ellingsen-Dalskau, Pedersen & de Boer, 2019; Finnanger Garshol, Ellingsen-Dalskau & Pedersen, 2019; Ibsen & Eriksen, submitted; Strandli et al., 2016; Sudmann & Borsheim, 2017). Activity engagement and required physical effort to partake in activities at care farms are usually higher than in activities in regular care institutions (de Boer et al., 2017; de Bruin et al., 2009; de Bruin, Oosting, van der Zijpp, et al., 2010; Ellingsen-Dalskau, Pedersen & de Boer, 2019). Furthermore, participants and their family caregivers experience less stigmatizing because of dementia since the care farm environment is a homelike noninstitutional kind of place. Instead, people with dementia feel and are treated as a volunteer or employee rather than a patient with cognitive and functional impairments. People with dementia additionally feel recognized, understood, and seen as people who can deliver a meaningful contribution. The studies further reveal that care farms can also promote respite, more personal time, and fewer feelings of guilt among family caregivers. Family caregivers additionally indicate that care farms provide care tailored to the individual needs of people with dementia (de Boer et al., 2017; de Boer et al., 2019; de Bruin et al., 2015; Sudmann & Borsheim, 2017). Based on these studies, it can be concluded that care farms have a wide range of benefits that might affect health and wellbeing of people with dementia and their family caregivers.

13.3.2 People with Mental Health Problems

Studies on care farming services for people with mental health problems have found that such services can be beneficial to users' quality of life and health. Studies have shown that participation in such farm offers can increase wellbeing (Leck, Evans & Upton, 2014), quality of life (Hemingway, llis-Hill & Norton, 2016; Leck, Evans & Upton, 2014), and increased cognitive capacity (Gonzalez et al., 2010), and have a positive impact on mental health, such as anxiety and depression (Berget et al., 2011; Gonzalez et al., 2009; Pedersen et al., 2012). The care farm services are mostly group-based and joint activities are often a starting point for developing social relations. Experiencing support from other users may create a sense of belonging and of being respected for who you are (Ellingsen-Dalskau, Berget et al., 2016; Ellingsen-Dalskau, Pedersen et al., 2016; Granerud & Eriksson, 2014). The farmer is particularly emphasized as central for initiating social activity and facilitating social relations between the users (Granerud & Eriksson, 2014; Hemingway, llis-Hill & Norton, 2016; Kogstad, Agdal & Hopfenbeck, 2014), and for providing social support to the user (Ellingsen-Dalskau, Berget et al., 2016; Ellingsen-Dalskau, Pedersen et al., 2016; Iancu et al., 2014; Pedersen et al., 2012). Increased social contact and the opportunity to be part of a social network is valued by the users (Elings & Hassink, 2008).

186   S. de Bruin, J. Hassink, and L.Vaandrager et al.

The importance of the animals and the nature surroundings of care farms are emphasized in several studies. Contact and work with livestock are seen as meaningful because it is about taking care of living beings (Granerud & Eriksson, 2014; Hassink et al., 2010). Additionally, it is experienced as a break from a stressful everyday life and a source of inner calm (Ellingsen-Dalskau et al., 2016; Pedersen et al., 2012). Nature experiences and green surroundings offer tranquility and opportunity to retreat and give a sense of belonging (Hassink et al., 2010; Iancu et al., 2014). The participants additionally emphasize being outdoors as positive, giving a sense of wellbeing and security (Kogstad, Agdal & Hopfenbeck, 2014). People with mental health problems further report an increase in their self-esteem, self-respect, perseverance, feelings of responsibility and physical condition. They appreciate the green environment, working with animals, being part of a community, the variety in activities, and personal guidance (Hassink et al., 2010).

These findings are in line with the growing recognition that green environments contribute to the wellbeing of people with mental health problems (Ellingsen-Dalskau et al., 2016; Kogstad, Agdal & Hopfenbeck, 2014).

13.3.3 Youngsters with Behavioral and Social Problems

Studies on care farms with youngsters with behavioral and social problems show that many of them were proud of being able to adapt to a new situation and to finish the program. Youngsters indicated that positive experiences, good contact with the farmer and family members, interaction with farm animals, physical and challenging activities, being on oneself away from family and friends and amusement, the green environment and time for reflection were the crucial elements for the success of the farm program. The youngsters learned to obey orders, to calm down, and think before acting and reflect on their lives. Their self-esteem increased and problem behavior decreased. These positive results remained also after a longer period and significant reductions in use of drugs, police contact, and drop-out from school were reported (Hassink et al., 2011; Schreuder et al., 2014).

13.4 Recommendations for Policy and Practice

This chapter illustrates that care farms offer a structure and opportunities for increased time outdoors in a supportive, safe, and enjoyable setting. A diversity of tailored and meaningful everyday activities for different groups are carried out which are characterized by a focus on abilities rather than on limitations of people. Experiences show that it is easy for the service provider to provide the activities and that the activities are easy for the user to join in. This links nicely with the settings approach for health promotion (Poland, Krupa & McCall, 2009), which moves beyond lifestyle-focused activities to promote physical exercise, to creating health-promoting places in which people live their lives and which allows them to actively use and shape their living environments (Dooris, 2013). An underlying quality of the health-promoting care farm setting is that the environment is predictable for users and it invites them to do everyday activities ("real activities") such as gardening or taking care of animals intuitively without any explicit emphasis on the health benefits of doing exercise. Also the social interactions and the person-centered approach result in people feeling better and as such also promote physical exercise. Many of the effective elements such as health-promoting physical environment, true involvement, and freedom of choice can be translated to other settings such as other health and social care institutions, workplaces, communities, schools, or hospitals.

As most care farms are located in rural areas, another possible future development is offering more nature-based services in urban areas. A recent study by Hassink et al. (2019) shows that there is a clear untapped potential in this area. Lessons learned from care farms also show the importance of the competencies of staff such as the ability to provide person-centered care and flexibility, which are often not yet part of the existing curricula of health and social care professionals. Those competencies are best acquired by learning by doing, such as working some days a week at a care farm to learn to provide care and promote health in a nonregular care environment.

References

Berget, B., Ekeberg, Ø., & Braastad, B. O. (2008). Animal-assisted therapy with farm animals for persons with psychiatric disorders: Effects on self-efficacy, coping ability and quality of life, a randomized controlled trial. *Clinical Practice and Epidemiology in Mental Health, 4*(9), doi: 10.1186/1745-0179-1184-1189.

Berget, B., Ekeberg, Ø., Pedersen, I., & Braastad, B. O. (2011). Animal-assisted therapy with farm animals for persons with psychiatric disorders: Effects on anxiety and depression, a randomized controlled trial. *Occupational Therapy in Mental Health, 27*(1), 50–64. doi: 10.1080/0164212X.2011.543641

de Boer, B., Beerens, H. C., Katterbach, M. A., Viduka, M., Willemse, B. M., & Verbeek, H. (2018). The physical environment of nursing homes for people with dementia: Traditional nursing homes, small-scale living facilities, and green care farms. *Healthcare, 6*(4). doi: 10.3390/healthcare6040137

de Boer, B., Hamers, J. P., Beerens, H. C., Zwakhalen, S. M., Tan, F. E., & Verbeek, H. (2015). Living at the farm, innovative nursing home care for people with dementia: Study protocol of an observational longitudinal study. *BMC Geriatrics, 15*, 144. doi: 10.1186/s12877-015-0141-x

de Boer, B., Hamers, J. P., Zwakhalen, S. M., Tan, F. E., Beerens, H. C., & Verbeek, H. (2017). Green care farms as innovative nursing homes, promoting activities and social interaction for people with dementia. *JAMDA, 18*(1), 40–46.

de Boer, B., Verbeek, H., Zwakhalen, S. M. G., & Hamers, J. P. H. (2019). Experiences of family caregivers in green care farms and other nursing home environments for people with dementia: A qualitative study. *BMC Geriatrics, 19*(1), 149. doi: 10.1186/s12877-019-1163-6 de Bruin, S. R., Buist, Y., Hassink, J., & Vaandrager, L. (2019). "I want to make myself useful": The value of nature-based adult day services in urban areas for people with dementia and their family carers. *Ageing & Society*, doi: 10.1017/S0144686X19001168.

de Bruin, S. R., de Boer, B., Beerens, H., Buist, Y., & Verbeek, H. (2017). Rethinking dementia care: The value of green care farming. *JAMDA, 18*, 200–203.

de Bruin, S. R., Oosting, S. J., Kuin, Y., Hoefnagels, E. C. M., Blauw, Y. H., De Groot, C. P. G. M., & Schols, J. M. G. A. (2009). Green care farms promote activity among elderly people with dementia. *Journal of Housing for the Elderly, 23*(4), 368–389.

de Bruin, S. R., Oosting, S. J., Tobi, H., Blauw, Y. H., Schols, J. M. G. A., & De Groot, C. P. G. M. (2010). Day care at green care farms: A novel way to stimulate dietary intake of community-dwelling older people with dementia? *The Journal of Nutrition, Health & Aging, 14*(5), 352–357.

de Bruin, S. R., Oosting, S. J., van der Zijpp, A. J., Enders-Slegers, M. J., & Schols, J. M. G. A. (2010). The concept of green care farms for older people with dementia: An integrative framework. *Dementia, 9*(1), 79–128.

de Bruin, S. R., Pedersen, I., Eriksen, S., Hassink, J., Vaandrager, L., & Grindal Patil, G. (2020). Care farming for people with dementia; what can healthcare leaders learn from this innovative care concept? *Journal of Healthcare Leadership, 12*, 11–18.

de Bruin, S. R., Stoop, A., Molema, C. C. M., Vaandrager, L., Hop, P., & Baan, C. A. (2015). Green care farms: An innovative type of adult day service to stimulate social participation of people with dementia. *GGM*, 1–10. doi: 10.1177/2333721415607833

Dooris, M. (2013). Expert voices for change: Bridging the silos – towards healthy and sustainable settings for the 21st century. *Health & Place, 20*, 39–50.

Dröes, R., Chattat, R., Diaz, A., Gove, D., Graff, M., Murphy, K., ... Johannessen, A. (2016). Social health and dementia: A European consensus on the operationalization of the concept and directions for research and practice. *Aging & Mental Health*, 1–14.

Elings, M., & Hassink, J. (2008). Green care farms, a safe community between illness or addiction and the wider society. *International Journal of Therapeutic Communities, 29*(3), 310–322.

Ellingsen-Dalskau, L., Berget, B., Pedersen, I., G., T., & Ihlebæk, C. (2016). Understanding how prevocational training on care farms can lead to functioning, motivation and well-being. *Disability and Rehabilitation, 38*(25), 2504–2513.

Ellingsen-Dalskau, L., Pedersen, I., & de Boer, B. (2019). *Farm based day care services for people with dementia – an observational study.* Paper presented at the 29th Alzheimer Europe conference, The Hague.

Ellingsen-Dalskau, L. H., Morken, M., Berget, B., & Pedersen, I. (2016). Autonomy support and need satisfaction in prevocational programs on care farms: The self-determination theory perspective. *Work, 53*(1), 73–85.

Finnanger Garshol, B., Ellingsen-Dalskau, L., & Pedersen, I. (2019). *Physical activity in day care services for people with dementia.* Paper presented at the 29th Alzheimer Europe conference, The Hague.

Garcia-Llorente, M., Rubio-Olivar, R., & Gutierrez-Briceno, I. (2018). Farming for life quality and sustainability: A literature review of green care research trends in Europe. *International Journal of Environmental Research and Public Health, 15*(6). doi: 10.3390/ijerph15061282

Gonzalez, M. T., Hartig, T., Patil, G. G., Martinsen, E. W., & Kirkevold, M. (2009). Therapeutic horticulture in clinical depression: A prospective study. *Research and Theory for Nursing Practice, 23*(4), 312–328.

Gonzalez, M. T., Hartig, T., Patil, G. G., Martinsen, E. W., & Kirkevold, M. (2010). Therapeutic horticulture in clinical depression: A prospective study of active components. *Journal of Advanced Nursing, 66*(9), 2002–2013.

Granerud, A., & Eriksson, B. G. (2014). Mental health problems, recovery, and the impact of green care services: A qualitative, participant-focused approach. *Occupational Therapy in Mental Health, 30*(4), 317–336.

Hassink, J., Agricola, H., Veen, E., Pijpker, R., de Bruin, S., Van der Meulen, H., & Plug, L. (2020). The care farming sector in the Netherlands: A reflection on its developments and promising innovations accepted by Sustainability.

Hassink, J., De Meyer, R., Van der Sman, P., & Veerman, J. W. (2011). Effectiviteit van ervarend leren op de boerderij. *Orthopedagogiek: Onderzoek en Praktijk, 50*, 51–63.

Hassink, J., Elings, M., Zweekhorst, M., Van Den Nieuwenhuizen, N., & Smit, A. (2010). Care farms in the Netherlands: Attractive empowerment-oriented and strengths-based practices in the community. *Health Place, 16*, 423–430.

Hassink, J., Hulsink, W., & Grin, J. (2012). Care farms in the Netherlands: An underexplored example of multifunctional agriculture – Toward an empirically grounded organization-theory-based typology. *Rural Sociology, 77*, 569–600.

Hassink, J., Hassink, J., Hulsink, W., & Grin, J. (2014). Farming with care: The evolution of care farming in the Netherlands. *68*, 1–11.

Hassink, J., Vaandrager, L., Buist, Y., & De Bruin, S. R. (2019). Characteristics and challenges for the development of nature-based adult day services in urban areas for people with dementia and their family caregivers. *International Journal of Environmental Research and Public Health, 16*(8), 1337. https://doi.org/1310.3390/ijerph16081337.

Hassink, J., Zwartbol, C., Agricola, H. J., Elings, M., & Thissen, J. T. N. M. (2007). Current status and potential of care farms in the Netherlands. *NJAS, 55*(1), 21–36.

Hassink, J., Zweekhorst, M., Elings, M., & Van den Nieuwenhuizen, N. (2010). Care farms attractive empowerment-oriented and strengths-based practices in the community. *Health Place, 16*, 423–430.

Haubenhofer, D. (2015). Kleines Land, grosse Wirkung! Green care und Soziale Landwirtschaft in Osterreich – *Green Care: Die Fachzeitschrift für naturgestützte Interaktion,* 14–16 https://georgeavenuefoundation.ch/wp-content/uploads/GreenCare_Sondernummer.pdf.

Hemingway, A., Ilis-Hill, C., & Norton, E. (2016). What does care farming provide for clients? The views of care farm staff. *NJAS - Wageningen Journal of Life Sciences, 79*, 23–29.

Iancu, S. C., Zweekhorst, M. B. M., Veltman, D. J., Van Balkom, A. J. L. M., & Bunders, J. F. G. (2014). Mental health recovery on care farms and day centres: A qualitative comparative study of users' perspectives. *Disability and Rehabilitation, 36*(7), 573–583.

Ibsen, I., & Eriksen, S. (2020). The experience of attending farm-based day care from the perspective of people with dementia; A qualitative study.

Ibsen, T. L., Eriksen, S., & Patil, G. G. (2018). Farm-based day care in Norway: A complementary service for people with dementia. *Journal of Multidisciplinary Healthcare, 11*, 349–358. doi: 10.2147/JMDH.S167135

190 S. de Bruin, J. Hassink, and L.Vaandrager et al.

Kogstad, R., Agdal, R., & Hopfenbeck, M. (2014). Narratives of natural recovery: Youth experience of social inclusion through green care. *International Journal of Environmental Research and Public Health, 11*(6), 6052.

Leck, C., Evans, N., & Upton, D. (2014). Agriculture – Who cares? An investigation of 'care farming' in the UK. *Journal of Rural Studies, 34,* 313–325.

Murray, J., Wickramasekera, N., Elings, M., Bragg, R., Brennan, C., Richardson, Z., ... Elsey, H. (2019). The impact of care farms on quality of life, depression and anxiety among different population groups: A systematic review. *Campbell Systematic Reviews,* https://doi.org/10.1002/cl2.1061.

Myren, G., Enmarker, I., & Hellzen, O. (2013). Relatives' experiences of everyday life when receiving day care services for persons with dementia living at home – "It's good for her and it's good for us". *Health, 5,* 1227–1235.

Myren, G., Enmarker, I., Hellzen, O., & Saur, E. (2017). The influence of place on everyday life: Observations of persons with dementia in regular day care and at the green care farm. *Health, 9,* 261–278.

Pedersen, I., Dalskau, L. H., Ihlebæk, C., & Patil, G. (2016). Content and key components of vocational rehabilitation on care farms for unemployed people with mental health problems: A case study report. *WORK: A Journal of Prevention Assessment & Rehabilitation, 53*(1), 21–30.

Pedersen, I., Ihlebæk, C., & Kirkevold, M. (2012). Important elements in farm animal-assisted interventions for persons with clinical depression – a qualitative interview study. *Disability and Rehabilitation, 34*(18), 1526–1534.

Pedersen, I., Martinsen, E. W., Berget, B., & Braastad, B. O. (2012). Farm animal-assisted intervention for people with clinical depression: A randomized controlled trial. *Anthrozoos, 25*(2), 149–160.

Pedersen, I., & Patil, G. (2018). *Farm based day care services in Norway for people with dementia – expert identified key components.* Paper presented at the 14th International People Plant Symposium, IPPS2018, Sweden.

Poland, B., Krupa, G., & McCall, D. (2009). Settings for health promotion: An analytic framework to guide intervention design and implementation. *Health Promotion Practice, 10*(4), 505–516.

Prestvik, A., Nebell, I., & Pettersen, I. (2013). *Aktør- og markedsanalyse av Inn på tunet. RAPPORT 2013-4.* Retrieved from: Norsk institutt for landbruksøkonomisk forskning (NILF) ISBN 978-82-7077-867-6 Series: NILF Rapport https://nibio.brage. unit.no/nibio-xmlui/handle/11250/2445501

Schreuder, E., Rijnders, M., Vaandrager, L., Hassink, J., Enders-Slegers, M. J., & Kennedy, L. (2014). Exploring salutogenic mechanisms of an outdoor experiential learning programme on youth care farms in the Netherlands: Untapped potential?. *International Journal of Adolescence and Youth, 19*(2), 139–152.

Strandli, E. H. A., Skovdahl, K., Kirkevold, Ø., & Ormstad, H. (2016). Inn på tunet – et helsefremmende tilbud-En studie om ektefellers opplevelse med dagaktivitetstilbud for personer med demens. *Tidsskrift for omsorgsforskning, 2*(3), 202–211.

Sudmann, T. T., & Borsheim, I. T. (2017). 'It's good to be useful': Activity provision on green care farms in Norway for people living with dementia. *International Practice Development Journal,* https://doi.org/10.19043/ipdj.19047SP.19008.

Yewon Cho, E. (2020). [Number of care farms in South Korea (personal communication)].

14 The Next Frontier: Wilderness Therapy and the Treatment of Complex Trauma

Graham Pringle, Will W. Dobud, and Nevin J. Harper

14.1 Introduction

What former generations called combat fatigue, shell shock or war neurosis is now known as Post-traumatic stress disorder (PTSD). Awareness for PTSD grew as researchers and practitioners began exploring the effect of non-combat traumatic experiences; however, PTSD did not explain similar symptoms in children and youth. Neuroimaging studies found differences, and similarities, in brain structures between abused and neglected children and concluded that rather than concentrating on events (or the absence of events) that "the age of exposure matters" when neurobiological harm is assessed (Teicher & Samson, 2016, p. 257). More recently definitions of complex trauma, often found in the therapy room, not only involve adverse events and neglect but now describe years of accumulated stress beginning in infancy. Practitioners began realizing that survivors, and specifically those who survived trauma when very young, made up the majority of people seeking clinical services, even in late adulthood (Greeson et al., 2011; Knight, 2014). We now know that one's history is as important as their symptoms.

Kezelman and Stavropoulos (2012) attempted to "tackle the last frontier of mental health and medical services" (p. ix) publishing *Practice Guidelines for Treatment of Complex Trauma and Trauma Informed Care and Service Delivery* and have released recent guidelines for clinical treatment for those with complex trauma (Kezelman & Stavropoulos 2019a; 2019b). Just as clinical language and diagnoses evolve, the literature on trauma-informed practice has also evolved over the past thirty years (Wilson, Pence, & Conradi, 2013). As with the early combat descriptions of PTSD, the definitions that guided early developments of trauma-informed practice focused on adverse *events*, instead of the impact of early-life trauma on hindbrain and limbic development. What is consistent, however, are the strong links between adverse childhood experiences such as neglect, abuse, or parental dysfunction, and "multiple risk factors for several of the leading causes of death in adults" (Felitti et al., 1998, p. 245). Along with advances in understanding psychological stress, alternative approaches to treatment have emerged and innovation in developing new approaches is welcomed

DOI: 10.4324/9781003154419-17

192   *W.W. Dobud, G. Pringle, and N.J.Harper*

(Kezelman & Stavropolous, 2019a; McGorry, 2015). It is this openness to alternatives that have led to growth in outdoor nature-based modalities (Shanahan et al, 2019).

Wilderness therapy is typically used for adolescents who may have not responded well to traditional therapy services (Gabrielsen et al., 2015; Norton et al., 2014). Though a diverse and developing field, wilderness therapy typically involves: (a) extended outdoor expeditions; (b) group settings; (c) individualized treatment plans; (d) the presence of a licensed mental health practitioner; and (e) the combination of traditional psychotherapy models with the natural environment (DeMille et al., 2018; Fernee et al., 2017; Russell & Farnum, 2004). There is variation in models of wilderness therapy across the globe in type of experience, duration, intensity, and inclusion of traditional psychotherapy practices (Harper, Gabrielsen, & Carpenter, 2018; Harper, Rose, & Segal, 2019). While wilderness therapy scholarship has increased, links to trauma-informed practice are few and far between (Norton et al., 2018; Norton et al., 2014), despite evidence that more than half of wilderness therapy participants in one study in the United States reported one or more recent adverse experiences (Bettmann et al., 2014). Though these wilderness therapy participants were typically referred for behavioral problems, such as disengaging from school or substance use, adverse experiences were amongst the most frequently reported concerns.

This chapter explores wilderness therapy practice through the lens of complex trauma in an attempt to map the application of theory to practice. We explore the question, if adverse experiences can shape the way a child's brain develops, can therapeutic experiences, in this case physically active experiences in natural environments, lead to changes that orient a person toward healing and recovery? For Perry (2009) and others, the short and long answers are 'yes' (Cozolino, 2002; Doidge, 2007; Kezelman & Stavropoulos, 2012; van der Kolk, 2000). Informed by practice and treatment guidelines (see Kezelman & Stavropoulos, 2012; 2019a; 2019b), a phased model is presented as to how wilderness therapy practitioners can implement trauma-informed practice to ensure physical and emotional safety, trustworthiness, collaboration, choice, and empowerment (Fallot & Harris, 2009). This, we offer, is the next frontier in the pursuit of safe, effective, and relational wilderness therapy practice.

14.1.1 Contextualizing Complex-Trauma

Trauma is often characterized as an experience; depicted by (a) its suddenness, (b) the lack of personal control, and (c) a negative emotional feeling toward the event. Complex trauma refers to the impact of such adverse experiences on a person's brain, mind, and body beginning "early in life" (Wamser-Nanney, 2016, p. 296). Complex trauma is created by adverse childhood experiences that are cumulative, repetitive, interpersonal, and developmental, yet the "trauma"' is not these events but rather their impact

The Next Frontier   193

on the person's development. Mistaking the event for the injury is common and skews treatment responses to dealing with the trauma event, (e.g., exposure-based treatments) rather than stabilizing and regaining developmental trajectory.

It is not surprising that household dysfunction and adverse experiences can disrupt a child's psychological wellbeing (Felitti et al., 1998), yet only recently has trauma-informed practice became prominent in mental health care. This may be due as much to (1) the failure to find genetic causes of mental illness (Johnstone & Boyle, 2018) and (2) growing awareness of the effectiveness of the physiological and systemic treatments in complex trauma treatment (Kezelman & Stavropoulos, 2012), as it is by (3) the realization that childhood adversity is in the etiology of most mental disorders (Allsopp et al., 2019). Green et al. (2010) calculated adversity is responsible for 45% of all childhood (aged 4–12 years) psychopathology and 26–32% of adolescent (aged 13–19 years) and adult (aged 20+ years) onset of psychopathology.

The effects and prevalence of complex trauma challenge some of our previously held understandings of mental health care, which is typically guided by paradigms of evidence-based practice and diagnostic criteria. Survivors of complex trauma have been diagnosed with major depressive disorder, oppositional defiant disorder, reactive attachment disorder, or attention-deficit/hyperactivity disorder, to name a few (Cook et al., 2005). These diagnoses capture little of the prolonged effects and developmental impacts of childhood trauma. Wilderness therapy, informed by the complex trauma literature, should seek broad health benefits as an alternative to narrow definitions and treatments focused on the limits of a diagnosis.

14.1.2 Treatment of Complex Trauma

Treatment of complex trauma begins with a *bottom-up* approach (Perry, 2006), which relates to neurosequential brain development and the processing of experiences. In general terms, newborns first learn to regulate their bodies (hindbrain), then seek relationships and social learning (limbic system) before acquiring cortical skills, such as language and abstract reasoning (forebrain). Early adversity can interfere with neurodevelopment in the lower brainstem, referred to as the hindbrain (observed in body dysregulation), and limbic system (relationship concerns), hence Perry's recommendation for bottom-up approaches. Although infants and young children may not remember early experiences of stress, their hindbrain and limbic system develop patterns of reaction and attachment and employs this information as its foundation for all future interactions.

Pervasive adverse experiences can create inflexible patterns of response. When a child responds to emotional arousal, their body is compelled to take action (van der Kolk, 2003) through the sustained activation of the autonomic nervous system (ANS) by the hypothalamic-pituitary-adrenal

194 W.W. Dobud, G. Pringle, and N.J.Harper

(HPA) axis. The HPA axis triggers brain and body chemicals and hormones to flee-fight-freeze and maintains this posture while danger is present. When the danger is a person living with a child, HPA activation over months and years can severally disrupt the development of brain and body and the person's ability to connect and relate. The HPA activation then becomes a permanent body-brain-mind state and persists even after the danger has passed or left the family. This results in a finely tuned system maintaining hypervigilance and chronic stress in endless and over-reactive feedback loops, effectively re-triggering the ANS upon the mildest sense of threat or change (Niermann et al., 2017). In these instances, there is a need for physical movement toward safety before the ANS and HPA can deactivate (Terpou et al., 2019) and make the higher brain areas in the cortex available for talk therapies (Mutluer et al., 2017). Therapeutic practices informed by the neuroscience and complex trauma literature seek to regulate the body and brainstem toward HPA deactivation and then to meet relationship needs before using the reasoning capacity of the cortical brain. The safe social environment of a wilderness therapy program, the physical activity, and the natural environment become tools for improving connections between brain, body, and the natural and social environment (Harper et al., 2019).

14.2 Phased Treatment of Complex Trauma in Wilderness Therapy

In this section, we provide a description of applying best practice guidelines for the treatment of complex trauma (Kezelman & Stavropoulos, 2012; 2019a) in wilderness therapy and we suggest that clinicians focus their attention on the 2019 Guidelines, while non-clinical practitioners may be more comfortable with the 2012 Guidelines. They are different texts rather than editions. The foundation of both guidelines is five core *domains*: safety, trustworthiness, choice, collaboration, and empowerment (Fallot & Harris, 2009; Kezelman & Stavropoulos, 2012; 2019a). While not sounding revolutionary, treating clients with dignity is the foundation of this approach. As Forner (2018) described, "*if we treat people with fierce, fierce dignity, we can't go wrong*" (emphasis in original). These five core principles, described further below, can be applied to all wilderness therapy interactions.

Emotional, relational, and physical safety is the priority in trauma-informed work. Although implementing adventurous activities in what clients may perceive as potentially frightening environments, it is the role of the wilderness therapy provider to ensure participants feel physically and psychologically safe throughout their experience, and the phased process, as described in this chapter, is recommended. A lack of safety may trigger deactivation of higher brain regions and activation of flee-fight-freeze responses in lower brain regions. While eliminating all triggers is impossible, attention is paid to forewarning about upcoming experiences, watching for early indicators of stress, and making frequent expressions of care as the foundations of safety.

Trustworthiness relates to informed consent, which is taken seriously in trauma-informed approaches because agency (individual choice) is perceived as the opposite of oppression and coercion. Consequently, we advocate that providers clearly outline the rationale for their program and enable fundamental participant choice, not merely with a signed document (Katz & Webb, 2016), but repeatedly, as each new activity is encountered (Gola et al., 2016).

Choice, and *challenge by choice* specifically, are common idioms in the wilderness therapy and outdoor education literature (Carlson & Cook, 2007; Gass, Gillis, & Russell, 2012). That said, common to wilderness therapy programming, decisions about how far to hike, the food provided, other participants included in the group, and when to go home are often predetermined or out of the adolescent's control. We acknowledge the difficulty in allowing adolescents to make every decision, but as much as possible, providers should make opportunities for participants to frequently and routinely exercise choice, no matter how small.

Collaboration and consensus between wilderness therapy providers and participants should be made around the purposes of the program and intended outcomes early in a program (Gargano & Turcotte, 2019). This effort involves complexity of decision making in the individual's best interest, not discomforting the group, and helps an adolescent to learn to share and to contribute (Norton et al., 2018; Tucker et al., 2016). The outdoor experiences should be shared *with* the participants as opposed to participants feeling the program is being done *to* or *for* them.

Empowerment and skill-building equip participants to make decisions and develop positive behavior. Where wilderness therapy has been rightly criticized at times for boot camp styled programming and behavior management approaches (Anderson, 2014; Kimball & Bacon, 1993; Russell & Hendee, 2000), a trauma-informed approach focuses on facilitating a "climate of competence" (Natynczuk, 2014), where clients feel their choice and feedback are taken seriously. Clients should feel essential to the team and that their contributions are valued.

These five domains need to be attended to throughout the wilderness therapy process, from admission to graduation. As stated previously, the key difference to this framework is the neurosequential *bottom-up* approach (Perry, 2006). The processing of traumatic experiences is a lower priority to physiological regulation and integration. We offer a three-phase process that addresses the bottom-up approach described previously.

14.2.1 Phase 1: Safety/Stabilization

Phase 1, safety, is the primary aim and can take time to establish (Cloitre et al., 2012). However, in our experience, and supported by informal polling

196   *W.W. Dobud, G. Pringle, and N.J.Harper*

of wilderness therapy practitioners, many programs seem to rapidly reach a level of safety and stability in the group within the space of days rather than weeks or months. This is thought to reflect the *green bubble* (Umbers, 2011), which occurs as isolated small groups experiences in natural environments. We note a social drive to be in harmony with others when faced with novel situations which may be the reason for rapid norming of behaviors in outdoor group programs (Richardson, Marsh, & Schmidt, 2010; Withagen, Araújo, & de Poel, 2017). Additionally, a growing body of evidence "supports the notion that contact with nature and physical activity in nature has a profound positive influence on human wellness" (Brymer, Cuddihy, & Sharma-Brymer, 2010, p. 24).

Wilderness therapy groups work through *flow* experiences, which occurs when a person is happily absorbed in an activity and not distracted by thoughts and sensations except those required for achieving the task. Flow reduces HPA activation by exercising the ANS and enabling the re-stabilization of the body's system while creating a deep sense of achievement and joy (Csikszentmihalyi & Csikszentmihalyi, 1990). In wilderness therapy, participants may experience instances of flow during adventurous activities while in a supportive group environment, facilitated by the leaders who aim to establish and maintain social and physical safety and rapidly resolve any conflict (Allan, McKenna, & Hind, 2012). This may be an unusual and attractive situation for participants and increases attachment through protection and care.

There is a range of physiological effects that occur in the wilderness therapy setting which can promote regulation and stability. For example, Porges' (2009) polyvagal theory (PVT) "provides a rich explanation of how play can produce transformative learning experiences" (Harper et al., 2019, p. 86). PVT focuses on the ANS controlling rest, digestion, heart rate, temperature, and other involuntary responses. The ANS consists of the sympathetic branch, which activates the flee or fight response, and the parasympathetic branch, which returns the organism to homeostasis, or the calm state. When stress activates the HPA axis and the ANS is aroused, people are drawn to physical action; either by fleeing a scene or preparing to fight. PVT explains that social connection and a sense of safety contribute to optimal arousal. Participants' bodies may be prepared for autonomic fight or flight responses during experiences that include risk, such as exposure to cold temperatures, remote locations or fast-running rivers, yet a strong social connection can dampen those responses and allow participants to experience potentially risky activities in a playful and social manner (Ackerman, 2011). In this case, the body is in a healing state while the person engages in the experiential activities and is later capable of processing the experience.

Another consideration for safety and stabilization is emotional and physiological regulation. For Perry (2009), repetitive, rhythmic, and sensory activities that link body to mind are essential to regulation. In wilderness therapy, participants may engage in hiking, paddling, stretching, yoga, mindfulness, or patterned breathing exercises. These rhythmic activities, taking place in a therapeutic climate, can help to regulate the brain stem and limbic system, which in turn helps participants prepare for the possibility of processing sensations, thoughts, and emotions.

Though these phases are outlined as if to be linear, the literature on the treatment of complex trauma is clear that safety and stabilization are central to care. The priorities of Phase 1 must be assessed and attended to throughout any experience, regardless of what phase providers perceive the group has achieved. When delivering this model of wilderness therapy, practitioners should attend to the physiological responses of the participant, such as the ability to focus attention, to process language, or whether there are signs of an elevated heart rate or breathing rate. Practitioners should take special care when introducing potentially risky activities and note when participants are entering a state of hyper- or hypoarousal.

14.2.2 Phase 2: Processing

Phase 2 is perhaps the most easily recognized of the three phases (Allan et al., 2012). Many group, family, and individual therapeutic processes are pursued through outdoor adventure contexts (Tracey, Gray, Truong, & Ward, 2018; Wai, 2005). Indeed, adventure experiences, in natural spaces, are found to be therapeutic in and of themselves (Adhémar, 2008; Avila, 2011; Carpenter & Harper, 2015; Harper et al., 2019; Pryor, Carpenter, & Townsend, 2005). The processing of experience and schemas can be led through many methods (Griswold, 2014), and typically groups are gathered for regular reflection (Tucker et al., 2016).

Although we are providing a model for the phased treatment of complex trauma in wilderness therapy, we find it important to point out that there are many ways practitioners help participants to process, and they all work equally well (Wampold & Imel, 2015). Likewise, the decision to take participants outside has not been evidenced to alter treatment outcomes (Dobud & Harper, 2018), but may harness the soothing aspect of natural spaces and enable a deeper connection to, or as, the therapeutic process (Avila, 2011; Ewert et al, 2014; Mantler & Logan, 2015; Schweitzer, Glab & Brymer, 2018). Each practitioner uses different tools for processing experiences, such as cognitive-behavioral, dialectical-behavioral, solution-focused, or acceptance and commitment therapy, and in this framework, practitioners are urged not to process in detail until Phase 1 has been achieved. It is in Phase 2 when the incorporation of various empirically supported psychotherapeutic practices is indicated.

Therapists are cautioned with regard to common approaches to talk therapy in the context of complex trauma. Kezelman and Stavropoulos (2019a) addressed the use of established treatments for this population, warning that complex trauma is neither normal nor typical, and that

198   *W.W. Dobud, G. Pringle, and N.J.Harper*

well-intended and routine practices may be unhelpful. Remembering that complex trauma occurs in the context of relationships that do not ensure safety, our practices must be intensely relational. Simply pointing to the "therapeutic relationship" is insufficient as young people with complex trauma are unlikely to have a coherent sense of self and a deep distrust of relationships, even to the point that a deepening relationship itself may come to feel threatening and reminiscent of predatory behavior or experiences of role confusion. Other standard approaches to be re-evaluated include "*I*" statements, a focus on "feelings," "will power," "inner strengths," "following the client," and rigid boundaries. In short, existing therapeutic practices and techniques may inadvertently harm those with complex trauma who require experiences that engender safety and dignity, and then build skills and abilities that we otherwise assume are present amongst children and adolescents.

Despite these cautions, there are many typical wilderness therapy practices that lend themselves to therapeutic processes in Phase 2. For example, group debrief circles allow young people to hear the experiences of peers and adults and to compare to their own understanding of the day's events. To understand that other's experience of the same event may be legitimately different to one's own is to mentalize. According to Schmid, Petermann, and Fegert (2013), mentalizing is required before empathy can be experienced by participants. However, this opportunity to develop mentalizing and empathy may be missed if we demand that young people contribute in debrief circles. Interdependence rather than independence should be the aim of the group work and safety requires that a young person be permitted to listen without the anxiety of contributing and being judged by others for their contribution or lack thereof.

Complex trauma typically includes many experiences of violations, throughout childhood and even into late adulthood. The complex adolescent may not understand boundaries and testing boundaries should be understood as part of the therapy process and not "resistance." With this in mind, we agree with de Shazer (1984) with his original call to remove concepts of resistance from therapy practice. Creating safety requires giving power to the participant. This approach includes honoring their dissent and responding non-violently as a lived experience of the ebb and flow of being in a close relationship (Bloom, 2018). What wilderness therapy can provide is the empathetic give and take of being in a platonic relationship where the participant can be both the giver and receiver of care, and for-given for transgressions while also provided with explicit and kind coaching on social and conflict skills. These are not new practices and we find it useful to reflect on Clifford Knapp's (1988) work on creating humane climates in the outdoors.

Knapp described the benefit of attending to non-verbal communications rather than relying on talk as the transformative process. Moments of absorption in scenic views, interesting natural phenomena, weather, adventure activity, or the informal fireside chat should be encouraged. This requires that time constraints and program structure be re-evaluated. Such moments seem rare for young people with complex trauma and enable the HPA and CNS to re-set. Such experiences should not be forced or timetabled tightly (e.g., solo day), as such rigidity is coercive and likely to return the individual and group into Phase 1 (Safety). Practitioners should be responsive to the moment by moment opportunities for young people to discover for themselves the comfort of normative behavior. A rigid model may be more of a hindrance to a humane, trauma-informed, empathetic, and well-grounded practitioner.

This approach to processing experience may delight some and horrify others. Where the skilled practitioner is oriented to the phased approach and to the development of both individuals and group without the constraints of rigid plans, levels, rules, and traditions, they are able to attend to needs and opportunities and can respond and lead through providing invitations for positive behavior and self-determination. This is the idealized process and yet must be balanced with the reality that the experience will be lived differently for each person and may not be achievable for some.

Where a young person is distressed by severing their attachment to family or community, they are not indicated for wilderness therapy that removes them from their home environment. Because a young person may become distressed by the merest hint of danger, and complex young people may have lived in a perpetual state of imminent terror, a trip to a local park may be the limit of their capacity. Program providers should focus their attention on the suitability of referrals based on the type of outdoor experiences their organization provides rather than on privileging their program's structure or model of therapy. Practitioners and managers are advised to "fail successfully" (Duncan, Miller, & Hubble, 2007) by ensuring that where a therapeutic experience seems unlikely that they maintain that person's dignity to provide choices of other practitioners and programs that may be more suitable. The analogy of "square pegs and round holes" comes to mind and we should expect and cater for the fact that not every young person is a candidate for wilderness therapy programs (Harper, Mott, & Obee, 2019).

A self-reflective practitioner, enabled to facilitate client-directed experiences and provided the freedom to respond to the processing of these experiences, requires supervision and support. Re-enactments of past trauma and chaotic interpersonal dynamics make the achievement of Phase 1 (Safety) and the work of Phase 2 (Processing) intense and challenging. However, the best "tool" in wilderness therapy is the practitioner and that tool requires care and maintenance. While some forms of wilderness therapy programming include therapists "parachuting" into the group to conduct more traditional talk therapy sessions, these practitioners might be absent from client-initiated flow experiences. Simply put, wilderness therapy practitioners should be there when the moments arrive.

200   W.W. Dobud, G. Pringle, and N.J.Harper

Qualifications may be less important than the "good enough" adult empowered toward responsive healing experiences. Where these adults are supported by a multidisciplinary team of expert supervisors and case managers, they can be maintained in their "good enough" role, through the ups and downs that is processing the experience for adolescents with complex trauma. Wilderness therapy clinicians are advised to re-evaluate their role and to center their work upon the adults living with the participants (McLoughlin & Gonzalez, 2014).

14.2.3 Phase 3: Integration

In Phase 3 (Integration), practitioners aim to provide closure to the wilderness therapy program, enabling participants to make meaning of their experience. Splitting Phase 3 into two, *Integration During Program* and *Integration After Program*, seems appropriate to draw practitioners' attention to the immediate integration processes which they can lead in person and those that may need to be enacted in their absence by the participant after the program. The practitioner is dual focused on enhancing positive change within the individual and how these changes are sustained in the home environment. Though it is common for adolescents in wilderness therapy to be referred to ongoing residential treatment in the United States (Bolt, 2016), we view a positive outcome as a successful return to the participant's family and community.

Phase 3a (Integration During Program) prepares the participant to return to their old environment, appropriately grieving the loss of the unique relationship experienced on the program (Gath, 2009) and consolidating potentially helpful changes to old routines. The emphasis is on the participant enacting health changes with, and without, social support with the goal of creating or influencing a safe and comfortable ecological niche rather than returning to a coercive situation and powerlessly complying. Time away in wilderness therapy can break patterns of negative interaction, allowing opportunity for a "fresh start" (Riddell, 2014) and readiness to engage in positive interactions post-program.

In Phase 3b (Integration After Program), program leaders may be involved in follow up processes in great detail working with the family or employ mentors who may, or may not, have attended the program (Chapman et al., 2017). Conversely, the leaders may be entirely absent post-program, however, this does not absolve them from providing artifacts to, and professional communication, with the participants' social supports. This may be in the form of reports, photos and video footage, social media communication, letters and emails, or in-person attendance at family therapy, celebratory events, and reunions as best suits the capacity and processes of follow up support systems (Bettmann et al., 2016; DeMille et al., 2018). Each participant may benefit from a different set of follow up opportunities and one size never fit all. Maintaining responsibility for

Phase 3b prompts the program leaders to assist the participant, and their social supports, to introduce the behaviors and learnings taken from the wilderness therapy experience into their normal environment rather than ceasing their commitment at admission to the program.

14.3 Discussion

In this chapter, we introduced the phased treatment of complex trauma in wilderness therapy, and we have colloquially referred to this as *The Next Frontier*. Wilderness therapy has a checkered history, suffering from claims of abusive and neglectful practices resulting in legal action, and potentially traumatizing practices, such as involuntary admission (Becker, 2010; Tucker et al., 2015; 2018). The likelihood of complex trauma impacting many young people entering wilderness programs around the world is cause to adopt a new lens. This lens delivers an alternative narrative for wilderness therapy, by incorporating knowledge of neurological and physiological responses gleaned from the literature in the pursuit of humane and inclusive practice. As advocates and practitioners of this exciting field, we feel that the next frontier in wilderness therapy should center on safety, dignity, respect, empowerment, and choice.

There are many people working in the outdoors with populations likely to have experienced complex trauma and adverse childhood experiences. Importantly, we do not find this work isolated to practicing mental health professionals, such as psychologists or social workers, but all those working with people in the outdoors activity sectors. For example, any school group is likely, on average, to contain several students with high exposure to adverse childhood experiences regardless of socio-economic background (Burke Harris, 2018). An expedition or center-based adventure activity will expose students to risk which may inadvertently overwhelm some who may not regularly exhibit outward behaviors of distress (Courtois, 2008). It is quite possible that participants can become triggered, dysregulated, and dissociative without leaders or peers noticing.

This chapter provides a new perspective on wilderness therapy practice by examining the physiological effects of complex trauma and how adventures in outdoor environments can facilitate neurobiological regulation and empowerment. Creating clear links to PVT (Porges, 1995), the neurosequential model (Perry, 2009), and best practice guidelines for the treatment of complex trauma (Kezelman & Stavropoulos, 2012, 2019b) are novel to the wilderness therapy literature and are worthy of future research. We believe that the frontier for wilderness therapy has moved as a result of this knowledge.

Studying the neurobiological and physiological effects could elicit a greater understanding of wilderness therapy participation. Providers can administer trauma symptom scales, such as the Adverse Childhood Experiences International Questionnaire (WHO, 2018), to measure the

202 *W.W. Dobud, G. Pringle, and N.J.Harper*

prevalence of participants arriving to wilderness therapy with symptoms of complex trauma. Daily participant feedback scales as well as physiological and biofeedback tools can be utilized to understand the impact of the experience and to individualize wilderness therapy programs based on the responses of participants in real time (Dobud, Cavanaugh, & Harper, 2020).

Like any approach to working with clinical populations in therapeutic settings, limitations exist. While trauma-informed approaches, and particularly those acknowledging the prevalence of complex trauma, are becoming more popular in mental and behavioral health care, wilderness and other outdoor therapies have been slow to examine and adopt such approaches. If wilderness therapy practitioners focus on the cognitions, the bottom-up approach we have stressed throughout this chapter may be disregarded. That said, we argue for future research to investigate the model we have presented.

Trauma-informed approaches are becoming mainstream (Kezelman & Stavropoulos, 2012) and ideas of empowerment and safety are obviously nothing new to therapeutic approaches to working with young people. What is new, particularly in the United States, and may be challenging to many instances of wilderness therapy practice, is that addressing complex trauma requires models of care that allow for adolescent choice. Choice may include not being in wilderness therapy. We, as practitioners and researchers of wilderness therapy, strongly advocate for a review of practices and policies in programs, to bring them into alignment with the next frontier wilderness therapy mapped by what is now known regarding complex trauma and the benefits of an ethic of dignity.

References

Ackerman, D. (2011). Deep play. New York, Vintage.

Adhémar, A. J. (2008). Nature as clinical psychological intervention: Evidence, applications and implications. University of Arhus, Denmark.

Allan, J. F., McKenna, J., & Hind, K. (2012). Brain resilience: Shedding light into the black box of adventure processes. *Australian Journal of Outdoor Education, 16*(1), 3–14.

Allsopp, K., Read, J., Corcoran, R., & Kinderman, P. (2019). Heterogeneity in psychiatric diagnostic classification. *Psychiatry Research, 279,* 15–22

Anderson, S. (2014, August 12). When wilderness boot camps take tough love too far. *The Antlantic.* Retrieved from https://www.theatlantic.com/health/archive/2014/08/when-wilderness-boot-camps-take-tough-love-too-far/375582/

Avila, M. A. (2011). *Connection to nature as an intervention for children exposed to trauma.* (3460622 Psy.D.), Alliant International University, Ann Arbor, MI.

Bettmann, J. E., Tucker, A. R., Tracy, J., & Parry, K. J. (2014). An exploration of gender, client history, and functioning in wilderness therapy participants. *Residential Treatment for Children & Youth, 31*(3), 155–170.

Bettmann, J. E., Tucker, A. R, Behrens, E., & Vanderloo, M. (2016). Changes in late adolescents and young adults' attachment, separation, and mental health during wilderness therapy. *Child and Family Studies,* 1–12.

Bloom, S.L. (2018). The sanctuary model and sex trafficking: Creating moral systems to counteract exploitation and dehumanization. In *Social work practice with survivors of sex trafficking and commercial sexual exploitation* (pp. 241–273). Columbia University Press; US

Bolt, K. L. (2016). Descending from the summit: Aftercare planning for adolescents in wilderness therapy. *Contemporary Family Therapy, 38*(1), 62–74.

Brymer, E., Cuddihy, T. F., & Sharma-Brymer, V. (2010). The role of nature-based experiences in the development and maintenance of wellness. *Asia-Pacific Journal of Health, Sport and Physical Education, 1*, 21–27.

Burke Harris, N. (2018). *The deepest well: Healing the long-term effects of childhood adversity*. New York, NY: Houghton Mifflin Harcourt.

Carlson, K. P., & Cook, M. (2007). Challenge by choice: Adventure-based counseling for seriously ill adolescents. *Child and Adolescent Psychiatric Clinics of North America, 16*(4), 909–919.

Carpenter, C., & Harper, N. J. (2015). Health and wellbeing benefits of activities in the outdoors. In B. Humberstone, H. Prince, & K. Henderson (Eds.), *Routledge international handbook of outdoor studies* (pp. 56–59). Abingdon,UK: Routledge International Press.

Chapman, C., Deane, K., Harré, N., Courtney, M., & Moore, J. (2017). Engagement and mentor support as drivers of social development in the Project K youth development program. *Journal of Youth & Adolescence, 46*(3), 644–655.

Cloitre, M., Courtois, C. A., Ford, J. D., Green, B. L., Alexander, P., Briere, J. N., Herman, J. L., Lanius, R. A., Stolbach, B. C., Spinazzola, J., van der Kolk, B. A., & van der Hart, O. (2012). The ISTSS expert consensus treatment guidelines for complex PTSD in adults. Retrieved from http://istss.org.

Cook, A., Spinazzola, J., Ford, J., Lanktree, C., Blaustein, M., Cloitre, M., DeRosa, R., Hubbard, R., Kagan, R., Liautaud, J., Mallah, K., Olafson, E., & van der Kolk, B. A. (2005). Complex trauma in children and adolescents. Psychiatric Annals, *35*(5), 390–398.

Courtois, C. A. (2008). Complex trauma, complex reactions: Assessment and treatment. *Psychological Trauma: Theory, Research, Practice, and Policy, 41*(1), 86–100.

Cozolino, L. (2002). The neuroscience of psychotherapy: building and rebuilding the human brain (norton series on interpersonal neurobiology). New York, NY: WW Norton & Company.

Csikszentmihalyi, M., & Csikszentmihalyi, I. S. (1990). Adventure and the flow experience. In J.C. Miles & S. Priest (Eds.), *Adventure Education*. Pennsylvania: Venture.

DeMille, S. M., Tucker, A. R., Gass, M. A., Javorski, S., VanKanegan, C., Talbot, B., & Karoff, M. (2018). The effectiveness of outdoor behavioral healthcare with struggling adolescents: A comparison group study a contribution for the special issue: Social innovation in child and youth services. *Children and Youth Services Review, 88*, 241–248.

de Shazer, S. (1984). The death of resistance. *The Family Process, 23*, 11–17.

Dobud, W. W., & Harper, N. J. (2018). Of dodo birds and common factors: A scoping review of direct comparison trials in adventure therapy. *Complementary Therapies in Clinical Practice, 31*, 16–24.

Doidge, N. (2007). The brain that changes itself: Stories of personal triumph from the frontiers of brain science. New York, NY. Viking Press.

Duncan, B. L., Miller, S. D., & Hubble, M. A. (2007). How being bad can make you better. *Psychotherapy Networker, 57*, 36–45.

204   W.W. Dobud, G. Pringle, and N.J.Harper

Ewert, A., Mitten, D., & Overholt, J. (2014). Natural environments and human health. Wallingford: CABI.

Fallot, R. D., & Harris, M. (2009). Creating cultures of trauma-informed care (CCTIC): A self-assessment and planning protocol. Washington, DC: Community Connections.

Felitti, V. J., Anda, R. F., Nordenberg, D., Williamson, D. F., Spitz, A. M., Edwards, V., Koss, M. P., & Marks, J. S. (1998). Relationship of childhood abuse and household dysfunction to many of the leading causes of death in adults. *American Journal of Preventive Medicine, 14*(4), 245–258.

Fernee, C. R., Gabrielsen, L. E., Andersen, A. J. W., & Mesel, T. (2017). Unpacking the black box of wilderness therapy. *Qualitative Health Research, 27*(1), 114–129.

Forner, C. & Kate, M. A. (2018). Dissociation 101: A comprehensive exploration into the field of dissociation and complex trauma. Retrieved from https://secure.ce-credit.com/courses/102301/dissociation-101-a-comprehensive-exploration-into-the-field-of-dissociation-and-complex-trauma

Gabrielsen, L. E., Fernee, C. R., Aasen, G. O., & Eskedal, L. T. (2015). Why randomized trials are challenging within adventure therapy research: Lessons learned in Norway. *Journal of Experiential Education, 39*(1), 5–14.

Gargano, V., & Turcotte, D. (2019). Helping factors in an outdoor adventure program. *Journal of Social Work, 0*(0), 1–19.

Gass, M. A., Gillis, H. L., & Russell, K. C. (2012). *Adventure therapy: Theory, research, and practice.* New York: Routledge.

Gath, S. (2009). *Adventure and therapy: A training guide for adventure facilitators.* Ann Arbor: Prescott College.

Gola, J. A., Beidas, R. S., Antinoro-Burke, D., Kratz, H. E., & Fingerhut, R. (2016). Ethical considerations in exposure therapy with children. *Cognitive and Behavioral Practice, 23*(2), 184–193.

Green, J., McLaughlin, K. A., Berglund, P. A., Gruber, M. J., Sampson, N. A., Zaslavsky, A. M., & Kessler, R. C. (2010). Childhood adversities and adult psychiatric disorders in the national comorbidity survey replication I: Associations with first onset of DSM-IV disorders. *Archives of General Psychiatry, 67*(2), 113–123.

Greeson, J. K., Briggs, E. C., Kisiel, C. L., Layne, C. M., Ake, G. S., Ko, S. J., & Fairbank, J. A. (2011). Complex trauma and mental health in children and adolescents placed in foster care: Findings from the National Child Traumatic Stress Network. *Child Welfare, 90*(6), 91–108.

Griswold, J. (2014). Mental health professionals' use of adventure therapy with couples and families, St. Catherine University, Saint Paul, MN.

Harper, N. J., Gabrielsen, L. E., & Carpenter, C. (2018). A cross-cultural exploration of 'wild' in wilderness therapy: Canada, Norway and Australia. *Journal of Adventure Education and Outdoor Learning, 18*(2), 148–164.

Harper, N. J., Mott, A. J., & Obee, P. (2019). Client perspectives on wilderness therapy as a component of adolescent residential treatment for problematic substance use and mental health issues. *Children and Youth Services Review, 105*, 104450.

Harper, N. J., Rose, K., & Segal, D. (2019). *Nature-based therapy: A practitioners guide to working outdoors with children, youth, and families.* Canada: New Society Publishers.

Johnstone, L., & Boyle, M. (2018). The power threat meaning framework: Towards the identification of patterns in emotional distress, unusual experiences and troubled or troubling behaviour, as an alternative to functional psychiatric diagnosis. In J. Cromby, J. Dillon, D. Harper, P. Kinderman, E. Longden, D. Pilgrim, & J. Read (Eds.). Leicester: British Psychological Society.

Katz, A. L., & Webb, S. A. (2016). Informed consent in decision-making in pediatric practice. *Pediatrics, 138*(2), 1–16.

Kezelman, C.A., & Stavropoulos, P.A. (2019b). *Complimentary guidelines to practice guidelines for clinical treatment of complex trauma.* Sydney: Blue Knot Foundation.

Kezelman, C.A., & Stavropoulos, P.A. (2019a). *Practice guidelines for clinical treatment of complex trauma.* Sydney: Blue Knot Foundation.

Kezelman, C.A., & Stavropoulos, P.A. (2012). Practice guidelines for treatment of complex trauma and trauma informed care and service delivery. Sydney: ASCA.

Kimball, R. O., & Bacon, S. B. (1993). *The wilderness challenge model.* In M. A. Gass (Ed), Adventure therapy: Therapeutic applications of adventure programming, (pp. 11–41). Dubuque, IA: Kendall Hunt.

Knapp, C.E. (1988). *Creating humane climates outdoors: A people skills primer.* ERIC Clearinghouse on Rural Education and Small Schools, Las Cruces, NM.

Knight, C. (2014). Trauma-informed social work practice: Practice considerations and challenges. *Clinical Social Work Journal, 43*(1), 25–37.

Mantler, A., & Logan, A.C. (2015). Natural environments and mental health. *Advances in Integrative Medicine, 2*(1), 5–12.

McGorry, P. D. (2015). Early intervention in psychosis: Obvious, effective, overdue. *Nervous and Mental Diseases, 203*(5), 310–318.

McLoughlin, P.J., & Gonzalez, R. (2014). Healing complex trauma through therapeutic residential care: The lighthouse foundation therapeutic family model of care. *Children Australia, 39*(3), 169–176.

Mutluer, T., Şar, V., Kose-Demiray, Ç., Arslan, H., Tamer, S., Inal, S., & Kaçar, A. Ş. (2017). Lateralization of neurobiological response in adolescents with Post-Traumatic Stress Disorder related to severe childhood sexual abuse: the Tri-Modal Reaction (T-MR) model of protection. *Trauma & Dissociation, 19*(1), 108–125.

Natynczuk, S. (2014). Solution-focused practice as a useful addition to the concept of adventure therapy. *InterAction, 6*(1), 23–36.

Niermann, H.C.M., Figner, B., Tyborowska, A., van Peer, J.M., Cillessen, A.H.N., & Roelofs, K. (2017). Defensive freezing links Hypothalamic-Pituitary-Adrenal-axis activity and internalizing symptoms in humans. *Psychoneuroendocrinology, 82,* 83–90.

Norton, C. L., Tucker, A. R., Farnham-Stratton, M., Borroel, F., & Pelletier, A. (2018). Family enrichment adventure therapy: A mixed methods study examining the impact of trauma-informed adventure therapy on children and families affected by abuse. *Journal of Child & Adolescent Trauma, 12,* 85–95.

Norton, C. L., Tucker, A. R., Russell, K. C., Bettmann, J. E., Gass, M. Gillis, H. L. & Behrens, E. (2014). Adventure therapy with youth. *Journal of Experiential Education, 37,* 46–59.

Perry, B. D. (2006). Applying principles of neurodevelopment to clinical work with maltreated and traumatized children: The neurosequential model of therapeutics. In N. B. Webb (Ed.), *Social work practice with children and families: Working with traumatized youth in child welfare* (p. 27–52). The Guilford Press.

206   W.W. Dobud, G. Pringle, and N.J.Harper

Perry, B.D. (2009). Examining child maltreatment through a neurodevelopmental lens: Clinical applications of the Neurosequential Model of Therapeutics. *Loss and Trauma, 14,* 240–255.

Porges, S. W. (1995). Orienting in a defensive world: Mammalian modifications of our evolutionary heritage. A polyvagal theory. *Psychophysiology, 32*(4), 301–318.

Porges, S. W. (2009). The polyvagal theory: new insights into adaptive reactions of the autonomic nervous system. *Cleveland Clinic Journal of Medicine, 76*(Suppl 2), S86.

Pryor, A., Carpenter, C., & Townsend, M. (2005). Outdoor education and bush adventure therapy: A social-ecological approach to health and wellbeing. *Australian Journal of Outdoor Education, 9*(1), 3–13.

Richardson, M. J., Marsh, K. L., & Schmidt, R. C. (2010). Challenging the egocentric view of coordinated perceiving, activing, and knowing. *The Mind in Context,* 307–333.

Riddell, J. K. (2014). The development of self in relationships: Youths' narratives of change through a residential, wilderness and family therapy intervention. Unpublished Master's Thesis, Toronto, ON: York University.

Russell, K. C., & Farnum, J. (2004). A concurrent model of the wilderness therapy process. *Adventure Education & Outdoor Learning, 1,* 39–55.

Russell, K. C., & Hendee, J. C. (2000). Outdoor behavioral healthcare: Definitions. common practice, expected outcomes, and a nationwide survery of programs. *Technical Report # 26.* Moscow, Idaho: Idaho Forect, Wildlife and Range Experiment Station.

Richardson, M. J., Marsh, K. L., & Schmidt, R. C. (2007). Challenging the egocentric view of coordinated perceiving, acting, and knowing. In The Mind in Context (307–333), New York, Guilford Press.

Schmid, M., Petermann, F., & Fegert, J.M. (2013). Developmental trauma disorder: Pros and cons of including formal criteria in the psychiatric diagnostic systems. *BMC Psychiatry, 13*(1), 3.

Schweitzer, R. D., Glab, H. L., & Brymer, E. (2018). The human-nature experience: A phenomenological-psychoanalytic perspective. *Frontiers in Psychology, 9*(969), 1–12.

Shanahan, D. F., Atell-Burt, T., Barder, E. A., Brymer, E., Cox, D. T., Dean, J., Depledge, M., Fuller, R. A., Hartig, T., Irvine, K. N., Jones, A., Kikillus, H., Lovell, R., Mitchell, R., Niemelä, J., Nieuwenhuijsen, M., Pretty, J., Townsend, M., van Heezik, Y., Warber, S., & Gaston, K. J. (2019). Nature–based interventions for improving health and wellbeing: The purpose, the people and the outcomes. *Sports, 7*(6), 141.

Teicher, M. H., & Samson, J. A. (2016). Annual research review: Enduring neurobiological effects of childhood abuse and neglect. *Journal of Child Psychology and Psychiatry, 57*(3), 241–266.

Terpou, B. A., Harricharan, S., McKinnon, M. C., Frewen, P., Jetly, R., & Lanius, R. A. (2019). The effects of trauma on brain and body: A unifying role for the midbrain periaqueductal gray. *Neuroscience Research. 0*(0), 1–31.

Tracey, D., Gray, T., Truong, S., & Ward, K. (2018). Combining acceptance and commitment therapy with adventure therapy to promote psychological wellbeing for children at-risk. *Frontiers in Psychology, 9,* 1565.

Tucker, A. R., Bettmann, J. E., Norton, C. L., & Comart, C. (2015). The role of transport use in adolescent wilderness treatment: Its relationship to readiness to change and outcomes. *Child & Youth Care Forum, 44*(5), 671–686.

Tucker, A. R., Combs, K. M., Bettmann, J. E., Chang, T. H., Graham, S., Hoag, M., & Tatum, C. (2018). Longitudinal outcomes for youth transported to wilderness therapy Programs. *Research on Social Work Practice. 28*(4), 438–451.

Tucker, A. R., Norton, C., DeMille, S. M., & Hobson, J. (2016). The impact of wilderness therapy: Utilizing an integrated care approach. *Experiential Education, 39*(1), 15–30.

Tucker, A. R., Beale, B., & Norton, C. L. (2018). *Ohio adventure therapy collaborative: A pilot study.* Paper presented at the 2018 Symposium on Experiential Education Research. Jacksonville, FL.

Tucker, A. R., Norton, C. L., Itin, C. M., Hobson, J., & Alvarez, M. A. (2016). Adventure therapy: Nondeliberative group work in action. *Social Work with Groups, 39*(2–3), 194–207.

Umbers, A. (2011). The green bubble: Narrative, time away in the bush, and restoring personal agency after hard times. *International Journal of Narrative Therapy & Community Work, 2*, 23–32.

van der Kolk, B. A. (2000). Posttraumatic stress disorder and the nature of trauma. *Dialogues in Clinical Neuroscience. 2*(1), 7–22.

van der Kolk, B. A. (2003). The neurobiology of childhood trauma and abuse. *Child and Adolescent Psychiatric Clinics of North America. 12*(2), 293–317.

Wai, K. L. K. (2005). From adventure to therapy: A model for healing. *INTI, 1*(5), 417–431.

Wampold, B. E., & Imel, Z. E. (2015). *The great psychotherapy debate: The evidence for what makes psychotherapy work (2nd ed,).* New York: Taylor & Francis.

Wamser-Nanney, R. (2016). Examining the complex trauma definition using children's self-reports. *Child & Adolescent Trauma, 9*(4), 295–304.

Wilson, C., Pence, D., & Conradi, L. (2013). Trauma-informed care. *Encyclopedia of Social Work.*

Withagen, R., Araújo, D., & de Poel, H. J. (2017). Inviting affordances and agency. *New Ideas in Psychology, 45*, 11–18.

World Health Organization [WHO]. (2018). Adverse childhood experiences internationoal questionnaire (ACE-IQ). *World Health Organization.* Retrieved from https://www.who.int/violence_injury_prevention/violence/activities/adverse_childhood_experiences/en/

15 What Can We Learn About Nature, Physical Activity, and Health from *parkrun?*

Gareth Wiltshire and Stephanie Merchant

15.1 Introduction

The relationship between nature and health has become an important topic of research interest. There now exists a large literature base contributing to conceptual developments associated with therapeutic landscapes (Hartig et al., 2014; Bell et al., 2015; Thomas, 2015; Merchant, 2017), green space (e.g. parks, woodlands, countryside) (De Vries et al., 2003; Maas et al., 2006) and blue space (e.g. lakes, rivers and coasts) (Coleman and Kearns, 2015; Foley, 2015) which help us understand the interactions between human health and the environment. Interest in these topics has been drawn from diverse literature works spanning the likes of health geography, medical sociology, environmental studies and health psychology to the extent that the evidence base for the impact of nature is considered to be well-established and is being taken seriously as a matter of public health promotion (DEFRA, 2017; Bowler et al., 2010). Less well-established is our understanding of how physical activity can play a complementary role in facilitating the relationship between nature and health or, indeed, how nature can augment the experience of physical activity and potentially contribute to its maintenance as an important lifestyle practice for health and wellbeing.

While all advances within the literature on nature, physical activity and health are undoubtedly necessary and valuable, it is crucial to take seriously the ways in which our new understandings play out in the "real-world"; that is, outside of abstract theorizing, experimental conditions and research-specific contexts. An appreciation for concrete, tangible and empirical phenomena within the realm of nature, physical activity and health aligns with the emphasis on translational and impactful research increasingly being embraced across research agendas (Ogilvie et al., 2009). Indeed, the real world can often expose theoretical explanations to contextual complexities and a "messiness" that otherwise would be missing from idealized accounts about the relationship between nature, physical activity and health. Furthermore, we take particular interest in investigating real-world phenomena in order to offer meaningful examples of

DOI: 10.4324/9781003154419-18

how complex ideas can manifest in mundane, everyday practices that can be communicated with policy-makers and publics as well as within research communities (Mirvis, 2009). In this way, bringing the real world into focus can bring ideas to life and offer a vision for how nature, physical activity and health can matter for people in their own lived experiences.

With these ambitions in mind, this chapter explores the weekly 5-km running initiative "*parkrun*" as an opportunity to join up the emerging interest in nature, physical activity and health with an ambition of learning from real-world practices. For readers unfamiliar with *parkrun*, the chapter will first provide an outline of the key features and characteristics of the initiative before reviewing the published research literature on *parkrun* that has emerged over the last 5-years. We then draw on the key theoretical and conceptual contributions that we see as pertinent to understanding *parkrun* in an attempt to illuminate new ways of understanding the initiative and, in turn, explore how *parkrun* can illuminate new ways of understanding the relationship between nature and human health.

15.2 Contextualizing *Parkrun* as an Opportunity for Physical Activity in Nature

parkrun began as a weekly time-trial opportunity for a small group of local runners at a single public park in the UK in 2004. Due to growing popularity by 2007, the organizers had set up seven separate events with several hundred participants taking part. In 2019, the *parkrun* website reported 656 registered events in the UK, hosting an average of 206 participants at each site per week (*parkrun*, 2019). Furthermore, *parkrun* now has an international reach, with over 4 million runners having taken part in 20 different countries. Several key features of *parkrun* characterize the event that is important to understand before attempting to explore the relationship between nature, health and *parkrun*.

Taking part in *parkrun* consists of running, jogging or walking a 5-km course. This first characteristic is important to note for a number of reasons, not least because it is inherently a physical challenge requiring effort beyond the routine requirements of everyday life. As a relatively demanding physical activity easily categorized as moderate-to-vigorous in reference to public health guidelines (DoHSC, 2019), it is likely to mean that taking part in *parkrun* will be somewhat psychologically demanding too, often requiring motivation to initially attend, to complete the course and even more so to improve on previous performances.

Despite being unavoidably challenging, much emphasis is placed on being open to all abilities. "It's for everyone" is declared on the homepage of the website along with the statement that "you will never come last" in acknowledgment of the policy that every team of marshals at *parkrun* events will include a "tail walker" who is responsible for completing the course with or behind the slowest participant (*parkrun*, 2019). The average time taken to complete the 5-km course is 28 minutes (about double the time of the women's 5 km world record). Indeed, as many participants walk the courses, the slowest finishing time is inevitably far slower than the 28 minute average. Reece et al. (2019) note that in 2017, there were 64,888 instances of runners taking over 50 minutes to complete a *parkrun* which represents an increase of 88% compared with the previous year meaning that *parkrun* is generally getting slower. This apparent growing appeal to less-able participants has led to the suggestion that "what started as a community time trial, is now a global movement encouraging mass participation in physical activity with excellent public health potential" (Reece et al., 2019, p.326).

The second characteristic of *parkrun* events is that they predominantly take place in public parks. This has been a feature of *parkrun* from its inception and continues to be a key part of the *parkrun* branding and marketing material with, for example, the website landing page featuring an image of a tree in the logo, as well as green spaces and woodland animals.

As a core aspect of *parkrun*, taking place in public parks is likely to leave participants exposed to diverse weather conditions, potentially challenging terrain as well as many other natural elements of interest to this chapter. Indeed, with often hundreds of participants at each event and no agreed exclusivity of access, this aspect of *parkrun* may also invite confrontation from other park users and even political challenges from local government authorities who fund the upkeep of parks (this was the case for one location in Stoke Gifford, UK). Furthermore, holding events in public parks opens up questions around geographical barriers and health inequalities as parks are more likely to be located in more affluent areas. Notwithstanding these issues, the fact that *parkrun* most commonly remains in public parks means that natural environments largely characterize the experience of taking part and that *parkrun* can significantly contribute to exercise in outdoor, natural settings as an emerging area of research.

Another central component to *parkrun* is that performances are timed and recorded. Before taking part for the first time, participants are required to register online and print off a unique barcode. Upon completing the run, marshals will scan runners' barcode that links the participant with the finishing position and a performance time. This is recorded on the *parkrun* website along with other data including finishing position, age-group ranking, personal best, total number of completed runs and affiliated club (if applicable). The expectation of quantification appears to be in line with recent trends in physical activity participation, which includes practices such as recording step counts and GPS data through wearable technologies, accessible on digital platforms (Millington, 2014). Although the insistence of quantification within physical activity contexts has received much criticism for enabling obsessive self-monitoring and social comparisons, the age-group ranking system could arguably help act against the tendency to marginalize and repudiate aging bodies (Tulle,

2008). For example, Nettleton (2013, p.200) argues that within age-group running classifications "the tyranny of youthful bodies dissipates as some runners even look forward to moving into older age categories precisely because this can generate new opportunities."

The final characteristic of *parkrun* that ought to be highlighted here is that it is free to attend for participants. The organization is an expanding not-for-profit limited company with numerous charitable and commercial partners. However, as *parkrun* has a relatively small number of paid staff (21 in the UK, for example) to oversee its operations and a modest annual budget, the weekly events can only be made possible through the volunteer labor of local participants themselves who occasionally marshal instead of taking part in the spirit of reciprocity. According to the UK *parkrun* annual report in 2016, this labor was the equivalent to over £5 million in that year (*parkrun*, 2016).

While there are costs associated with *parkrun* events such as barcode scanners, signage and high-visibility clothes for marshals, these costs are often covered through small start-up grants when groups of local organizers apply to initiate an event. However, the ongoing costs are minimal because each event is organized by the local volunteers who carry out safety briefings, set up the course signage, guide participants along the route, take photographs and record times. There are a number of implications that follow on from the event being free. First, it ostensibly removes cost as a key barrier to physical activity and reduces exclusivity on financial grounds, and second, it alters the relationship between participants and organizers from one defined by financial transaction to one of camaraderie and cooperation. The "high-vis heroes" are appreciated and celebrated by the runners, and volunteers report positively on the sense of community that they feel from giving back to the event.

15.3 An Overview of Research on Parkrun

Over the last 5 years, there has been growing interest in *parkrun* from researchers across numerous disciplines including public health, sociology, psychology and leisure studies. Indeed, with *parkrun*'s ambition to be proactive in engaging with research, they have worked closely with the Advanced Well-being Research Centre at Sheffield Hallam University (UK) that manages the numerous applications to engage with *parkrun* for research. The resulting literature adds much to what we know about *parkrun* and has implications for our understanding of how nature is implicated.

First, the evidence is emerging of the health and wellbeing benefits of taking part in *parkrun*. Grusuit et al. (2017) found that participants reported a transition from being a non-exerciser to a regular exerciser as a result of *parkrun* which is an important finding given that the greatest health gains are realized when moving from being inactive to active, and there is a dose-response relationship between exercise and health.

212   G. Wiltshire and S. Merchant

Stevinson and Hickson (2018) similarly found significant reductions in body mass index, with a weight loss of 1.1% in their study sample and 2.4% among overweight participants, as well as a 12% increase in fitness. Although this appears to be positive for previously inactive participants, Linton and Valentin (2018) recognize that new runners get injured more frequently than experienced runners which could lead to drop-out. Mental health has been studied too, with Grusiet et al. (2017) reporting that *parkrun* has the potential to improve overall personal well-being and Stevinson and Hickson (2018) reported modest increases in happiness and decreases in perceived stress. In Morris and Scott's (2018) study, "all participants reported that *parkrun* was beneficial to his/her mental health, helping to reduce isolation, depression, anxiety and stress, and increasing confidence as well as giving participants space to think" (p.114).

As a result of these health benefits, there is medical interest in "prescribing" *parkrun* to patients through GP referrals. One GP published a testimonial to this effect, encouraging the prescription of *parkrun*:

> I used to think that inspirational stories were rare and unique, but as time has gone on I've realised just how common tales like these are. It's actually the commonness and not the unusualness that's astonishing. I've seen the wonderful power of how *parkrun* can transform lives and I am convinced that it's the best sort of medicine I can prescribe (Tobin, 2018, p.588).

Research also suggests that *parkrun*'s claim to be "for everyone" is a somewhat reasonable claim, with numerous reports about its inclusivity. An early publication on *parkrun* (Stevinson et al. 2015) noted that perceived inclusivity was evident from interview data, asserting that "the diversity of participants in terms of age, background, and running ability, made *parkrun* feel equally welcoming to all members of the community" (p.172). A participant in their study said,

> It does not allow me to use the barrier "Oh I'm not going to be good enough" because it's so inclusive by involving everyone, and I know there are people who are slower that finish last every week, but still go and try (p.173).

This finding has also been found quantitatively using survey data from new participants, with Cleland et al. (2019) reporting that *parkrun* appears to attract a diversity of participants, including those harder to engage in physical activity such as women, those overweight or obese, and those with poorer health. Indeed, according to Morris and Scott (2018), *parkrun* participants feel a sense of "genuine equality" at *parkrun* between the fastest and slowest runners which helped to avoid novice participants feeling that they were less important than more experienced others. This was summarized by one of their participants who said,

> You can be a runner regardless of whether you can get around in 10 minutes or an hour and 10 minutes. You're exactly the same as those elite runners because you've all set off at the same time and you've all done that course (p.117).

Another key finding from the published literature on *parkrun* is that it is social. Masters' (2014) account describes *parkrun* as "a group activity where you can meet like-minded people" and a participant in Sharman et al.'s (2019, p.166) study observed, "you make contacts then you make friends with people who go [to *parkrun*] and so your social activity instead of going to have a glass of wine is getting up early and going for a run". Notions of "community spirit" were also talked about in Sharman et al.'s (2019) study which is a finding echoed in Hindley's (2018) research into *parkrun* as a "third place" in people's lives, serving an important role distinct from the home and the workplace. For Hindley (2018, p.1), "*parkrun* acts as a temporary public space that is conducive for incidental and casual social interaction." The social aspect of *parkrun* can also be recognized in the way that participants often initially attend with friends, family, colleagues and neighbors and go on to invite others to attend with them.

Wiltshire and Stevinson's (2018) paper on *parkrun* and social capital suggests that *parkrun* participants are likely to be socially connected to *parkrun* prior to attending and that those individuals may, in turn, mobilize other existing social ties to invite and encourage others in their network to attend. This was also found by Sharman et al. (2019), with one participant describing herself as "evangelical" about *parkrun*. Other publications have emphasized that this social aspect is instrumental psychologically because it can increase confidence and motivation among runners which, interestingly, enhances the desire and importance for offering the same support to others (Stevinson et al., 2015). Fostering a sense of community in this way, participants in Morris and Scott's (2018) study saw themselves as being "in it together" with other participants in reference to the experience of sharing the physical act of running and a sense of accomplishment. Wiltshire et al. (2018) took this idea further and suggested that *parkrun* can be viewed as a "health practice" – rather than the more individualistic idea of a personal "behaviour" – through being an opportunity to perform bodywork in a collective context; what was termed "collective body-work."

In addition to research illuminating that *parkrun* can have positive health outcomes, that it is inclusive and social, several studies have reported the impact of *parkrun* on the identity of participants too. In Wiltshire et al.'s (2018) paper, identity (or "subject position") was discussed as a topic of interest because many participants were previously inactive prior to *parkrun* and did not consider themselves to be particularly able runners. One of

214 *G. Wiltshire and S. Merchant*

their participants described herself as, "a person who runs. I'm definitely not a runner because I'm not very good at it" and another said, "a jogger, a jogger. I'm too slow to be a runner. Yeah, I'm too slow to be a runner." In this way, these participants articulated a split between their own embodied subjectivities (health desiring, feeling old or overweight) and the subject position of being a "runner," despite regularly engaging in the activity of running itself. However, as participants become more engaged in *parkrun*, there is research to suggest that they begin to feel more comfortable with identifying as a "runner." For Hindley (2018), qualitative data suggested that *parkrun* fosters a sense of belonging and identity which blurred into other aspects of individuals' social lives, recognizing that identities are inherently social. Further, over a third of Stevinson et al.'s (2015, p. 175) participants reported that *parkrun* had led to the development of a new identity as a runner and had encouraged them to enter races or join a club. Indeed, Stevens et al. (2019, p.227) claim that their findings "indicate positive relationships between individuals developing strong social identities in exercise settings." Returning to Wiltshire et al.'s (2018) paper, they explain this transition by suggesting that *parkrun* offers up an opportunity to identify as a "parkrunner" instead of a "runner" which illustrates that "the social context of *parkrun* allows participants to tentatively reconcile the paradox of being an 'unfit-runner' through their participation" (p.12).

Despite this groundswell of research in recent years, relatively little research has been reported about the experience of *parkrun* as an opportunity to engage in physical activity in natural settings. McCartney (2015, p.1) published a short commentary noting that "running in a park involves none of the vile mirrors that haunt me in gyms; instead, you are surrounded by trees and grass and encouraged by marshals to keep going." Additionally, Stevinson et al. (2015) reported that over half of the participants in their interviews discussed how "being outdoors in the fresh air among beautiful scenery brought additional pleasure to the experience that increased the desire to return each week" (p.175). These examples are useful starting points, but there exists a gap in understanding how the natural context shapes *parkrun* and a need to further unpack, theorize and understand this relationship.

15.4 *Parkrun* and Nature

As we begin to consider the relationship between *parkrun* and nature, it is important to account for the contemporary socio-historical context in which the event has emerged. Offering a different perspective to much of the research on *parkrun* to date, we are interested in drawing out the ways in which *parkrun* can be seen as a reaction to – and sometimes a reflection of – a breadth of issues arising out of the contemporary social conditions associated with neoliberalism and postmodernity. That is, it is possible to view parkrun as a "tonic," in that it tackles a variety of the ills afforded

What Can We Learn About Nature 215

to contemporary "western" cultures in urbanized and sub-urbanized geographies. These built environments afford: an increased distancing from natural environments or green spaces; a rise in occularcentric, sedentary lifestyles associated with screen-based desk work and forms of entertainment, and; a reduction in a sense of community spirit, accentuated by increasingly digitized/mediated forms of communication and human-human connection. With this socio-historical context in mind, in this section, we situate *parkrun* at the nexus of several theoretical debates and offer three explanatory accounts that help advance an understanding of how *parkrun* can enable the potential health benefits of nature and, indeed, how nature can help maintain people's engagement with physical activity. These are: (1) affective green space, (2) affect and the senses and (3) affective communities.

15.4.1 Parkrun Enables Access to Affective "Green Space"

It has been widely reported that exercising in green spaces offers a variety of psychological, biochemical, physiological and social benefits to the practitioner (Gladwell et al., 2013). This "green exercise" – in contrast to exercise in built environments – is believed to account for higher exercise adherence rates, more significant effects on blood pressure levels and greater impact on emotional wellbeing (Little, 2017). Indeed, Howe and Morris (2008) conceptualize "natural" space as a gymnasium, clinic and shrine for runners, whose mobile engagements with green landscapes serve as physiological, rehabilitative and spiritual purposes, respectively. A cursory tour of a few *parkruns* illustrates that the degree to which true "nature" exists in *parkrun*'s landscapes can vary significantly. However, the prevalence of green or even blue space within them does tend to be markedly more prevalent than the day-to-day spaces frequented by postmodern urbanites. Relatedly, a range of studies has detailed the fact that the restorative effects of "nature" are not confined to lengthy exposures to wilderness settings. Indeed, Bratman et al. (2015) suggest that even though brief encounters with nature, the evidence in favor of the positive impact of nature experience on psychological functioning is widespread and robust. Situating oneself in one of *parkrun*'s urban parks, beach trails or country estates then, for the duration of the run, would certainly remain significant.

From a theoretical perspective, such benefits of green exercise have been attributed to the closer ties humans have had with natural environments throughout the evolutionary period (until recently). According to Ulrich (1981; 1979), experiencing nature through the senses activates the human parasympathetic nervous system, which, in turn, lessens stress levels and autonomic arousal (Bratman et al., 2015). Formalized in his "Stress Reduction Theory" (SRT), Ulrich (1981) argues that this is a result of humans' innate association of certain natural features with advantageous

216   G. Wiltshire and S. Merchant

opportunities, for example, refuge, foraging and safety. In line with recent academic applications of theories of affect (although arguably at odds with Non-Representational approaches that denounce attempts to quantify affect), SRT posits that viewing/experiencing natural features, such as those that dominate urban parklands, affectively triggers human physiology (e.g. lowering cortisol secretion, skin conduction and heart rate), in a positive and measurable way.

Not only does *parkrun* enable an exposure to nature which otherwise might have been absent in the weekly routines of many people in contemporary cultures, but it is quite conceivable that green exercise helps maintain regular physical activity by virtue of being in nature. Many of the responses associated with SRT and Non-Representational approaches to affect are felt phenomenologically and subjectively by participants. While it may be unclear whether such experiences are immediately conscious or unconscious, the sense of pleasure which has commonly been self-reported following experiences of physical activity in natural settings strongly suggests that participants themselves are far from ignorant of affect. This is important to point out because pleasure is a key, if frequently overlooked, aspect of people's motivation to maintain physical activity (Phoenix and Orr, 2014). Simply put, if *parkrun* elicits pleasant experiences, then it is more likely that participants will come back next week, especially in the contemporary moment in which such experiences are increasingly scarce.

15.4.2 Parkrun Provides an Affective and Sensory Experience

The different "ratios of sense" that make up the sensuous and perceptual means by which we come to understand and dwell in space are said to be dependent on shared cultural norms and consequently vary according to social context and geographical location (Howes, 1991). Postindustrial "western" society is argued to have alienated itself from nature, so too has it alienated itself from the more proximate senses of smell, touch, proprioception, viscerality and vestibular, while heightening the role of vision (Marks, 2000). As Buck-Morss (1992) argues, even within modernity, development and culture are uneven and complex enough that habitual practices and performances result in different forms of sensory knowledge. Illustrating this, Marks (2000, p.206) explains that cooks, musicians and blind people develop "specialized configurations" of their "sensoria," the sum of their interpreted perception of an environment. So too then can parkrunners specifically, and runners more generally. These "specialized configurations" are what we consider to be particularly important to the study of the body in relation to nature, since parks for leisure foster alternative "ways of being" to the "everyday" spaces of the home or the workplace. Such distinct leisure and sporting practices would similarly result in Marks's (2000) claim that some senses are heightened over others.

What Can We Learn About Nature 217

Running in green space can magnify a variety of challenges for the body, from terrain textures to meteorological conditions, all conditional on the ebbs and flows of the seasons. Giving the body regular opportunities to experience the sensations associated with *parkrun* is, thus, emblematic of a more-than-visual engagement with space in which the body is literally at the whim of the elements. As an example, Brown's (2017) work on the affective capacities of ground textures (mud, roots, inclines, wet rocks, scree, gravel etc.) truly highlights the power of alighting the sense of touch (and to a lesser extent proprioception) through exposure to distinct landscapes of running. As Brown states (2017, p.312), "sensing the terrain through bodily touch, or ground-feel, can play a fundamental role in generating a range of valued affects."

In line with Paterson's (2005) work on the therapeutic capacities of human-human based touch, Brown (2017, p.312) argues that "natural" landscapes of running, and by extension many *parkrun* settings foster a more-than-human notion of "feeling with" the "grain, consistency and shape of the terrain." These experiences are therapeutic in the sense that they offer opportunities to reconnect with the inner ludic desires that postmodern humans so rarely are afforded opportunities to express. For Brown (2017), the "playability" of becoming one with mud and rain and creatively using the ground's inclines to generate speed, determine foothold, bodily angles, or test physical capacities are all aspects of running experience that contribute to conceptualizing distinct landscapes of leisure as salutogenic.

Beyond enabling this otherwise absent sensory experience which has benefits in and of itself, we further suggest that sensory experiences can play a part in maintaining adherence to physical activity as a health-enhancing practice too. First, the senses can serve to access experiences of pleasure through offering an opportunity for the playfulness described above as well as aspects of novelty, nostalgia and exploration. Indeed, participants at *parkrun* are likely to find a common sense of enjoyment in sensing, for example, the warmth of sunshine, the sight of blue skies and the sound of birdsong (although these are, of course, subject to context and individual preference). However, less obvious is the potential for participants to find appreciation for the challenges associated with finding balance when running in strong winds, exposing the skin to cold temperatures and feeling the wetness of rain on the hair, face, body and feet. Yet, in the context of otherwise highly standardized and controlled sensory lives, it is certainly possible that parkrunners report positively on these experiences both as individuals and having experienced them as a collective.

15.4.3 *Parkrun Fosters Affective Communities*

Closely aligned to the notion of sensory (re)awakening and, by extension, sport-specific bodily awareness and mastery is the idea that runners gain capital from the effort and skill they exhibit in distinct running contexts.

It is clear that participating in *parkrun* can yield Bourdieu's (1978) commonly studied concepts of social, cultural, symbolic and even economic capital (e.g. improved fitness resulting in increased workplace productivity) (Wiltshire et al., 2018). However, of particular value in relation to an "affective" sense of connection to other parkrunners is the notion of existential capital. To overcome weather conditions, the impact of these on the material landscape (e.g. mud, ice, groundwater) and significant gradients, taps into some inherent human condition that according to Nettleton (2013, p.197) "cements relations in the sporting field [... and] dilutes other aspects of social inequality." Whilst Nettleton's work concentrates specifically on fell running, she offers many points of departure for thinking about the social aspects of *parkrun*, including the value of social connection in postmodern urban communities that are characterized by a breadth of inequalities. As a free, regular and inclusive event, *parkrun* is a rare physical activity offering within the health and fitness industry, which in theory can bring together people from a wide array of socio-economic backgrounds. Paradoxically, by drawing on Bourdieu's conceptualizations of "fields" and "capital," Nettleton (2013) offers a way of thinking about the power of shared embodied understanding or "existential capital" to better understand how runners (often from different backgrounds/life stages) unite rather than differentiate from each other. In this way, parkrunners become emotionally bonded as part of a somewhat primal "tribe" not merely through engaging in the same activity but by virtue of that activity taking place within a natural landscape.

Understanding affective communities in this way ties the field of *parkrun* to exercise adherence, not purely from the perspective of maintaining health goals, but rather through an augmentation and complication of "other considerations of mental and emotional wellbeing, sociality and confidence" (Little 2017, p.327). Existential capital, argues Nettleton (2013, p.207), "accrues value that is not obviously exchanged for financial reward or symbolic status [... but] has an immediate, fluid and yet enduring quality created within the process of running. The gains therefore are quite abstracted and intrinsic." This form of capital, then, is valued for its own sake (e.g. camaraderie, shared existential understanding, solidarity) and not on the basis of its exchange value (Nettleton, 2013, p.208), a notion further at odds with postmodern capitalist society.

15.5 Implications and Conclusion

In this chapter, we have introduced the increasingly popular 5-km running initiative, "*parkrun*," as a real-world example of how physical activity, health and nature are related to each other in important and interesting ways. After highlighting some of the key characteristics of *parkrun* (it is relatively physically strenuous; it takes place in public parks; it is timed; it is free) we outlined four commonly reported research findings from the

What Can We Learn About Nature 219

growing body of literature on the initiative. This literature provides an evidence base illuminating that *parkrun* (1) can positively impact health and wellbeing, (2) is ability-inclusive, (3) has positive social and community benefits and (4) can impact participants' identities. In an attempt to extend this literature in order to more adequately address emerging debates about nature and health, we have put forward some possible explanatory accounts for understanding the relationship between *parkrun*, nature and health. Setting our arguments within the contemporary socio-historical context, we have suggested that three of the main reasons why people engage, and indeed continue to engage, with *parkrun* are because: i) it enables access to affective "Green Space"; *ii)* it provides an affective and sensory experience; iii) it fosters affective communities. Whilst the theoretical perspectives drawn on to make these arguments (stress reduction theory, phenomenology and Bourdieu's updated take on Capital respectively) are not inherently theories of affect, they each share a notion of the body being subconsciously re-awakened to a primal and shared state through its active engagement with the landscape. For the context of this chapter, that landscape is populated with "green" or "natural" elements that are increasingly edited out of everyday human exposure. Additionally, the activity is that of running – a physical form of exercise that similarly is being supplanted, in this case by sedentary and occularcentric ways of being.

Learning from the success of *parkrun* and from our growing understanding of why it is successful leads to some important implications for policymakers and practitioners working in domains related to physical activity, health and nature. In line with the implicit assumptions of this book, *parkrun* strongly suggests that humans would be foolish to neglect our natural capabilities and inclinations as biological organisms that have emerged as part of, and inseparable from, our natural environment. In order to avoid such neglect, an obvious clarion call would be to support the availability and maintenance of natural environments – particularly in urban and sub-urban areas and particularly in low socioeconomic areas with limited access to opportunities for green exercise. Importantly, our discussion in this chapter has highlighted that many of the positive benefits of *parkrun* are not attributable to nature alone, but rather positive experiences are emergent properties of other phenomena (e.g. sensory experiences and community bonding) occurring in combination with, and in the context of, nature. Furthermore, as we have framed *parkrun* as a "tonic" that can remedy some of the ill effects of living in contemporary western capitalist economies, another broad implication of our chapter is that it is important to continue considering alternative ways of organizing societies in which initiatives like *parkrun* are less appealing, novel and therapeutic because the needs of human societies are more regularly and satisfactorily met in our everyday lives. Nevertheless, *parkrun* represents an exciting avenue for continued investigations into these debates as well

220 G. Wiltshire and S. Merchant

as providing meaningful health-enhancing opportunities to a significant mass of people on a weekly basis across the world.

References

Bell, S. L., Phoenix, C., Lovell, R., & Wheeler, B. W. (2015). Seeking everyday wellbeing: The coast as a therapeutic landscape. *Social Science & Medicine, 142*, 56–67.

Bourdieu, P. (1978) Sport and class. *Social Science Information, 17*(6), 819–840.

Bowler, D. E., Buyung-Ali, L. M., Knight, T. M., & Pullin, A. S. (2010). A systematic review of evidence for the added benefits to health of exposure to natural environments. *BMC Public Health, 10*(1), 456.

Bratman, G. N., Daily, G. C., Levy, B, J., & Gross, J, J. (2015). The benefits of nature experience: improved affect and cognition. *Landscape and Urban Planning, 138*, 41–50.

Brown, K. M. (2017). The hapstic pleasures of ground-feel: The role of textured terrain in motivating regular exercise. *Health & Place, 46*, 307–314.

Buck-Morss, S. (1992). Aesthetics and anaesthetics: Walter Benjamin's artwork essay reconsidered. *October, 62*, 3–41.

Cleland, V., Nash, M., Sharman, M. J., & Claflin, S. (2019). Exploring the health-promoting potential of the "parkrun" phenomenon: What factors are associated with higher levels of participation? *American Journal of Health Promotion, 33*(1), 13–23. http://doi.org/10.1177/0890117118770106

Coleman, T., & Kearns, R. (2015). The role of bluespaces in experiencing place, aging and wellbeing: Insights from Waiheke Island, New Zealand. *Health & Place, 35*, 206–217.

Cutforth, C. (2017). So much more than a run in the park. *The Leisure Review, 84*. Retrieved from http://www.theleisurereview.co.uk/articles17/cutforth_parkrun.html

De Vries, S., Verheij, R., Groenewagen, P., Spreeuwenberg, P., 2003. Natural environments e healthy environments? An exploratory analysis of the relationship between greenspace and health. EnvironMent and Planning A, 35, 1717e1731.

Department for Environment, Food and Rural Affairs (2017) Evidence statement on the links between natural environments and human health, available online accessible here: https://ore.exeter.ac.uk/repository/handle/10871/31598.

Department of Health and Social Care (2019) Physical activity guidelines: UK Chief Medical Officers' report, available at: https://www.gov.uk/government/publications/physical-activity-guidelines-uk-chief-medical-officers-report.

Foley, R. (2015). Swimming in Ireland: Immersions in therapeutic blue space. *Health & Place, 35*, 218–225.

Gladwell, V., Brown, D., Wood, C., Sandercock, G. & Barton, J. (2013). The great outdoors: how a green exercise environment can benefit all. *Extreme Physiology & Medicine, 2*, 1–7.

Hartig, T., Mitchell, R., De Vries, S., & Frumkin, H., 2014. Nature and health. Annual Review Public Health, 35, 207e228.

Hindley, D. (2018). "More than just a run in the park": An exploration of parkrun as a shared leisure space. *Leisure Sciences, 0400*, 1–21. http://doi.org/10.1080/01490400.2017.1410741.

What Can We Learn About Nature 221

Howe, P. & Moriss, C. (2008). An exploration of the co-production of performance running bodies and natures within "running taskscapes". *Journal of Sport and Social Issues, 33*, 308–330.

Howes, D. (1991) *Varieties of Sensory Experience.* Toronto: Toronto University Press.

Linton, L., & Valentin, S. (2018). Running with injury: A study of UK novice and recreational runners and factors associated with running related injury. Journal of Science and Medicine in Sport, 21(12), 1221–1225. https://doi.org/10.1016/j.jsams.2018.05.021

Little, J. (2017) Running, health and the disciplining of women's bodies: The influence of technology and nature. Health and Place, 46, 322–327.

Maas, J., Verheij, R., Groenewegen, P., De Vries, S., Spreeuwenberg, P., 2006. Green space, urbanity, and health: how strong is the relation? Journal of Epidemiology Community Health, 60, 587e592.

Marks, L. (2000) *The Skin of the Film: Intercultural Cinema, Embodiment, and the Senses.* London: Duke University Press.

Masters, N. (2014). Parkrun eases the loneliness of the long-distance runner. *British Journal of General Practice, 64*(625), 408. http://doi.org/10.3399/bjgp14X681025.

Merchant, S. (2017) Therapeutic movement/leisure practices. In Silk, M., Andrews, D. & Thorpe, H. *Routledge Handbook of Physical Cultural Studies.* London: Routledge (pp. 72–83).

Millington, B. (2014). Amusing ourselves to life: Fitness consumerism and the birth of bio-games. *Journal of Sport and Social Issues, 38*(6), 491–508.

Mirvis, D. M. (2009). From research to public policy: An essential extension of the translation research agenda. *Clinical and Translational Science, 2*(5), 379–381.

Morris, P., & Scott, H. (2018). Not just a run in the park: A qualitative exploration of parkrun and mental health. *Advances in Mental Health, 17*, 110–123. http://doi.org/10.1080/18387357.2018.1509011

Nettleton, S. (2013). Cementing relations within a sporting field: Fell running in the english lake district and the acquisition of existential capital. *Cultural Sociology, 7*(2), 196–210.

Ogilvie, D., Craig, P., Griffin, S., Macintyre, S., & Wareham, N. J. (2009). A translational framework for public health research. *BMC Public Health, 9*(1), 116.

Parkrun (2016). parkrun UK: Annual run report 2016, available at: https://blog.parkrun.com/uk/2017/04/27/parkrun-uk-2016-run-report/.

Parkrun (2019). parkrun.com, available at: www.parkrun.com.

Paterson, M. (2005). Affecting touch: towards a felt phenomenology of therapeutic touch. In Davidson, J., Bondi, L. & Smith, M. *Emotional geographies.* Ashgate, Aldershot: Hants (pp. 161–176.)

Phoenix, C., & Orr, N. (2014). Pleasure: A forgotten dimension of physical activity in older age. *Social Science & Medicine, 115*, 94–102.

Reece, L. J., Quirk, H., Wellington, C., Haake, S. J., & Wilson, F. (2019). Bright spots, physical activity investments that work: Parkrun; A global initiative striving for healthier and happier communities. *British Journal of Sports Medicine, 53*(6), 326–327. http://doi.org/10.1136/bjsports-2018-100041.

Sharman, M. J., Nash, M., & Cleland, V. (2019). Health and broader community benefit of parkrun—An exploratory qualitative study. *Health Promotion Journal of Australia, 30*(2), 163–171. http://doi.org/10.1002/hpja.182.

222   G. Wiltshire and S. Merchant

Stevens, M., Rees, T., & Polman, R. (2019). Social identification, exercise participation, and positive exercise experiences: Evidence from parkrun. *Journal of Sports Sciences, 37*(2), 221–228.

Stevinson, C., & Hickson, M. (2018). Changes in physical activity, weight and wellbeing outcomes among attendees of a weekly mass participation event: a prospective 12-month study. *Journal of Public Health, 41*, 807–814. http://doi.org/10.1093/pubmed/fdy178

Stevinson, C., Wiltshire, G., & Hickson, M. (2015). Facilitating Participation in Health-Enhancing Physical Activity: A Qualitative Study of parkrun. *International Journal of Behavioral Medicine, 22*(2), 170–177. http://doi.org/10.1007/s12529-014-9431-5

Thomas, F. (2015). The role of natural environments within women's everyday health and wellbeing in Copenhagen, Denmark. *Health & Place, 35*, 187–195.

Tobin, S. (2018). Life & times prescribing parkrun. *British Journal of General Practice, 68*(677), 588. http://doi.org/10.3399/bjgp18X700133

Tulle, E. (2008) *Ageing, the body and social change.* London: Routledge.

Ulrich, R. S. (1979) Visual landscapes and psychological well-being. *Landscape Research, 4* (1), 17–23

Ulrich, R. S. (1981) Naturak versus urban scenes: Some psychophysiological effects. *Environment and Behaviour, 13*(5), 523–556

Wiltshire, G. R., Fullagar, S., & Stevinson, C. (2018). Exploring parkrun as a social context for collective health practices: Running with and against the moral imperatives of health responsibilisation. *Sociology of Health and Illness, 40*(1), 3–17. http://doi.org/10.1111/1467-9566.12622

Wiltshire, G., & Stevinson, C. (2018). Exploring the role of social capital in community-based physical activity: qualitative insights from parkrun. *Qualitative Research in Sport, Exercise and Health, 10*(1), 47–62. http://doi.org/10.1080/2159676X.2017.1376347.

16 Students' Appropriation of Space in Education Outside the Classroom. Some Aspects on Physical Activity and Health from a Pilot Study with 5th-Graders in Germany

Christoph Mall, Jakob von Au, and Ulrich Dettweiler

16.1 Space Appropriation in Educational Settings

The quality of students' space appropriation and the respective influence on their knowledge acquisition, behavior change, PA and health is strongly connected to the properties of the teaching environments and the pedagogical concepts, which has been widely discussed in academic disciplines such as philosophy and aesthetics (Böhme, 2000; 2002), school architecture (Böhme, 2009), education (Nugel, 2014) and public health (Völker, Matros, & Claßen, 2016). Böhme, for instance, understands space in states of aesthetic atmospheres which he describes as standing "between subjects and objects" and create, thus, the emotional experiences of the objective world. Nugel, on the other side, asks from a critical constructivist perspective what kind of knowledge about space is generated in narrative scientific discourses, and what significance such discourses have for pedagogical space theory and practice. Both understand space as a value-loaded concept, which suggests the relevance of space in educational settings. The children's "co-curating of relational spaces" (Thiel, 2018) or concepts compatible with a comprehensive understanding of children's mobility in (urban) open spaces, such as place attachment, affordances, wayfinding and prospect-refuge (Johansson, Mårtensson, Jansson, & Sternudd, 2020) have become the focus of research in order to support children's independent and active mobility. One promising approach to combine meaningful learning opportunities, PA and well-being with an explicit concept of space is the "Education Outside the Classroom" (EOtC) movement. EOtC can be described as regular weekly or bi-weekly compulsory school and curriculum-based education in a natural or cultural setting outside the school building (Bentens et al., 2009). EOtC is mainly based on teaching concepts called udeskole or uteskole from Denmark and Norway and can be considered a grassroots movement initiated by enthusiastic teachers. It has, therefore, by nature, different shades in its meanings and practise.

DOI: 10.4324/9781003154419-19

224   *C. Mall, J.v. Au, and U. Dettweiler*

In this context, EOtC can provide meaningful opportunities for students to explore different natural and cultural places, to learn *about*, *from* and *within* them, and to be physically active in the appropriation of space.

16.2 Education Outside the Classroom – EOtC

During EOtC, lessons are in accordance with the syllabus and regularly take place outside the school building. The focus is on student-centered teaching, interdisciplinary learning, practical learning and the conscious use of natural and cultural places (Bentsen, Mygind, & Randrup, 2009). The meaning of "regularly" differs depending on regional aspects and specific school environments. Especially in Scandinavia and the United Kingdom, different forms of EOtC are widely practised. These forms also include different age groups in relation to different school systems. EOtC or *udeskole (Denmark)/uteskole (Norway)* can be described as a grassroots movement and began in the 1990s in Denmark with a handful of motivated teachers. Barfod et al. (2016) conducted a representative, nation-wide survey and conclude that in 2014, 17.9% of all Danish public schools and 19.4% of all independent and private schools practice EOtC with at least one class, which is an increase from 14% of public and independent/private schools in 2007. That describes a potential shift from traditional indoor teaching towards more variety and the use of places outside the classroom. In our systematic literature review (Becker, Lauterbach, Spengler, Dettweiler, & Mess, 2017), we evaluated the possible effects of regular outdoor teaching. We found that EOtC can have positive effects on students' academic learning, social interaction, PA and mental health. However, the average methodological quality of the 13 evaluated scientific studies was mediocre and, therefore, the scientific evidence was rather limited until spring 2016. Recently published and methodologically more reliable studies indicate that EOtC can lead to an improvement in reading performance (Otte et al., 2019), learning motivation (Bølling, Otte, Elsborg, Nielsen, & Bentsen, 2018), social behavior (Bølling, Niclasen, Bentsen, & Nielsen, 2019), as well as well-being (Jørring, Bølling, Nielsen, Stevenson, & Bentsen, 2019) and, importantly, increased PA among boys (Schneller et al., 2017; Schneller, Schipperijn, Nielsen, & Bentsen, 2017). For students with comparatively low socioeconomic status, an inverse correlation between EOtC and hyperactivity-inattention and peer problems has been reported (Bølling et al., 2019). During outdoor classes, high levels of light PA (LPA) are associated with a health-related reduction of their cortisol level (Becker et al., 2019; Dettweiler, Becker, Auestad, Simon, & Kirsch, 2017), and in addition, breaks and rest periods during outdoor lessons seem to have a positive effect on stress reduction (Mygind, Stevenson, Liebst, Konvalinka, & Bentsen, 2018). These specific findings sit within a body of research that suggests natural green or blue environments, i.e. landscapes covered by forests, meadows, rivers or lakes, generally provide great potential to enhance students' health (Mygind et al., 2018; Roberts, Hinds, & Camic, 2019).

Research has found that increasing numbers of teachers see EOtC has great potential to improve students' learning outcomes and everyday competences (Mygind, Bølling, M., & Barfod, K.S.). From the educational or pedagogical perspective, it facilitates inquiry-based teaching and, therefore, student-centered learning with cognitive challenges (Barfod & Daugbjerg, 2018), and fosters school and teaching development processes in terms of cross-curricular lessons, testing of new methods and extension of multifaceted competencies (Sahrakhiz, 2017).

With respect to the students' strategies to deal with space in EOtC, an early phenomenological study from Norway by Tordsson (2003) described the different ways children and adolescents understand spatial qualities of natural places. Tordsson was especially interested in the *affordance* of natural environmental "objects" as trees or open meadows, in that he portrayed the *objects' qualities or properties that defined their possible uses*. He elucidated how environments and "objects" offer opportunities to children to perform certain actions: the tree affords to be climbed, the meadow to be played in. Tordsson suggests that we (children) have a common understanding to respond to certain spatial properties and qualities. In another Norwegian study, Fiskum and Jacobsen (2013) found that EOtC offered an increased variability of such affordances compared to indoor classes, and that compared to girls, boys more often used natural elements, which *might* indicate that boys are relatively more connected to the specific outdoor environments, thereby predisposing them to more explorative approaches to appropriating the space. Based on interviews with primary school students, Sahrakhiz, Harring, & Witte (2017) argued that EOtC, which most often takes place in natural green environments, provides learning opportunities and challenges and involves students physically, cognitively, perceptually and socially. Space appropriation is especially promoted in play through movement and exploration. Hereby, the student-led activities seem to promote motivation and contentment, whereas teacher-led activities were partially perceived with lack of interest or disaffirmation (Armbrüster et al., 2016). In summary, EOtC practice, which is often based in natural green and blue spaces, offers several opportunities for student developments during compulsory school time: it can promote PA, wellbeing and learning motivation.

During EOtC, the characteristics of place and space, as well as the pedagogical concepts, are essential for the aforementioned benefits; the appropriation of space seems to play a crucial part in modeling the benefits of EOtC. In the following section, we provide insights from data collected at a school practicing EOtC in Germany. The data focus on the relevance of students' PA and health with respect to space appropriation.

16.3 Research Example of Education Outside the Classroom from Heidelberg, Germany

In this example, we were interested in comparing the PA levels and students' perceptions of PA, social relations, learning and place of 5th-grade students (ages 10–11) who took part in EOtC classes, with students who took part in regular classroom classes (5th- and 6th-grade students, ages 10–12). The EOtC students studied the subjects of biology, geography, natural phenomena and physical education, in one compulsory school day per week mostly in a nearby forest. Our data collection took place in the school year 2014–2015 and three classes were enrolled in the EOtC class. Students from a regular (non-EOtC) class served as a control group. The EOtC teachers' focus was to facilitate student-centered, hands-on and experimental learning situations and to promote education for sustainable development in the outdoor setting. Different opportunities for problem-solving, co-operation, experimentation and to be physically active on pupils' free choice were enabled by the out-of-classroom setting. Across the entire school year, specific places in the forest were visited on a regular basis.

In order to understand certain aspects of students' health, academic learning and their social relations, we measured students' physical activity via accelerometry during the fall, spring and summer season. We also conducted focus interviews with specific focus regarding students' perceptions of physical activity, social relations, learning and place. We translated the interviews from German to English. For further details regarding the overall study aims, design and results, see our peer-reviewed published articles that are partially based on data sets discussed in this chapter (Becker et al., 2019; Dettweiler et al., 2017).

We analyzed students' PA according to the Compositional Data Analysis approach (Chastin, Palarea-Albaladejo, Dontje, & Skelton, 2015), and our results from this are descriptively presented in ternary plots (Figure 16.1). Ternary plots enable graphic presentation of data from human behavior that is perfectly co-dependent (i.e. interrelated, not independent of each other), such as students' sedentary behavior, LPA and moderate-vigorous PA (MVPA), measured during a school day. A reduction of the amount of time spent in one behavior automatically leads to an increase in at least one of the other behaviors. Therefore, to acknowledge the inherent relationship or co-dependency between sedentary behavior and physical activity is crucial to derive health recommendations.

16.3.1 Findings, Discussion and Future Directions

The analysis shows that the EOtC students exhibited relatively lower relative amounts of sedentary behavior and completed relatively more of LPA and MVPA in comparison to the regular classroom students.

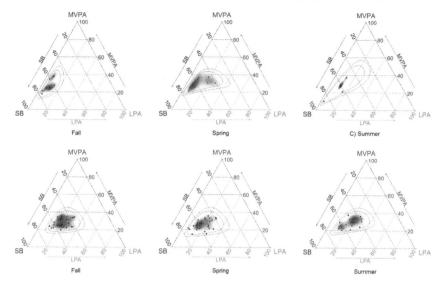

Figure 16.1 Ternary plots of the compositions of students' mean time spent in sedentary behavior (SB), light physical activity (LPA), and moderate-to-vigorous physical activity PA (MVPA). Panel A shows the regular classroom students; panel B shows the EOtC students; both panels are segregated by season (fall; spring; summer). A) Regular classroom students B) EOtC students

Figure 16.1 shows ternary plots of students' sedentary behavior, LPA and MVPA for the regular classroom students (in panel A) and the EOtC students (in panel B), each segregated by season (fall, spring and summer). Ternary plots are used the visually present the distribution of the sample composition and can, therefore, be understood as scatterplots of compositions. The black dots represent the measured behavior of every student in relation to sedentary behavior, LPA and MVPA during one school day. The blue shades indicate the density of similar behaviors within the group; the more intense the color the higher the density. The circles represent the 95% and 99% probability regions of all students. One potential confounder for students' PA during school time is the season of the year. That is because weather conditions such as temperature, precipitation and wind vary in the Heidelberg region and one could hypothesize that students are less active during unpleasant conditions. The 95% and 99% probability regions for the EOtC students are closer to the center of the ternary plot.

Our analysis of students' sedentary behavior and PA indicates that students sit less and are more active during EOtC in comparison to normal indoor classes. This is an important empirical hint that EOtC taking place in natural green and blue environments seems to be beneficial for students' PA and health. We discuss the meaning of students' PA in relation to their appropriation of space by means of the conducted focus interviews. In these interviews, the students described in rich detail what they have explored at specific places in the forest, how it is connected to the learned content and compare it to similar situations during normal indoor classes. They describe their possibilities to be physically active during lessons of biology, geography and natural phenomena that are traditionally not associated with high levels of PA, as the indoor classroom naturally limits the available space.

> And here it is just like this, if we do an experiment then we can really do it. For example, if we do something with water, then it is great with the stream down there and in school, there is no such thing. And then we only do it with such glasses, and with some you can't do it at all, because you really need such a small river.

The student describes an experiment with the aim to measure and understand flow velocity. In the outdoor setting, it has a meaning as a natural phenomenon. From the students' perspective, it would not make sense to transfer the experiment to an indoor setting, as the practical relevance and the phenomenon by itself would get lost. The experiment was closely connected to students' PA, as they needed to walk or run between different stations while developing boats, measurement tools and gathering information by talking to the teachers and classmates.

> I'm more immune, I haven't been out in the fresh air that much yet, and now I am. My immune system was strengthened, so I was less ill. And it was really nice once when a man came who knew mushrooms really well and then we looked for mushrooms and then he told us what they were called and what they could do. And in the end we cooked the edible mushrooms and ate them together. And he showed us mushrooms that are poisonous. And if you can see them only on pictures, then you cannot remember that as well as if you see them in real.

The student reflects about his health conditions reasoning that the fresh air during EOtC was beneficial for his immune system, probably recalling some conversations with his parents or teachers. Furthermore, he describes an incident in which an expert helped the students find and identify mushrooms. The combined active process of walking around in the forest searching for mushrooms, comparing edible and poisonous ones, and the group experience of outdoor cooking enables long-term memory. The rather inactive method of working with pictures of mushrooms in a book would hardly be able to provide such rich experiences and to have an – subjectively observed – impact on students' health.

> We can even walk during class. In principle, we always move, except when we write something down or talk about something. And you can imagine everything much better.

> For some children it is much easier to understand, because here you can explain it well and sometimes when we talk about something, then we also look for animals that look like this. For some children showing thinks helps much more.

Student's report that they are able to be physically active during class. They walk or run to different places within the forest and the nearby environment of the forester's lodge. Seeing and getting in touch with these place and talking about the experiences can be especially helpful to better understand the contents.

The students furthermore spoke about their ability to concentrate in relation to PA and the environment.

> But from the concentration I find it better on a forest day, because there we are a lot outside and there you can walk a bit and then you can concentrate again.
>
> I also think you can't concentrate so well in the forest. But the good thing about the forest is, you can see the examples, you can watch them live.
>
> I also think it's a bit harder to concentrate in the forest because you're distracted from other things like birds or ants or something like that, but in the forest you're much freer and I like everything except the forester's lodge.

These examples demonstrate different experiences, as for some students the outdoor environment seems to be better place for concentration, whereas for others it involved many distractions. Students' encounter and interaction with original examples of the world, which are explicit parts of the EOtC concept, seem to be challenging and promoting students' cognitive functions at the same time. From a general perspective, PA in children is associated with positive psychophysiological effects, e.g. more efficient brain activity, better scholastic achievements and higher cognitive performance (Erickson, Hillman, & Kramer, 2015; Mandolesi et al., 2018; Sibley & Etnier, 2003). Rasberry et al.'s (2011) systematic literature review found that 50.5% of studies reported statistically significant positive associations between students' PA and academic achievement (48% reported no statistically significant associations and only 1.5% reported statistically significant negative associations). This indicates the relevance of students' PA in relation to their being able to concentrate during school time. However, students' academic achievement within EOtC needs to be further investigated.

As a conclusive remark, we can say that the relatively more-open learning situation in EOtC invites the children to more physical active compared to "normal" indoor schooling.

The mere lack of classroom walls and the increased opportunity to encounter natural objects seems to inspire students to ask new questions and to solve problems in unconventional and creative ways. That is in concordance with the discussed observations by Fiskum & Jacobsen (2013) and Johansson et al. (2020). Furthermore, many students use the "physical freedom" that comes with open learning spaces to interact with students that they rarely meet in rigid classroom situations and to satisfy their need for movement during complicated understanding processes. Even though we still see a shortage in reliable studies on learning outcomes in EOtC, our strong impression as researchers and practitioners in this field is that children can highly benefit from EOtC in physical as well as in social, methodical and personal dimensions. The presented results from Heidelberg offer insights into one approach in the evolving field of EOtC research. We expect that many different viewpoints will shed further light on the potential benefits and barriers of taking students outside the classroom.

In conclusion, the quality of and variety of students' appropriation of space in educational settings is highly important for their individual learning experience. EOtC, which often takes place in natural green and blue environments, offers very rich opportunities for appropriation of space. This seems to be beneficial to the students' social interaction, academic achievement, and physical and psychological health. Yet, future research in EOtC should examine those relationships more solidly with larger longitudinal studies.

References

Armbrüster, C., Gräfe, R., Harring, M., Sahrakhiz, S., Schenk, D., & Witte, M. D. (2016). Playing, Moving, Exploring – Primary School Children's Practices of Appropriating Space in the German Draußenschule. *Discourse. Journal of Childhood and Adolescense Research, 4*, 473–489. doi:10.3224/diskurs.v11i4.25605

Barfod, K., & Daugbjerg, P. (2018). Potentials in Udeskole: Inquiry-Based Teaching Outside the Classroom. *Frontiers in Education, 3*. doi:10.3389/feduc.2018.00034

Barfod, K., Ejbye-Ernst, N., Mygind, L., & Bentsen, P. (2016). Increased Provision of Udeskole in Danish Schools: An Updated National Population Survey. *Urban Forestry & Urban Greening, 20*, 277–281. doi:10.1016/j.ufug.2016.09.012

Becker, C., Lauterbach, G., Spengler, S., Dettweiler, U., & Mess, F. (2017). Effects of Regular Classes in Outdoor Education Settings: A Systematic Review on Students' Learning, Social and Health Dimensions. *International Journal of Environmental Research and Public Health, 14*(5), 485. doi:10.3390/ijerph14050485

Becker, C., Schmidt, S., Neuberger, E. W. I., Kirsch, P., Simon, P., & Dettweiler, U. (2019). Children's Cortisol and Cell-Free DNA Trajectories in Relation to Sedentary Behavior and Physical Activity in School: A Pilot Study. *Frontiers in Public Health, 7*(26). doi:10.3389/fpubh.2019.00026

Bentsen, P., Mygind, E., & Randrup, T. B. (2009). Towards an Understanding of Udeskole: Education Outside the Classroom in a Danish context. *Education, 37*(1), 29–44. doi:10.1080/03004270802291780

Students' Appropriation of Space 231

Berndt, C., Kalisch, C., & Krüger, A. (2016). *Räume Bilden – Pädagogische Perspektiven Auf Den Raum*. Bad Heilbrunn: Verlag Julius Klinkhardt.

Böhme, G. (2000). Acoustic Atmospheres. A Contribution to the Study of Ecological Aesthetics. *Soundscapes, 1*(1), 14–18.

Böhme, G. (2002). *Die Natur vor uns. Naturphilosophie in Pragmatischer Hinsicht [Nature in front of ourselves. Nature Philosophy from a Pragmatist Point of View]*. Zug: Die Graue Edition.

Böhme, J. (2009). *Schularchitektur im Interdisziplinären Diskurs*. Wiesbaden: Springer.

Bølling, M., Niclasen, J., Bentsen, P., & Nielsen, G. (2019). Association of Education Outside the Classroom and Pupils' Psychosocial Well-Being: Results From a School Year Implementation. *Journal of Scoolh Health, 89*(3), 210–218. doi:10.1111/josh.12730

Bølling, M., Otte, C. R., Elsborg, P., Nielsen, G., & Bentsen, P. (2018). The Association Between Education Outside the Classroom and Students' School Motivation: Results from a One-School-Year Quasi-Experiment. *International Journal of Educational Research, 89*, 22–35. doi:10.1016/j.ijer.2018.03.004

Chastin, S. F. M., Palarea-Albaladejo, J., Dontje, M. L., & Skelton, D. A. (2015). Combined Effects of Time Spent in Physical Activity, Sedentary Behaviors and Sleep on Obesity and Cardio-Metabolic Health Markers: A Novel Compositional Data Analysis Approach. *PLoS One, 10*(10), e0139984. doi:10.1371/journal.pone.0139984

Dettweiler, U., Becker, C., Auestad, B. H., Simon, P., & Kirsch, P. (2017). Stress in School. Some Empirical Hints on the Circadian Cortisol Rhythm of Children in Outdoor and Indoor Classes. *International Journal of Environmental Research and Public Health, 14*(5), 475. doi:10.3390/ijerph14050475

Erickson, K. I., Hillman, C. H., & Kramer, A. F. (2015). Physical activity, brain, and cognition. *Current Opinion in Behavioral Sciences, 4*, 27–32. doi:10.1016/j.cobeha.2015.01.005

Fiskum, T. A., & Jacobsen, K. (2013). Outdoor education gives fewer demands for action regulation and an increased variability of affordances. *Journal of Adventure Education and Outdoor Learning, 13*(1), 76–99. doi:10.1080/14729679.2012.702532

Johansson, M., Mårtensson, F., Jansson, M., & Sternudd, C. (2020). Chapter Twelve - Urban space for children on the move. In E. O. D. Waygood, M. Friman, L. E. Olsson, & R. Mitra (Eds.), *Transportation and Children's Well-Being* (pp. 217–235). Amsterdam, Netherlands: Elsevier.

Jørring, A. H., Bølling, M., Nielsen, G., Stevenson, M. P., & Bentsen, P. (2019). Swings and Roundabouts? Pupils' Experiences of Social and Academic Well-Being in Education Outside the Classroom. *Education 3–13*, 1–16. doi:10.1080/03004279.2019.1614643

Mandolesi, L., Polverino, A., Montuori, S., Foti, F., Ferraioli, G., Sorrentino, P., & Sorrentino, G. (2018). Effects of Physical Exercise on Cognitive Functioning and Wellbeing: Biological and Psychological Benefits. *Frontiers in Psychology, 9*, 509–509. doi:10.3389/fpsyg.2018.00509

Mygind, E., Bølling, M., & Seierøe Barfod, K. (2018). Primary Teachers' Experiences with Weekly Education Outside the Classroom During a Year. *Education, 47*(5), 599–611. doi:10.1080/03004279.2018.1513544

232 *C. Mall, J.v. Au, and U. Dettweiler*

Mygind, L., Stevenson, M., Liebst, L., Konvalinka, I., & Bentsen, P. (2018). Stress Response and Cognitive Performance Modulation in Classroom versus Natural Environments: A Quasi-Experimental Pilot Study with Children. *International Journal of Environmental Research and Public Health, 15*(6), 1098. doi:10.3390/ijerph15061098

Nugel, M. (2014). *Erziehungswissenschaftliche Diskurse über Räume der Pädagogik.* Wiesbaden: Springer.

Oelkers, J. (1993). Erziehungsstaat und pädagogischer Raum: Die Funktion des idealen Ortes in der Theorie der Erziehung. *Zeitschrift für Pädagogik, 39,* 631–648.

Otte, C. R., Bølling, M., Stevenson, M. P., Ejbye-Ernst, N., Nielsen, G., & Bentsen, P. (2019). Education Outside the Classroom Increases Children's Reading Performance: Results from a One-Year Quasi-Experimental Study. *International Journal of Educational Research, 94,* 42–51. doi:10.1016/j.ijer.2019.01.009

Rasberry, C. N., Lee, S. M., Robin, L., Laris, B. A., Russell, L. A., Coyle, K. K., & Nihiser, A. J. (2011). The Association between School-Based Physical Activity, Including Physical Education, and Academic Performance: A Systematic Review of the Literature. *Preventive Medicine, 52,* S10–S20. doi:10.1016/j.ypmed.2011.01.027

Roberts, A., Hinds, J., & Camic, P. M. (2019). Nature Activities and Wellbeing in Children and Young People: a Systematic Literature Review. *Journal of Adventure Education and Outdoor Learning,* 1–21. doi:10.1080/14729679.2019.1660195

Sahrakhiz, S. (2017). The 'Outdoor School' as a School Improvement Process: Empirical Results from the Perspective of Teachers in Germany. *Education, 46*(7), 825–837. doi:10.1080/03004279.2017.1371202

Sahrakhiz, S., Harring, M., & Witte, M. D. (2017). Learning Opportunities in the Outdoor School–Empirical Findings on Outdoor School in Germany from the Children's Perspective. *Journal of Adventure Education and Outdoor Learning, 18*(3), 214–226. doi:10.1080/14729679.2017.1413404

Schneller, M. B., Duncan, S., Schipperijn, J., Nielsen, G., Mygind, E., & Bentsen, P. (2017). Are Children Participating in a Quasi-experimental Education Outside the Classroom Intervention more Physically Active? *BMC Public Health, 17*(1), 523. doi:10.1186/s12889-017-4430-5

Schneller, M. B., Schipperijn, J., Nielsen, G., & Bentsen, P. (2017). Children's Physical Activity During a Segmented School Week: Results from a Quasi-Experimental Education Outside the Classroom Intervention. *International Journal of Behavioral Nutrition and Physical Activity, 14*(1), 80. doi:10.1186/s12966-017-0534-7

Sibley, B. A., & Etnier, J. L. (2003). The Relationship between Physical Activity and Cognition in Children: A Meta-Analysis. *Pediatric Exercise Science, 15*(3), 243–256. doi:10.1123/pes.15.3.243

Thiel, J. J. (2018). 'A Cool Place Where We Make Stuff': Co-curating Relational Spaces of Muchness. In C. M. Schulte and C. M. Thompson (Ed.), *Communities of Practice: Art, Play, and Aesthetics in Early Childhood* (pp. 23–37). Cham: Springer.

Tordsson, B. (2003). *Å Svare på Naturens Åpne Tiltale.* Oslo: Institutt for samfunnsfag.

Völker, S., Matros, J., & Claßen, T. (2016). Determining Urban Open Spaces for Health-Related Appropriations: A Qualitative Analysis on the Significance of Blue Space. *Environmental Earth Sciences, 75*(13), 1067. doi:10.1007/s12665-016-5839-3

von Au, J. (2018). Draußentage - Lernen mit Herz, Hand und viel Verstand. *Pädagogik, 4,* 10–13. doi:10.3262/PAED1804010

17 Outdoor and Adventurous Activities in Supporting Wounded, Injured and Sick Military Personnel and Veterans

Christopher William Philip Kay and Rebecca Jena Sutton

Interventions that positively influence the mental and physical well-being of wounded, injured and sick military personnel (WIS-MP) are now found across the globe (Bauer, Newbury-Birch, Robalino, Ferguson, & Wigham, 2018; Caddick & Smith, 2018; Dietrich, Joye, & Garcia, 2015; Straits-Tröster et al., 2011). Many of these interventions are based on Outdoor and Adventurous Activities (OAA) precisely because they offer unique opportunities for mental health benefits, additional to those of physical activity alone (Buckley, Brough, & Westaway, 2018; Lawton, Brymer, Clough, & Denovan, 2017; Niedermeier, Hartl, & Kopp, 2017; Pasanen, Tyrväinen, & Korpela, 2014).

In recent years, an increasing focus has been placed on understanding, and more extensively evidencing, the impact of OAA for individual beneficiaries and society. As an example, the European Network of Outdoor Sport recently included an adaptive sport and adventurous activity course that supports WIS-MP and veterans in their project, 'The Benefit of Outdoor Sport for Society' (Gregory et al. 2019).

Here we outline how OAA are being/have been used to support military personnel and veterans around the world. In this, we highlight how the unique features of OAA are being used to release the adaptive well-being capacities of WIS-MP. Our evidence can be used to better inform any level of decision-making around policy and funding. The body of evidence we present represents an important new collation of the positive impact OAA can have on people's lives. This extends beyond the rich day-to-day experiences that will be familiar to practitioners. We also describe how to establish practice-based evidence that will generate a compelling case to support investment.

17.1 Current Initiatives Utilizing OAA to Improve the Well-Being of Serving and Ex-Military Personnel

17.1.1 US and Canada

Using OAA to support veterans has been most enthusiastically adopted in the US. Reflecting the diversity of program content, water-sport expeditions

DOI: 10.4324/9781003154419-20

234   *C.W.P. Kay and R.J. Sutton*

have used oar boats, paddle boats, rafts and kayaks for river running as well as fly-fishing trips (Anderson, Monroy, & Keltner, 2018; Dustin, Bricker, Arave, & Wall, 2011; Mowatt & Bennett, 2011). The US features over 800 therapeutic recreation specialists who deliver veterans' programs within the Veterans Affairs Health Care System (Petersen 2017). That support is driven by a far-reaching appreciation among practitioners that OAA in naturalistic settings can help address basic, yet still controversial, questions about emotions and enhanced emotional control (Anderson et al., 2017).

OAA interventions are being used as an adjunct to formal, but over-stretched, clinical services. Indeed, in the US, formal clinical support for military veterans has been insufficient (Berman et al., 2018). To under-line the scale of demand, even though services were expanded in 2017 to secure more than seven million veteran visits, 28% (238,000 of 847,0000) of veterans who applied for health care services died before receiving care (Berman et al., 2018).

As a precursor to OAA, Wilderness experience programs were one of the earliest documented forms of recreational therapy, deployed in the 19th century. In this approach, "camp cures" were prescribed for mentally exhausted or distressed individuals, located in forests or on ranches. In the US the belief was that breathing fresh air and living close to nature would replenish participants 'nervous energy' (Dietrich et al., 2015; Schuster, 2003). Modern-day wilderness expeditions, such as the Warrior Hike Program (WHP), which consists of a 6-month hike of the Appalachian Trail, aim to provide a positive therapeutic effect by immersing partici-pants in the natural environment. The WHP also aimed to enhance the psychological well-being of US combat veterans presenting with symptoms of war-originating Post-Traumatic Stress Disorder (PTSD) (Hyer et al., 1996). Capitalising on a strong physical demand, the WHP also aims to facilitate further purposeful change by establishing bonds with other combat veterans and by gradually re-socializing participants into society. Recent research identified four key themes in veteran's accounts of their WHP experiences: improved social reconnection, life-improving change, inner peace and psychological healing, processing and reflection (Dietrich et al., 2015). Similarly, in a 9-day climb of Mt Kilimanjaro, physically injured Canadian veterans experienced increased self-determination, coping skills and perceived increase of social support during the experience, fostering psychosocial resources. The longitudinal impact however remains to be studied (Burke & Utley, 2013).

In some OAA, veterans are immersed in nature along with therapists. This approach has successfully reduced symptoms of PTSD in many attendees during interventions (Hawkins et al., 2016). In one expedition, riverside camping, day hikes and night-time campfires were part of the approach, although the intervention featured no formal therapy or dis-cussion sessions in the day-to-day routines. Instead, the focus was on con-necting with nature and being encouraged to relax and "take-in" nature. Written journal responses from participating veterans indicated decreases

Outdoor and Adventurous Activities 235

in hyperarousal, increased ability to reflect on life events in the natural environment and increased positive mood (Dustin et al., 2011). In an interesting departure from physically demanding programs, research into the effectiveness of fly-fishing experiences also revealed reductions in participants' symptoms of stress and perceived stress as well as improved sleep quality (Vella et al., 2013).

Team Red, White and Blue (TRWB) is a non-profit organization, formed in 2010, which aims to enrich the lives of America's veterans through physical and social activity and connecting them to their community. TRWB uses OAA provision within a wide portfolio of offerings. They target the "reverse culture shock" some veterans experience after leaving the military. This "shock" results from adjusting to the differences between military and civilian lifestyle, leaving many feeling isolated and overwhelmed. With an almost total absence of social connection, psychological ill-health can follow. TRWB aims for beneficiaries to reclaim their sense of belonging to a socially cohesive community (Angel et al., 2018).

TRWB is based on volunteers providing an inclusive and consistent support structure embedded within local communities. Volunteer leadership teams provide daily-to-weekly sporting physical and social engagements for members. The activities they use accent social engagement, including one-to-one "eagle engagements" over a coffee allowing quiet time to chat, team-specific athletic events such as functional fitness sessions and social events.

As an older provider, initiated in 1967, Disabled Sports USA also works to improve the lives of wounded veterans, youths and adults with disabilities through sport and recreational opportunities (Wilson & Clayton, 2010). They cater for veterans with visual impairments, amputations, neuromuscular/orthopaedic conditions and cognitive disabilities. Through participation in up to 50 sports including archery, cross-country skiing, rafting, rock climbing, snowboarding and snowshoeing, they provide opportunities for individuals to develop confidence, fitness and independence. Over 70,000 beneficiaries are served through the nationwide program, delivered in more than 40 states and over 135 communities.

Programme Insights - EquiCenter

Text by Jonathan Friedlander, President & CEO of EquiCenter, Inc.

The need for hope and purpose is crucial and one organisation offering that is the New York EquiCenter, a non-profit organisation utilising horses to aid healing for US veterans through a therapeutic equestrian programme where US veterans participate in hands-on experiences with horses, both mounted and ground based.

The center offers a variety of programmes to veterans. The latest of which is Mission Mustang, that brings together veterans and previously unhandled mustangs in the hope of helping both groups. The Mission Mustang is a 10-week pilot programme, developed after veteran demand outgrew the Centre's capacity in 2018. A partnership with the Bureau of Land Management saw the introduction of a new breed of therapy; a partnership between recently gathered mustangs and veterans, with the objective of a mutual experiential development. The unification of a 'hypervigilant prey animal' with an often hypervigilant veteran can immediately generate a strong sense of relatedness; both are often experiencing acute stress, anxiety and loss in an unfamiliar environment with a need to transition and fit into their new herd or society respectively. One veteran described the strength of relatedness they felt on the mustangs' arrival; "I'm watching them [the wild mustangs], and I realised that I was seeing the same symptoms I have experienced. We all ... just said, 'Oh, my God, that's us.'"

Under the guidance of two nationally acclaimed mustang trainers the pilot programme commenced with 10 veterans working one-to-one with a trainer and a horse, to gain the mustangs' trust through self-awareness and moderation of body language. The programme facilitated development of basic horsemanship qualities such as, learning to calm the animal, training the mustang to stand for grooming, to wear a halter and lead, load onto a trailer and have its feet handled; all of which greatly increase the mustangs' chances of adoption.

The most visible benefit is seen during the initial raw stage of arrival; this is when both horse and veteran experience the pinnacle of fear and power of connection. The veterans report having a new purpose, pride and accomplishment in learning how to calm and train their horses. There is currently a waiting list of veterans wanting to take part in the programme, and 48,000 mustangs in BLM-holding facilities. With thousands of veterans needing help, the EquiCenter is hoping Mission Mustang will be a model for others to follow.

Programme Insights – Adventure Not War

Text by Stacy Bare, Founder of Adventure Not War.

I came home after a year in Baghdad with the United States Army in 2007. My intention was not to be a veteran. That was a technical designation I could otherwise ignore. Unfortunately, I was unable to cope with the traumas I had experienced directly in war, or the traumas that I had mostly avoided prior to deployment.

I was an alcoholic and a cocaine addict within weeks of my return. I fantasized and planned my own death numerous times. Two years later, discussing my options of suicide or returning to the US Military, a friend I had served with asked me to go rock climbing instead. I put off my suicide for a couple of weeks and went to climb with him on September 20th, 2009.

That climb gave me a sense of purpose, focus, and the ability to live in the moment for the first time since returning from war. I rappelled off that climb a changed man; in the ensuing months, I embraced my veteran identity and worked to bring more veterans into the healing power of nature. I soon began to think about the possibility of applying the healing power of nature directly to the places where I had been an active participant in the military; cleaning up after war or had plans for deployment. I started to socialize this idea with friends and colleagues. I wanted to replace a personal narrative of pain, fear, and loss in these places with one of beauty, adventure, and generosity.

"You want to go ski in Iraq?!? You're crazy! You'll get beheaded" sums up the average response. 2013 was the year I got married, it was a big year. My wife provided the loudest voice of support for me to go back and experience places like Bosnia, Angola, Abkhazia in the Republic of Georgia, Iraq, and Afghanistan. She told me that if I needed to go back so I could come home, she was all in. A chance meeting with Alex Honnold a year later kickstarted the project. He told me if I planned it, he'd come climb with me in Angola and, without a real plan or idea about what would happen after that, we went in the fall of 2015. In 2017, I returned with two friends, Matt Griffin and Robin Brown, who had also served in Iraq, and film makers Max Lowe and Mack Fischer. We were fortunate to be the first recorded team to ski Mt. Halgurd. I returned home from Iraq emotionally exhausted—but more whole than when I left.

In future years I'd like to be able to take groups of veterans to the regions, if not the exact place, where they fought or served to help add beauty and generosity into their narrative of places that may have only held pain and fear before.

17.1.2 UK

In 1949, the UK initiated its first National Park as part of the nation's postwar reconstruction. This is one of the earliest examples of governmental acknowledgment of the appreciation of the societal benefits that access to nature yields. As a post-war response, National Parks provided recreational opportunities for the public and those returning from war as well as preserving and enhancing the natural beauty of park environments. Lewis Silkin, UK Minister for Town and Country Planning, described it as "...the most exciting Act of the post-war Parliament" (Parks 2018). This appreciation of the benefits of experiences in natural surroundings has continued to grow. While large numbers of people have activated the potential of the

238   *C.W.P. Kay and R.J. Sutton*

National Parks for their well-being, they were insufficient – in their own right – to do this for many veterans. For them, the move has been toward bespoke, population-specific OAA provision (Greer & Vin-Raviv, 2019)

A number of supportive OAA programs and experiences are now available for veterans in the UK. Charities and organizations such as Help For Heroes, Outpost Charity, High Tide Adventure, Adventure Quest, Veterans in Community, Royal Yachting Association and The Royal British Legion (TRBL) provide OAA programs of varying lengths that focus on adventure training, wilderness therapy and adaptive adventure for veterans. Only one OAA course is mandatory for WIS-MP in the British Army and Royal Air Force; the Multi-Activity Course (MAC). This is delivered by Carnegie Great Outdoors of Leeds Beckett University on behalf of TRBL at The Battle Back Centre.

Walking with the Wounded is a UK charity that supports injured veterans and their families by empowering them to regain their independence and connect with their communities. Established in 2010, the charity has organized outdoor expeditions around the world for WIS-MP, including walks of America, Britain, South Pole and Everest. Their aim is to inspire and remind WIS-MP of their capability for leading fulfilling lives and achieving at the highest levels.

Founded in 2007, The Warrior Programme initially aimed to help homeless people in the UK to cope better and regain control of their lives. After a partnership with TRBL in 2009 and a successful pilot programme specifically for veterans, the Warrior team now focuses on military personnel (The Royal British Legion, 2019). The Warrior Programme features a 3-day residential motivation and training foundation course, followed by 12 months of structured signposting and support (Verey, Keeling, Thandi, Stevelink, & Fear, 2016). Run across England and Wales, the program supports veterans and their families struggling with the transition to civilian life through coaching of practical coping-oriented skills.

In 2019, The Warrior Programme partnered with Walking With The Wounded to form The Northern Care Coordination Partnership (NCCP). The NCCP started a 2-year pilot project in the North East and North West of England. The aim of the program is to reduce the stresses of arranging treatment services and provide positive, quicker treatment journeys for veterans referred by the NHS Mental Health Services. This provision is responding to a core problem affecting mental support for veterans, speed of access.

As in the US, UK provision has integrated physical activity with aquatic environments to positively influence well-being. Here the aim is to create a "blue gym in order for them to make a safe return back into the armed forces, or a smooth transition into civilian life" (Caddick, Smith, & Phoenix, 2015; Smith et al., 2012; Surf-action, 2017). OAA, such as surfing, have helped veterans shift their mindset and attention to the present moment, ceasing ruminations about past traumatic incidents (Caddick et al., 2015). In the 8-week Ocean Therapy Course, comprising of weekly three-hour sessions delivered by Surfing GB instructors, sessions use the surfing experience to activate group developmental discussions to foster transitional skills (Surf-action 2017). Participants reported a fulfilling sense of absorption in the activity; some participants extended the surfing analogy to comment that their PTSD symptoms were "washed out of their system" (Caddick et al., 2015).

Some organizations have used OAA not only to help participants physically and psychosocially but also vocationally. Adventure Quest UK Community Interest Company (AQ) is an adventure therapy service for veterans experiencing serious and complex mental ill-health. AQ offers individually tailored and therapeutic support and training. Many of their hundreds of beneficiaries have obtained the Mountain Leader qualification and over 60% of those who qualified, secured work within the outdoor industry. AQ provides a two-tier 12-month program based on need, current ability and mental resilience. Tier one represents a general well-being program conducted in mountainous environments of the UK, delivered using a person-centered psycho/social-educational approach. Tier two is a Mountain Leader development pathway, providing the necessary knowledge and experience for beneficiaries to develop the skills and competencies to secure an outdoor national qualification – the Mountain Leader (summer) Award. To date, AQ has had a 100% success rate in its beneficiaries qualifying as Mountain Leaders, which compares favorably to the current industry average of 72%.

17.2 A Review of Evidence of the Effectiveness of Outdoor and Adventurous Interventions for Serving and Ex-Military Personnel

A significant volume of research has already addressed the effectiveness of OAA programmes. Just as the US dominates the delivery landscape, it does the same in the academic literature. UK-based research, however, is on the rise, including research with recently affected, still-serving armed forces WIS-MP. Despite this, more clarity is required regarding a range of psychosocial impacts. There is a need to generate evidence that justifies the use of OAA to secure well-being and, especially, to show how OAA compare with other types of interventions (Routzahn, 2019; Shirazipour et al., 2019).

An established research approach immerses research staff into OAA programs alongside recovering WIS-MP and veterans. Here the aim is to provide an informal context, where the researcher can be honest about their identity and purpose, generating a more natural situation to report upon (Erlandson, Harris, Skipper, & Allen, 1993).However, it remains an ongoing challenge to embed researchers into programs so the programs, and the participants, continue as normal. Yet, normalizing the presence of researchers within programs is important for establishing program impacts and for investigating attribution.

240   *C.W.P. Kay and R.J. Sutton*

Special Editions of journals such as *The Therapeutic Recreation Journal* have focussed on using OAA to support veterans (Van Puymbroeck & Lundberg, 2011). This body of work evidenced how multi-day OAA trips facilitated decreased symptoms of post-traumatic stress during the excursions (Dustin et al., 2011). Placing researchers alongside practitioners have provided opportunities to gather key evidence into the benefits for participants. These benefits included promoting recovery, alleviating symptoms and assisting with psychological well-being. This immersion approach has gained traction more recently, across a number of OAA sporting contexts including surfing, fishing, river boarding, hiking, climbing, horse riding, mountain biking, kayaking & mountaineering (Angel, & Armstrong, 2016; Bennett, Piatt, & Van Puymbroeck, 2017; Burke & Utley, 2013; Caddick & Smith, 2017; Dustin et al., 2011; Hooker, 2018; Joshi & Goldman, 2019; Peacock, McKenna, Carless, & Cooke, 2019; Poulsen, Stigsdotter, & Davidsen, 2018; Walter et al., 2019).

17.3 Expedition Research and Mission Himalaya 2018

Several recent research studies have noted that veterans' interaction with nature was more central to behavior change outcomes than was using therapeutic techniques (Mowatt & Bennett 2011, Hawkins et al., 2016). Longer-term experiences, such as multi-week trips ensure prolonged exposure to the natural environment. While few long-term programs have involved WIS-MP and veterans, still fewer expedition-style programs have been researched. In those that have, many, but not all participants experience positive psychological outcomes. The stress of the expedition environment, for example, may result in post-expedition psychological growth (Smith et al., 2017). Data from 83 mountaineers suggested that perceived stress and personality dimensions of agreeableness and openness influenced post-expedition growth (Smith et al., 2017). Growth following these experiences was also associated with initial well-being, suggesting some level of pre-existing suitability for activating expedition effects. Expeditions can also cultivate key psychosocial elements of self-determination, active coping and social support. As was found on a two-and-a-half-week expedition to Kilimanjaro with four veterans through participant Interviews and observations. This work highlighted the capacity of meaningful and challenging activities for improving the experience of recovery after serious injury (Burke & Utley, 2013). Research like this, questions the assumption of "universal effects" for participants and proposes the need for closer consideration of how any expedition can be better developed and supported to ensure more people benefit, more often.

Some studies are addressing long-term developmental experiences attributable to OAA expeditions. Mission Himalaya 2018 is an ongoing research study led by Leeds Beckett University into the long-term influence of an expedition intentionally designed to support veteran well-being. The expedition involved 28-days of trekking in Nepal and a weather-impeded attempt to summit Mera Peak (6476 m). The mountaineering staff were also health coaches from the Battle Back Centre; all were experienced in facilitating supportive conversations regarding experiential learning and how to intentionally transfer learning to home contexts beyond the expedition.

Interviews were conducted prior to, during and after the month-long expedition with 10 participants (nine male, one female). Findings highlight widely varying and individualized notions regarding expeditions and how participating veterans define a "successful" expedition. The experience improved measures of well-being and hope as well as positively influencing participants' ability to be more empathetic. It helped some to generate new perspectives of their own ability in returning to work and in managing life and recovery. Importantly, the evaluations identified a powerful and obvious "cliff-edge" experience following the expedition; the extensive and rich support of the expedition was contrasted to the relative void of such experiences when returning to home contexts. This research is longitudinal and due to continue until 2023, five years after the expedition (Kay, 2019).

17.4 Battle Back Centre Research

Established in 2011, the Battle Back Centre facilitates the recovery of UK wounded (battle casualties), injured (non-battle casualties) and sick (mental or physical illness) military personnel. This is achieved through the delivery of bespoke MACs which use adaptive sport and adventurous activities as a context for personal development and growth. Distinctively, the MAC is currently the only mandatory course for British Army and Royal Air Force WIS-MP which involves adaptive sport and adventurous training (MoD, 2016).

The bespoke tailored courses are dynamically adapted by staff to suit the needs of the participants and to enhance inclusivity. During the five-day MAC, each day commences with an educational session wherein the expert coaching staff introduce new psychological concepts or strategies (e.g. motivation, attitude, goal setting) and finishes with encouraging reflective discussions aimed at developing participants' understanding of behavior change and their own personal development. This teaching content is then activated through various adventurous sports including kayaking, archery, mountain biking, hill walking, rock climbing and caving. High levels of participation in every activity are enabled, regardless of individual circumstances, by the presence of a full-time Technical Advisor and the extensive array of equipment available at the Centre. The combination of educational sessions and a person-centered approach positively influences participants' mental well-being, physical health and helps improve their ability to better manage aspects of daily life.

242   C.W.P. Kay and R.J. Sutton

Battle Back courses are designed around Self Determination Theory (SDT). An on-going process evaluation assesses both delivery quality, and overall programme outcomes, against the three central tenets of SDT: Autonomy, Competence and Relatedness. The theory suggests that optimal psychological well-being may only be achievable when these three basic needs are supported (Peacock, Carless, & McKenna, 2018; Ryan & Deci, 2000). Importantly, these elements of SDT are theorized as universal human concerns and they map well against the widely reported concerns of existing WIS and of veterans about returning to civilian life regarding fitting in, restoring confidence in personal resourcefulness and for building a strong sense of personal purpose and meaning.

This MAC was regularly refined because it was designed using a "developmental evaluation" approach. In this approach, embedded evaluators engaged with all MAC activities, reporting key – often minute-by-minute – findings to delivery staff each week. This approach normalized the evaluators' presence and helped both staff and clients appreciate the role evaluators played. Additionally, as evaluators were mindful of the need for sensitivity to participants' likely ongoing concerns about psychological safety and anxieties around the use of surveillance, this process showed that evaluators posed no threat. For staff, the knowledge that every session was assessed against three clear SDT criteria (autonomy, competence and relatedness) helped ensure their focus and priority. This approach continues today; every MAC (over 150 courses to date, supporting over 4,000 participants) has been evaluated in this way.

Despite being delivered to in-service staff, a "challenge by choice" approach prevails in all MAC activities and processes. This develops Autonomy; participants choose their level of engagement in each adventurous activity. With a ratio of one instructor for every three clients, the MAC offers unrivaled opportunities to master sport-based tasks. This also creates spontaneous chances for private discussions about how to manage the challenges of different activities and how to transfer learning to subsequent activities. All this supports positive thinking, helping participants to feel Competent (Kaiseler et al., 2019). Reflection sessions, conducted to debrief each day's activities and events, amplify this as participants' achievements in knowledge development, skills and meaningful tasks are highlighted and celebrated. Participation in the respective outdoor activities allows for a comfortable social environment to develop. Careful attention to these social processes and how they are best conducted has helped to address Relatedness (Ferrer & Davis 2019).

17.5 Research Findings from Battle Back Recovery Courses

MAC evaluations have been conducted with in-service UK WIS-MP at the Battle Back Centre since they began in 2011. Now, a substantial evidence base exists regarding the positive impacts of these interventions. Between

2012 and 2015, 971 participants showed an average increase of 15.9% in positive mental well-being over the duration of the 5-day course (Peacock et al., 2019). This reliably reproducible effect has also been reported in 759 participants between 2017 and 2018 (Kay & McKenna 2021). Across both time periods, Autonomy, Competence and Relatedness also significantly increased during the course. By 2015, the findings from Battle Back suggested that, in the short term at least, involvement in the MAC had positive outcomes for the psychological well-being and the wider development of participants (Carless & Douglas, 2016). More recently, Kaiseler et al. (2019) qualitatively investigated the long-term impact of the course on participants' ability to make positive changes. The behavior changes reported by participants six months after attending a MAC were aligned with improved psychological well-being (Kaiseler et al., 2019). This substantial body of research identified the immediate effects of the MACs on participants' well-being and basic psychological needs. Critically, since 2016 longitudinal research has been conducted to better understand the lasting impact of the intervention. This research has found that mental well-being substantially improved in military personnel who completed the MAC (i.e., above the civilian national average). It also showed mental well-being gradually declined for these personnels over the 12-months preceding the MAC. However, the mental well-being of these personnels at 12 months was still higher than before they participated in the MAC (Figure 17.1).

As for positive need satisfaction, all three aspects of psychological need satisfaction (i.e., feelings of competency, autonomy, relatedness) increased

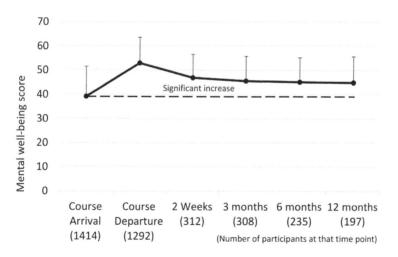

Figure 17.1 Sustainable improvements in participant's positive mental well-being 12 months after a multi activity course.

244　C.W.P. Kay and R.J. Sutton

by the end of the MAC. Over time, psychological need satisfaction and the sense of competence tended to decrease over time but remained higher than pre-MAC, 12 months after. Relatedness & autonomy, however, gradually returned to levels comparable to pre-MAC levels.

More individualised, qualitative research has also been conducted with MAC participants. MACs stimulate a balance of present- and future-oriented psychosocial outcomes. Through daily activities, participants recreated aspects of themselves lost through injury or illness; many used these experiences as a springboard to reconsider their lives as having new horizons of possibility (Carless, Peacock, McKenna, & Cooke, 2013). Further, narrative study evidenced a predominance of transformation in participants' personal narrative during the courses (Carless, 2014; Carless, Sparkes, Douglas, & Cooke, 2014). These transformations held positive consequences for the participants' health and well-being.

17.6　Conclusion

Important gaps remain in our understanding of how to optimize OAA for WIS and/or veterans. With a need for more randomized controlled trials, to establish cause and effect relations, there is also a need to explore the optimum exposure to clarify dose-response relationships. More longitudinal research (to address transfer of learning and sustainability of intervention), diversification of the types of OAA interventions (e.g., residential versus home-based), consideration of systemic influences, representativeness of study samples, examination of diverse psychosocial constructs and consideration of program implementation options are also needed. However, despite these limitations, OAA interventions for WIS and veterans are emerging as uniquely powerful interventions.

References

Anderson, C., Monroy, M., & Keltner, D. (2017). Emotion in the Wilds of Nature: The Coherence and Contagion of Fear During Threatening Group-Based Outdoors Experiences. *Emotion, 18*, 355–368. doi:10.1037/emo0000378

Anderson, C., Monroy, M., & Keltner, D. (2018). Awe in Nature Heals: Evidence From Military Veterans, At-Risk Youth, and College Students. *Emotion, 18*, 1195–1202. doi:10.1037/emo0000442

Angel, C., & Armstrong, N. J. (2016). *Enriching Veterans' Lives Through an Evidence Based Approach: A Case Illustration of Team Red, White & Blue.* Retrieved from https://ivmf.syracuse.edu/wp-content/uploads/2018/03/EnrichingVeterans LivesThroughAnEvidenceBasedApproach.ACaseIllustrationofTeamRWB_ ExecutiveSummaryACC_02.23.18.pdf

Angel, C. M., Woldetsadik, M. A., Armstrong, N. J., Young, B. B., Linsner, R. l. K., Maury, R. V., & Pinter, J. M. (2018). The Enriched Life Scale (ELS): Development, Exploratory Factor Analysis, and Preliminary Construct Validity for U.S. Military Veteran and Civilian Samples. *Translational Behavioral Medicine, 10*(1), 278–291. doi:10.1093/tbm/iby109

Bauer, A., Newbury-Birch, D., Robalino, S., Ferguson, J., & Wigham, S. (2018). Is Prevention Better Than Cure? A Systematic Review of the Effectiveness of Well-Being Interventions for Military Personnel Adjusting to Civilian Life. *PLOS One, 13*(5), e0190144. doi:10.1371/journal.pone.0190144

Bennett, J. L., Piatt, J. A., & Van Puymbroeck, M. (2017). Outcomes of a Therapeutic Fly-Fishing Program for Veterans with Combat-Related Disabilities: A Community-Based Rehabilitation Initiative. *Community Mental Health Journal, 53*(7), 756–765. doi:10.1007/s10597-017-0124-9

Berman, N., Berman, D., & Davis-Berman, J. (2018). Outdoor Programs as Treatment for PTSD in Veterans: Issues and Evidence. Best Practices in Mental Health: An International Journal, *14*, 9–20.

Buckley, R. C., Brough, P., & Westaway, D. (2018). Bringing Outdoor Therapies Into Mainstream Mental Health. *Frontier Public Health, 6*, 119 doi:10.3389/fpubh.2018.00119

Burke, S. M., & Utley, A. (2013). Climbing Towards Recovery: Investigating Physically Injured Combat Veterans' Psychosocial Response to Scaling Mt. Kilimanjaro. *Disabil Rehabil, 35*(9), 732–739. doi:10.3109/09638288.2012.707743

Caddick, N., & Smith, B. (2017). Combat Surfers: A Narrative Study OF Veterans, Surfing, and War Trauma. *Movimento, 23*(1), 25–38.

Caddick, N., & Smith, B. (2018). Exercise is Medicine for Mental Health in Military Veterans: A Qualitative Commentary. *Qualitative Research in Sport, Exercise and Health, 10*(4), 429–440. doi:10.1080/2159676X.2017.1333033

Caddick, N., Smith, B., & Phoenix, C. (2015). The Effects of Surfing and the Natural Environment on the Well-Being of Combat Veterans. *Qualitative Health Research, 25*(1), 76–86. doi:10.1177/1049732314549477

Carless, D. (2014). Narrative Transformation Among Military Personnel on an Adventurous Training and Sport Course. *Qualitative Health Research, 24*(10), 1440–1450. doi:10.1177/1049732314548596

Carless, D., & Douglas, K. (2016). Narrating embodied experience: sharing stories of trauma and recovery. Sport, Education and Society, 21(1), 47–61. doi:10.1080/13573322.2015.1066769

Carless, D., Peacock, S., McKenna, J., & Cooke, C. (2013). Psychosocial Outcomes of an Inclusive Adapted Sport and Adventurous Training Course for Military Personnel. *Disability and Rehabilitation, 35*(24), 2081–2088. doi:10.3109/09638288.2013.802376

Carless, D., Sparkes, A. C., Douglas, K., & Cooke, C. (2014). Disability, Inclusive Adventurous Training and Adapted Sport: Two Soldiers' Stories of Involvement. *Psychology of Sport and Exercise, 15*(1), 124–131. doi:https://doi.org/10.1016/j.psychsport.2013.10.001

Dietrich, Z. C., Joye, S. W., & Garcia, J. A. (2015). Natural Medicine: Wilderness Experience Outcomes for Combat Veterans. *Journal of Experiential Education, 38*(4), 394–406. doi:10.1177/1053825915596431

Dustin, D., Bricker, N., Arave, J., & Wall, W. (2011). The Promise of River Running as a Therapeutic Medium for Veterans Coping with Post-Traumatic Stress Disorder. *Therapeutic Recreation Journal, 45*, 326–340.

Erlandson, D., Harris, E., Skipper, B., & Allen, S. (1993). Doing Naturalistic Inquiry: A Guide to Methods (1st ed.): SAGE Publications.

Ferrer, M., & Davis, R. (2019). Adapted Physical Activity for Wounded, Injured, and Ill Military Personnel: From Military to Community. *Palaestra, 33*(2), 6.

246 C.W.P. Kay and R.J. Sutton

Greer, M. & Vin-Raviv, N. (2019) Outdoor-Based Therapeutic Recreation Programs Among Military Veterans with Posttraumatic Stress Disorder: Assessing the Evidence. Military Behavioral Health, 7(3), 286–303. doi: 10.1080/21635781.2018.1543063

Gregory, M., Davies, L., Ramachandani, G., McClure, M., & Geddes, J. (2019). *BOSS: Testing of methodology to value social benefits of outdoor sport.* Retrieved from Brussels: https://outdoorsportsbenefits.eu/wp-content/uploads/2020/03/BOSS-Stage-3-Report.pdf

Hawkins, B., Townsend, J., & Garst, B. (2016). Nature-Based Recreational Therapy for Military Service Members: A Strengths Approach. *Therapeutic Recreation Journal, 50* (1). 55–74 doi:10.18666/TRJ-2016-V50-I1-6793

Hooker, T. (2018). *Equine Assisted Programs for Military Service Members: A Program Evaluation Using Importance-Performance Analysis.* All Theses. (2844).

Hyer, L., Summers, M. N., Boyd, S., Litaker, M., & Boudewyns, P. (1996). Assessment of Older Combat Veterans with the Clinician-Administered PTSD Scale. *Journal of Traumatic Stress, 9*(3), 587–593. doi:10.1007/BF02103667

Joshi, M., & Goldman, J. Z. (2019). Endure, Evolve, Achieve: Stakeholder Perspectives on the Effectiveness of the Swamp Apes Program in Restoring Biopsychosocial Functioning of American Veterans. *Cogent Psychology, 6*(1). doi:10.1080/2331190 8.2019.1584081

Kaiseler, M., Kay, C., & McKenna, J. (2019). The Impact of an Outdoor and Adventure Sports Course on the Wellbeing of Recovering UK Military Personnel: An Exploratory Study. *Sports, 7*(5). 112-121 doi:10.3390/sports7050112

Kay, C. (2019). *Mission Himalaya 2018 Research.* Retrieved from https://www.leedsbeckett.ac.uk/cgo/-/media/files/cgo/mission-himalaya-research-article.pdf

Kay, C., & McKenna, J. (2021). The enduring well-being impacts of attending the Battle Back Multi Activity Course for the lives of recovering UK armed forces personnel. *Submitted to Military Psychology.*

Lawton, E., Brymer, E., Clough, P., & Denovan, A. (2017). The Relationship between the Physical Activity Environment, Nature Relatedness, Anxiety, and the Psychological Well-being Benefits of Regular Exercisers. *8.* -. doi:10.3389/fpsyg.2017.01058

MoD. (2016). *UK Armed Forces Recovery Capability: Wounded, Injured and Sick in the recovery pathway: 1 October 2010 to 1 October 2016* Retrieved from https://assets.publishing.service.gov.uk/government/uploads/system/uploads/attachment_data/file/517242/20160331-WIS_Official_Statistic-Oct2015_final_revised-O.pdf

Mowatt, R., & Bennett, J. (2011). War Narratives: Veteran Stories, PTSD Effects, and Therapeutic Fly-Fishing. *Therapeutic Recreation Journal, 45,* 286–308.

Niedermeier, M., Hartl, A., & Kopp, M. (2017). Prevalence of Mental Health Problems and Factors Associated with Psychological Distress in Mountain Exercisers: A Cross-Sectional Study in Austria. *8*(1237). doi:10.3389/fpsyg.2017.01237

Parks, N. (2018). History of the National Parks. Retrieved from https://www.nationalparks.uk/students/whatisanationalpark/history

Pasanen, T. P., Tyrväinen, L., & Korpela, K. M. (2014). The Relationship between Perceived Health and Physical Activity Indoors, Outdoors in Built Environments, and Outdoors in Nature. *6*(3), 324–346. doi:10.1111/aphw.12031

Peacock, S., Carless, D., & McKenna, J. (2018). Inclusive Adapted Sport and Adventure Training Programme in the PTSD Recovery of Military Personnel: A Creative Non-Fiction. *Psychology of Sport and Exercise, 35,* 151–159. doi: https://doi.org/10.1016/j.psychsport.2017.12.003

Peacock, S. M., McKenna, J., Carless, D., & Cooke, C. (2019). Outcomes from a One-Week Adapted Sport and Adapted Adventure Recovery Programme for Military Personnel. *Sports, 7*(6), 135.

Petersen, H. (2017). The Success of Recreation Therapy for Veterans. Retrieved from https://www.va.gov/HEALTH/NewsFeatures/2016/February/The-Success-of-Recreation-Therapy-for-Veterans.asp

Poulsen, D. V., Stigsdotter, U. K., & Davidsen, A. S. (2018). "That Guy, Is He Really Sick at All?" An Analysis of How Veterans with PTSD Experience Nature-Based Therapy. *Healthcare, 6*(2), 64.

Roberts, G., Arnold, A., Turner, R., James, E., Colclough, M., & Bilzon, J. (2019). A Longitudinal Examination of Military Veterans' Invictus Games Stress Experiences. *Frontiers in Psychology, 10*(1934). doi:10.3389/fpsyg.2019.01934

Routzahn, S. (2019). *Effects of Adventure Therapy versus Support Groups on Emotional Stability for Veterans with PTSD Transitioning into Civilian Life.* Paper presented at the Spring Showcase for Research and Creative Inquiry.

Ryan, R. M., & Deci, E. L. (2000). Self-determination Theory and the Facilitation of Intrinsic Motivation, Social Development, and Well-Being. *American Psychologist, 55*(1), 68–78.

Schuster, D. G. (2003). Neurasthenia and a Modernizing America. *JAMA, 290*(17), 2327–2328. doi:10.1001/jama.290.17.2327%J JAMA

Shirazipour, C. H., Tennant, E. M., Aiken, A. B., & Latimer-Cheung, A. E. (2019). Psychosocial Aspects of Physical Activity Participation for Military Personnel with Illness and Injury: A Scoping Review. *Military Behavioral Health, 7*(4), 459–476. doi:10.1080/21635781.2019.1611508

Smith, B., Harms, W. D., Burres, S., Korda, H., Rosen, H., & Davis, J. (2012). Enhancing Behavioral Health Treatment and Crisis Management Through Mobile Ecological Momentary Assessment and SMS Messaging. *Health Informatics Journal, 18*, 294–308.

Smith, N., Kinnafick, F., Cooley, S. J., & Sandal, G. M. (2017). Reported Growth Following Mountaineering Expeditions: The Role of Personality and Perceived Stress. Environment and Behaviour, *49*(8), 933–955. doi:10.1177/0013916516670447

Straits-Tröster, K. A., Brancu, M., Goodale, B., Pacelli, S., Wilmer, C., Simmons, E. M., & Kudler, H. (2011). Developing Community Capacity to Treat Post-Deployment Mental Health Problems: A Public Health Initiative. *Psychological Trauma: Theory, Research, Practice, and Policy, 3*(3), 283–291. doi: 10.1037/a0024645

Surf-action. (2017). *Evaluation Report: The Surf Action 'Health and Wellbeing Residential Week' held at Morwenstow near Bude.* Retrieved from http://www.surfaction.co.uk/Assets/PDFs/Evidential-Reports/Residential-Evaluation-Report-2017.pdf

The Royal British Legion. (2019, 22/03/2019). The warrior programme – residential motivation and training course for veterans. Retrieved from https://support.britishlegion.org.uk/app/answers/detail/a_id/1495/~/the-warrior-programme—residential-motivation-and-training-course-for-veterans

Van Puymbroeck, M., & Lundberg, N. (2011). Introduction to Veteran Issues: The Role of Therapeutic Recreation. *Therapeutic Recreation Journal, 45*(4) 265-267.

Vella, E. J., Milligan, B., & Bennett, J. L. (2013). Participation in Outdoor Recreation Program Predicts Improved Psychosocial Well-Being Among Veterans With Post-Traumatic Stress Disorder: A Pilot Study. *Military Medicine, 178*(3), 254–260. doi:10.7205/MILMED-D-12-00308

248 C.W.P. Kay and R.J. Sutton

Verey, A., Keeling, M., Thandi, G., Stevelink, S., & Fear, N. (2016). UK Support Services for Families of Wounded, Injured or Sick Service Personnel: The Need for Evaluation. *Journal of the Royal Army Medical Corps, 162*(5), 324–325. doi:10.1136/jramc-2015-000483

Walter, K. H., Otis, N. P., Glassman, L. H., Ray, T. N., Michalewicz-Kragh, B., Kobayashi Elliott, K. T., & Thomsen, C. J. (2019). Comparison of Surf and Hike Therapy for Active Duty Service Members with Major Depressive Disorder: Study Protocol for a Randomized Controlled Trial of Novel Interventions in a Naturalistic Setting. *Contemporary Clinical Trials Communications, 16*, 100435. doi:https://doi.org/10.1016/j.conctc.2019.100435

Wilson, P. E., & Clayton, G. H. (2010). Sports and Disability. *Pm r, 2*(3), S46–S54. doi:10.1016/j.pmrj.2010.02.002

18 Implications, Impact and Future Directions: Translation into Wider Policy and Practice

Jo Barton, Mike Rogerson, and Eric Brymer

Sustainable health has become an important issue across the globe as evidenced by the United Nations sustainability development goal 3, which focuses on good health and wellbeing for all. However, this will require widespread sustained behavior change, supported by policies, evidence of good practice and regulations that incentivize prompt uptake and commitment.

Physical activity plays a key role in promoting healthy lives and wellbeing. It is considered a primary prevention for a total of 35 different chronic diseases, which include colon cancer, breast cancer, endometrial cancer, accelerated biological aging/premature death, sarcopenia, obesity, insulin resistance, prediabetes, type 2 diabetes, non-alcoholic fatty liver disease, peripheral artery disease, hypertension, endothelial dysfunction, arterial dyslipidemia, hemostasis, deep vein thrombosis, osteoporosis, osteoarthritis, balance, bone fracture/falls, rheumatoid arthritis, gestational diabetes, preeclampsia, polycystic ovary syndrome, erectile dysfunction, pain, diverticulitis, constipation and gallbladder diseases (Booth, Roberts, & Laye, 2012). Physical activity has also been linked to improvements in mental health and wellbeing, such as cognitive dysfunction, depression and anxiety, though the evidence suggests the relationship is nuanced (Biddle, 2016) and related to the type of activity, the physical activity environment and also individual differences (Davids, Araujo, & Brymer, 2016). Physical activity has also been linked to more salutogenic wellbeing outcomes such as flourishing.

In recent years, there is increasing evidence that the physical activity environment has a considerable impact on human health and wellbeing beyond the impact of physical activity on its own. The natural environment provides vital health services as well as other ecosystem services (NEA, 2011; Kubiszewski et al., 2017). In 2019, the UK's government published a 25 Year Environment Plan (DEFRA, 2019) setting out six priorities. One of these key priorities was to *"connect people with environments to increase health and well-being"*, and there has been a substantial shift toward utilizing green spaces and natural habitats to improve the health of whole populations. The environments we live and work in, thus, shape our behavioral choices

DOI: 10.4324/9781003154419-21

and health and wellbeing outcomes. Green space close to residences reduces mortality (Rojas-Rueda et al., 2019) and stress hormones (Ward Thompson et al., 2019), increases levels of physical activity (Rogerson et al., 2015), changes dietary decisions and habits (Kim et al., 2016; Micha et al., 2017) and affects the longevity of the elderly (Ji et al., 2019). However, there are existing inequalities in terms of opportunities to access quality local greenspaces. Individuals living in the most economically deprived areas typically have fewer nearby public greenspaces but evidence shows that green spaces are equigenic and reduce health inequalities (Mitchell & Popham, 2008; WHO, 2016). The United Nations sustainability development goal 11 (Sustainable cities and communities) includes a target to *"provide universal access to safe, inclusive and accessible, green and public spaces, in particular for women and children, older persons and persons with disabilities, by 2030"*. There is clearly a recognition here that ensuring equitable all-inclusive access to green assets will significantly contribute to promoting sustainable health for all.

Chapters in this special edition provide 1) further research evidence that nature contact and activity in green spaces have the capacity to improve health and wellbeing, 2) informative frameworks to help designers and researchers and 3) examples of good practice. There is still space for research to understand the nuances and determine how best to enhance the human-nature relationship for the benefit of humans and the planet. However, it is now imperative that we learn from the overwhelming evidence base and apply this knowledge at a global level. The impact of these findings indicates that policy makers and health practitioners, for example, need to find ways to encourage and provide more physical activity in nature experiences across all seasons and access to environments where rich biodiversity can flourish. With widespread urban sprawl and less access to local pockets of greenspace, the minimal biodiversity found in these living environments is already under threat. Yet research evidences the importance of providing open spaces rich in diversity for public health. The urgency of this cannot be overemphasized and the need for multidisciplinary approaches to research and application is imperative.

The implications of these issues are also financial as evidence has shown that physical activity in nature provides a good return on investment. Nature-based interventions can improve life satisfaction/happiness (LS/H; Pretty & Barton, 2020). Although it is generally challenging to achieve movements of more than 1 point on the LS/H scale naturebased interventions reported consistent margins of change greater than one. The economic benefits of these activities have also been calculated. The net present economic benefits per person from reduced public service use are £830–£31,520 (after 1 year) and £6450–£11,980 (after 10 years). This does not take into account the increased well-being benefits. It is now vital that governments, policy makers and practitioners across all sectors focus efforts on improving opportunities for physical activity in natural environments. Recognition of this is now international and reflected in responses to the United Nations Sustainable Development Goals (goal 3) (Chandra & Chand, 2018; Parsons et al., 2019; Peacock, & Brymer, 2018; Sharma-Brymer & Brymer, 2019), "One Health" models of human, environmental and wildlife health (Rabinowitz et al 2018) and clinical ecology (Nelson et al 2019).

Some argue that globalization, the rise in technology, population growth and the perceived diminution of nature's worth for human psychological, emotional and physical health have caused a disconnect between humanity and the rest of nature. As this disconnect continues and potentially grows, the prospects of achieving human wellbeing within the dominant economic development paradigm weaken. Vital alternative, sustainable and integrated development paradigms are being developed that aim to re-address the balance between the human system and the Earth system (Rockström, 2015).

Fortunately, research in this area continues to grow and we know a great deal more about the benefits of physical activity in nature and ways to facilitate it (e.g. Lumber et al, 2017). The chapters in this book clearly demonstrate this and provide hope that we will find a better way to relate to the rest of the natural world and consequently to ourselves.

It is now clear that the responsibility for mapping out the future for human health is not merely an issue for medicine and allied health. Perhaps more than any other issue affecting humanity, the future for the health of people and planet depends on multiple disciplines working together. This book reflects this notion with perspectives and evidence drawn from psychology, sport science, public health, environmental studies and others. Researchers who have contributed to this book herald from the UK, Australia, New Zealand, United States, Canada, Germany, The Netherlands and Norway providing a wide, inclusive and multidisciplinary insight to this research area.

Crucially, we need to understand more about how we can both enhance wellbeing through nature exposure and experiences in a sustainable manner. Continuing research in this area in an interdisciplinary and trans-disciplinary way is, therefore, vital. All too often researchers work within the safety of their own disciplines. Pioneers within this specialism should demonstrate (more often) how to work together across disciplines and showcase the fruits of their work widely and in ways that can be applied.

Despite the breadth of evidence, nature-based solutions remain inexplicably absent from the dominant models of health, health behavior change (e.g. Gritti, 2017) and workplace wellbeing (Richardson et al. 2017). Yet this book presents clear evidence of the benefits of human embeddedness within the natural world and a multidisciplinary approach. What also seems clear is that much depends on understanding the relationships between activity, individual characteristics and environmental characteristics. Future research should focus on two key areas:

252 *J. Barton, M. Rogerson, and E.Brymer*

i **Enhancing our understanding of the underpinning mechanisms, as this will help to inform decision-making processes.**

There is no human wellbeing without nature's well-being, and the threats to the living planet are present and severe. In order to maximize the opportunities for both humans and nature to thrive, further research is needed to understand how the human-nature relationship works and following on from this, how best to improve the human–nature relationship. This will require investigations that recognize and explore the complexities of the human–nature relationship, acknowledge the role of meaning and meaning-making and respond to this call for further research in a nuanced manner, avoiding reductionist or narrow tendencies. The continuation of interdisciplinary collaboration is, therefore, vital. Future research that provides a deeper understanding of the human–nature relationship has the potential to aid the development and improvement of these broader efforts. The continuation of current funding that supports these research needs and the expansion of funding opportunities to incorporate global collaborative large-scale income in this area is, therefore, needed if current crises in health, mental health and our planetary future are to be addressed.

ii **Practical application of targeted interventions and urban design by multi-disciplinary teams.**

There is an urgent need to find ways to improve the human–nature relationship through interventions, campaign activities, curricula, green infrastructure and urban design. Bringing together artists, planners, designers and researchers will enable the creation of more places that better-afford a connection to nature. Such research should go beyond understanding to offer more in terms of application, in part by creating accessible and effective tools for practitioners from all aspects of human–environment interaction to address the human–nature relationship. An exemplar and catalyst for this movement are provided in the Section 18.1.

18.1 Recommendations

There will always be a need for further research and understanding, but owing to the crises in wellbeing and biodiversity a new relationship with nature, where nature and wellbeing are central determinants of human development, is needed now. Therefore, the research featured in this book can be distilled into a number of recommendations that recognize the importance of multi-disciplinary collaboration, working partnerships, translation of knowledge, increasing accessibility and opportunity, and standardizing evaluation frameworks, so to better inform policy and practice.

18.1.1 Translation of Knowledge

The body of knowledge presented in this book should be of great interest to a broad range of governing bodies, organizations and decision makers, from local to national levels. However, to enhance the likelihood of impacts through such channels, it may be necessary to create further evidence and "present" it in ways that resonate more familiarly into those channels. For example, in the domain of health, the framework of decision makers' understanding is dominated by pharmaceutical approaches. Perhaps adopting principles, methods, and framing from pharmacy could further help integrate knowledge such as that in this book, into mainstream, systemic understanding. For example, like a nuanced development of pharmaceutical treatments, enhanced understanding of the dynamics between nature, physical activity and health, practices and experiences can be harnessed more specifically and efficaciously for health benefits.

18.1.2 Use of Technology

Ironically, in relation to the organic or "natural" phenomena of nature, physical activity and health, one important future avenue for furthering the understanding and presented across this book is likely to be that from technology. For example, further use of technology-driven measures from neuroscientific research can bring a new level of understanding of effects and mechanisms. Relatively simple electroencephalography measures have already examined brain patterns associated with acute green exercise participation. Functional magnetic resonance imaging measurements across longer time periods could provide a step toward data that compares with other intervention types within the domain of medical health.

Additionally, immersive and interactive virtual reality can bring nature soundscapes and imagery to individuals who have limited access to nature, due to living arrangements or ill health. Indeed, a chapter of this book has pointed toward the use of virtual reality to simulate nature environments. This could prove fruitful in terms of simulating both static presence in nature environments and undertaking physical activity in a virtual environment.

18.1.3 Use of Epidemiology and Social Return on Investments

Also, ironically – this time in relation to the intensely individualized and unique experience of physical activity in nature, other avenues of future interest that may more readily (relatively) impact on policy are those of epidemiology and analyzing "big data", as well as social return on investment analyses. Although there rightly remains a great calling to grow the pool of scientific understanding of experiential and other mechanisms of nature physical activity and health, the marriage of such evidence with that from the suggested additional approaches are more likely to impact policy, as

254   J. Barton, M. Rogerson, and E.Brymer

public budgets are squeezed and decision makers seek convincing business cases to access funding.

18.1.4 Improving Accessibility and Opportunities

Not only is proximity of greenspace and time spent in nature associated with better health and wellbeing, physical activity in natural environments also produces better health outcomes compared to activity in built or indoor environments. Being active outdoor builds social capital by facilitating social interaction and reducing loneliness. It also provides opportunities to encourage walking and exercise in nature in both residential and work contexts. However, acceptance of the knowledge presented across this book, in turn, points toward issues such as accessibility and opportunity. Increasing green infrastructure in public spaces, improving active travel routes and corridors, augmenting neighborhood walkability and enriching the quality of existing green space will all enhance access and opportunity and positively reach out to new target cohorts. The challenge is to develop, manage and promote these greenspaces in ways that engage groups with low participation rates, attract marginalized and socially excluded groups and meet the greenspace needs of new communities. To ensure sustained behavior change, such actions need to be accompanied by approaches to increase self-motivation, so habits are formed. This also requires an education component so that the public is more likely to incorporate seizing the benefits on offer into their lifestyle practices. Everyday experiences of nature matter. Thus, providing accessible green spaces, close to home and work, with opportunities and prompts for individuals across the lifespan to notice nature and its beauty is of great value.

18.1.5 Standardizing Evaluation Frameworks

An implication of research showing the efficacies of nature and physical activity for health is that this can and is having a positive impact on individuals' and organizations' practices to gain those demonstrated outcomes. Here, research needs to identify a wider range of outcomes to evidence the potential social and economical benefits in addition to those relating to health and wellbeing. To enable upscaling at both a national and international level, there is a need for more consistent metrics and standardized evaluation procedures, using sophisticated tools that are also culturally sensitive. Future research methodologies need to adopt a common system of evaluation so that research in different disciplines and countries can be evaluated as a body of work rather than a collection of disparate findings. Future research frameworks could also include positive wellbeing health measures, rather than solely focusing on ameliorating negative measures. For example, measuring the quality of life would be an ideal tool to use in future longitudinal studies and would also support economic analyses.

18.1.6 Biodiversity and the Seasons

We need to encourage a broader range of seasonal experiences in nature, of various durations, at various times, and we need to call on insight from a range of approaches to human–nature relationships (e.g. Stoic and Buddhist traditions; nature connectedness, indigenous knowledge). It is also important that habitats offer provision for a variety of wildlife. Biodiversity matters for human health and should be seen as a community service. Micro-variables such as birds, plants, wildlife, and native species create a bond between people and natural places. Providing isolated green spaces might provide some benefit, however, greater benefit will be obtained through culturally appropriate spaces rich in biodiversity.

18.1.7 Provision of Nature-Based Therapeutic Environments

Nature-based interventions are useful for the support of the therapeutic change. While there is still a need to better understand the nuances of intervention design in relation to therapeutic issues interventions are clearly successful. We need to provide appropriate environments for nature-based therapeutic interventions that are accessible to potential clients. This area is growing rapidly but needs social, political and policy support to ensure that people are provided with the best opportunities possible.

18.2 Implications for Policy Sectors

Chapters within this book collectively highlight some important implications for policymakers and practitioners working in this field. We know that our environmental and social context influences our health and well-being, so policies that positively shape these contexts will increase the likelihood that individuals will not only live longer but lead a better quality of life. Health and social care services are under immense pressure to manage the growing worldwide health problems and there are government drives to provide care in the local community. Early intervention studies of children whose adult health and well-being outcomes were improved when exposed to activities in natural places (such as playgrounds, gardens and woodlands) suggest a need for a more preventative approach (Bratman et al., 2012; Bratman et al., 2019; O'Brien et al., 2016). In affluent countries, the scale of healthcare costs has created a pressing need for changes to policy and investment priorities. In 2018, the UK's "Prevention Pays" policy was expanded and set ambitious targets for system-wide changes by 2040 (CMO, 2018 AMS, 2018). By protecting our health assets, we can slow the growth in healthcare demands to provide sustainable healthcare systems for future generations. This has implications for many sectors, suggesting the need for cross-disciplinary and sectoral strategies and action. In the current climate, it is more important than ever that we adopt a

256   *J. Barton, M. Rogerson, and E.Brymer*

strategic whole-systems approach that integrates a dynamic way of working. It requires collaborative working partnerships with multiple key agencies, including public health, social and healthcare providers, planning departments, parks and leisure management, transport providers, architects, artists, developers and community end-users. Bringing these stakeholders and communities together will enable them to develop "a shared understanding of the challenge" to increase the prospect of a longer-term systems change. Adopting a co-design and co-implementation approach by involving key stakeholders in the process will help increase the likelihood of communities welcoming green infrastructure changes.

In a post-Covid-19 world, where economic and social stresses on individuals and health systems will be higher, there is an urgent need to prioritize nature, physical activity and health on the international agenda to inform decision-making processes. Understanding how international policy and strategy levers can also feed into national and local policy will have the greatest health and wellbeing impact. This book highlights real-world examples of effective green exercise interventions. It also emphasizes the potential for translation to a wider range of settings, such as health and social care institutions, workplaces, communities, schools, hospitals, care homes and prisons if good practice can be shared.

Together the chapters in this book provide one bounded example of how interdisciplinary approaches to appreciating the nuances involved in uniting human and planetary health can help rethink the human–nature relationship and inform the international need for a perspective that positively impacts the wellbeing of human beings and our planet. The evidence is clear; the wellbeing of future populations and the planet depends on a cross-sector commitment and an authentic desire to refocus political and practical efforts on effective human-nature relationships. Across the chapters, a great deal of evidence for and understanding of the relationships between nature, physical activity and health has been presented. There appear to be overarching, highly generalizable and accessible aspects to these relationships, as well as aspects that are much more specific to cohorts and individuals.

Both the research findings and the suggested understanding of relationships between nature, physical activity and health, by definition, are limited by the disciplines, methods or contexts of their origins. This body of knowledge would now benefit from greater integration of inputs and approaches, and from being contributed to by an even wider spectrum of disciplines. Another origin-based noteworthy gap in the knowledge presented in this book is that of geography and culture. Understanding of nature, physical activity and health dynamics has been predominantly generated by academic researchers based in universities in developed countries, e.g. Europe, North America, Australia, and Japan, based on samples in those places. Little is known of the geographical or cultural generalizability of findings between these locations, let alone outside of them. Yet the cultural values attached to nature, physical activity and health vary greatly across the globe. Although this may be one avenue of interest for future research, this point also raises the question of whether geographical or cultural social norms may partly explain the academic focuses of this area. Even within academia, there are rising political and financial influences on motivation to undertake research on different topics, as well as on the pathways from knowledge generation to policy and practice. However, this should not deter us from immediate action; we need to act now to ensure that the future for people and planet is bright. Nature–based physical activity is a fundamental human need and provision of opportunities should be integrated across all human activities and, thus, policy sectors.

References

AMS (Academy of Medical Sciences). (2018) *Health of the Public in 2040*, AMS: London, UK, Available online: https://acmedsci.ac.uk/policy/policy-projects/health-of-the-public-in-2040 (accessed on 12th November 2020).

Biddle, S. (2016) Physical activity and mental health: evidence is growing. *World Psychiatry: Official journal of the World Psychiatric Association (WPA)*, 15(2), 176–177. https://doi.org/10.1002/wps.20331

Booth, F.W., Roberts, C.K., & Laye M.J. (2012) Lack of exercise is a major cause of chronic diseases. *Comprehensive Physiology*, 2(2), 1143–1211. http://dx.doi.org/10.1002/cphy.c110025

Bratman, G.N., Hamilton, J.P., & Daily G, C. (2012) The impacts of nature experience on human cognitive function and mental health. *Ann. N. Y. Acad. Sci. 1249*, 118–136 Annals of the New York Academy of Science Doi: 10.1111/j.1749-6632.2011.06400x.

Bratman, G.N., Anderson, C.B., Berman, M.G., Cochran, B., De Vries, S., Flanders, J., Folke, C., Frumkin, H., Gross, J.J., Hartig, T., et al. (2019) Nature and mental health: An ecosystem service perspective. *Sci. Adv. 5*, eaax0903.

Chandra, P.S., & Chand, P. (2018). Towards a new era for mental health. The Lancet, 392, (10157), 1495–1496. http://dx.doi.org/10.1016/ S0140-6736(18)32272-4

CMO (Chief Medical Officer). (2018). *Annual Report 2018: Better Health Within Reach*, UK Government: London, UK.

Davids, K., Araujo, D, Brymer, E. (2016). Designing affordances for health-enhancing physical activity and exercise in sedentary individuals. *Sports Medicine*, 46(7), 933–938. http://dx.doi.org/10.1007/s40279-016-0511-3.

DEFRA. (2019) *The 25 Year Environment Plan*, Department for Environment, Food and Rural Affairs: London, UK,

Gritti, P. (2017). The bio-psycho-social model forty years later: a critical review. *Journal of Psychosocial Systems*. 1(1), 36–41. https://doi.org/10.23823/jps.vlil.14

Ji, J.S., Zhu, A., Bai, C., Wu, C.D., Yan, L., Tang, S., Zeng, Y., & James, P. (2019). Residential greenness and mortality in oldest-old women and men in China: A longitudinal cohort study. *Lancet Planet. Health. 3*, e17–e25.

Kim, S.H., Kim, M.S., Lee, M.S., Park, Y.S., Lee, H.J., Kang, S.A., Lee, H.S., Lee, K.E., Yang, H.J., Kim, M.J., et al. (2016). Korean diet: Characteristics and historical background. *J. Ethn. Foods. 3*, 26–31.

258 *J. Barton, M. Rogerson, and E.Brymer*

Kubiszewski, I., Costanza, R., Anderson, S., & Sutton, P. (2017) The future value of ecosystem services: Global scenarios and national implications. *Ecosyst. Serv. 26,* 289–301.

Lumber, R., Richardson, M., & Sheffield, D. (2017). Beyond knowing nature: Contact, emotion, compassion, meaning, and beauty are pathways to nature connection. PloS One, 12(5), e0177186.

Micha, R., Peñalvo, J.L., Cudhea, F., Imamura, F., Rehm, C.D., & Mozaffarian, D. (2017). Association between dietary factors and mortality from heart disease, stroke, and type 2 diabetes in the United States. *JAMA, 317,* 912–924.

Mitchell, R.& Popham, F. (2008). Effect of exposure to natural environment on health inequalities: An observational population study. *Lancet, 372,* 1655–1660.

NEA. (2011) *National Ecosystem Assessment,* Defra: London, UK.

Nelson, D. H., Prescott, S. L., Logan, A. C., & Bland, J. S. (2019). Clinical ecology—transforming 21st-century medicine with planetary health in mind. Challenges, 10(1), 15.

O'Brien, L., Ambrose-Oji, B., Waite, S., Aronsson, J., & Clark, M. (2016) Learning on the move: Green exercise for children and young people. In Barton, J., Bragg, R., Wood, C., Pretty, J., (Eds.), *Green Exercise: Linking Nature, Health and Well-Being.* Routledge: Abingdon, UK.

Parsons, H., Houge Mackenzie, S., Filep, S., & Brymer, E. (2019) UN sustainable development goals of good health and wellbeing: Subjective wellbeing: Subjective wellbeing and leisure. In H.C. Filho (Eds.), Encyclopedia of the UN Sustainable Development Goals: Good Health and Wellbeing. Springer: New York, NY.

Peacock, S., & Brymer, E. (2018). Facilitating Mental Health. In H.C. Filho Eds. Encyclopedia of the UN sustainable development goals: Good health and wellbeing. Springer: New York, NY.

Pretty, J., & Barton, J. (2020) Nature-based interventions and mind–body interventions: Saving public health costs whilst increasing life satisfaction and happiness. International Journal of Environmental Research and Public Health., *17,* 7769. doi:10.3390/ijerph17217769

Rabinowitz, P. M., Pappaioanou, M., Bardosh, K. L., & Conti, L. (2018). A planetary vision for one health. BMJ Global Health, 3(5), e001137.

Richardson, M., Maspero, M., Golightly, D., Sheffield, D., Staples, V., & Lumber, R. (2017). Nature: A new paradigm for wellbeing and ergonomics. Ergonomics, 60(2), 292–305.

Rockström, J. "Bounding the Planetary Future: Why We Need a Great Transition", Great Transition Initiative (April 2015). https://www.greattransition.org/publication/bounding-the-planetary-future-why-we-need-a-great-transition.

Rogerson, M., Brown, D., Sandercock, G., Wooler, J., & Barton, J. (2015) A comparison of four typical green exercise environments and prediction of psychological health outcomes. *Perspectives Public Health,* 36 (3), 171–180.

Rojas-Rueda, D., Nieuwenhuijsen, M.J., Gascon, M., Perez-Leon, D., & Mudu, P. (2019) Green spaces and mortality: A systematic review and meta-analysis of cohort studies. *Lancet Planet. Health, 3,* e469–e477.

Sharma-Brymer, V., & Brymer, E. (2019). UN sustainable development goals of good health and wellbeing: Flourishing and eudemonic wellbeing. In H.C. Filho Eds. Encyclopedia of the UN Sustainable Development Goals: Good Health and Wellbeing, Springer: New York, NY.

Ward Thompson, C., Silveirinha de Oliveira, E., Tilley, S., Elizalde, A., Botha, W., Briggs, A., Cummins, S., Leyland, A.H., Roe, J.J., Aspinall, P., et al. (2019). Health impacts of environmental and social interventions designed to increase deprived communities' access to urban woodlands: A mixed-methods study. *Public Health Res.*, 7, 1–172.

World Health Organisation. (2016). *Urban Green Spaces and Health*. WHO Regional Office for Europe: Copenhagen, Denmark.

Index

Note: Page numbers in *italics* indicate figures and **bold** indicates tables in the text.

activities: adventure 148, 150–152, 194, 196; at a care farm 178–184; farming 177, 183; gait-related 51, 56; green gym 28; leisure 134; lifestyle-focused 186; nature-based 3; recreational 1; risky 196–197; student-led 225; teacher-led 225

adventure 150–154; and nature 149–150; and physical activity 149–150; psychological wellbeing benefits of 148–149; psychological wellbeing in 149–150

adventure recreation: outcomes of 153, *153*; psychological wellbeing frameworks for 147–155

Adventurous Physical Activities (APA) 63; building resilient brains 75–76; descriptive characteristics of students' resilience 69; as effective resilience-building intervention for young people 70, 73–75

affective benefits of nature interaction 7–17; benefits on physiology 8–11; benefits on self-reported affect 8–11; overview 7–8; policy and practice 16–17; studies in populations with mood disorders 14–16; theories for nature's mood effects 11–14

affective communities: *parkrun* fostering 217–218

affordances 113–116; defined 113; Gibson on 113; rich landscape, in nature 116–117

"Anthropocene syndrome" 35

application of green exercise concept 130–135

Attention Restoration Theory (ART) 3, 38, 95, 106

autonomic nervous system (ANS) 193–194, 196

autonomy: defined 75, 153; enhanced 149; psychological needs for 150–151, 153–154

basic psychological needs 150–154, 243

behavioral benefits: and immersive virtual nature 131; of virtual green exercise 127–142; and virtual reality 134

benefits: green exercise 36–37; of natural environments on physiology 8–11; of natural environments on self-reported affect 8–11

biodiversity and seasons 255

Biophilia Hypothesis 12

brain resilience and nature-based APA 70

calibration: defined 48; perceptual-motor 52

Camp Rating Scale (CRS) 71–72, *72*

care farms: activities at 178–184; around the world 178; cases 180–181, *180–181*; health-promoting context for client groups 177–187; impact on health and wellbeing 184–186; overview 177–178; people with dementia 179–182, 184–185; people with mental health problems 182–183, 185–186; recommendations for policy and practice 186–187;

Index 261

for youngsters with behavioral and social problems 183–184, 186
cognitive-behavioral therapy (CBT) 15
comorbidities: psychological 29; type 2 diabetes 23–24, 27, 29
competence, defined 75, 154
complex trauma: contextualizing 192–193; treatment of 193–194; wilderness therapy and treatment of 191–202
corporeality 89–90
COVID-19 pandemic 147
cyber sickness 139

"directed attention" 38

Ecological Dynamics Theory 28
ecological psychology 48, 103, 112
eco-phenomenology 84–85, 90–91
"Eco-Phenomenology" 90
education: adventure 149; campaigns 17; outside the classroom 226–230; over-reductive 64; psychological wellbeing frameworks for 147–155
"Education Outside the Classroom" (EOtC) movement 223–230
Environmental Preferences theory 13
Epidemiology 23; and social return on investments 253–254
eudaimonia 150–154; and wellbeing 160–161
exercise behavior: acute impacts on 133–134; long-term impacts on 134–135; and virtual green exercise 133–135

Facebook 127
future research: green exercise 39–41; physical activity in nature 120–122

gait interventions: falls as problem of perception and action 47–50; recommendations for research 54–57; situational taxonomy for designing and evaluating 47–57; situational taxonomy guiding green exercise research and practice 50–52; and STEPPING 52–54
Germany 223–230; discussion 226–230; education outside classroom 224–225; EOtC 224–225; findings 226–230; future directions

226–230; research example from Heidelberg, Germany 226–230; space appropriation in educational settings 223–224
Google Earth VR 127
green exercise: actively flourishing in nature 35–36; benefits 36–37; and comorbidities of type 2 diabetes 23–24, 27; and exercise adherence 26–27; forms of, for type 2 diabetes and barriers to participation 27–29; future research 39–41; green prescriptions 38; mechanisms 38–39; physical activity and type 2 diabetes 24–25; as treatment strategy for type 2 diabetes 23–29; type 2 diabetes, risk factors, and treatments 23–24; and vitamin D for type 2 diabetes 26–27
green exercise concept: application of 130–135; pathways to health and wellbeing 130–131; psycho-physiosocial benefits of virtual green exercise 131–133; strengths and limitations of evidence 135; virtual green exercise shaping behaviors 133–135
green exercise models 103–107
green exercise research: brief history of 95–96; situational taxonomy guiding 50–52
green prescriptions 38, 155

Haidt, Jonathon 64
head-mounted devices (HMDs) 129, 135
health: benefits, of virtual green exercise 127–142; impact of care farms on 184–186; and nature 1–3; and physical activity 1–3; two intertwining pathways to 130–131
Health for the World's Adolescents report 64
health promotion: designing IVN interventions for 135–141; and natural environments 116
hedonia 150–154; and wellbeing 160–161
Help For Heroes 238
High Tide Adventure 238
Hippocrates 42
Hoeve Klein Mariendaal 182–183

262 *Index*

human resilience 75
humans: and nature 112; and physical activity 112; and rest-of-nature 83
hypothalamic-pituitary-adrenal (HPA) axis 193–194, 196

immersion: defined 138; virtual reality 138
immersive virtual natural environments 129, 135–137
immersive virtual nature (IVN) 128–130, 129, 135–137; duration of exposure 140; effective experiences in virtual reality 138–139; enhancing indoor or green exercise behavior 133–135; future research on virtual green exercise 140–141; interventions for research and health promotion 135–141; and physical activity 137–138; technological nature 128–129; technology 140–141; and virtual reality 128–129
indoor or green exercise behavior: IVN enhancing 133–135
integrated conceptual green exercise models: brief history of green exercise research 95–96; conceptual models 102–103; developing 95–109; etiology 100–101; future directions 108–109; green exercise models 103–107; harnessing the models 107–108; nature and health models 96–100; overview 95
International Diabetes Federation 23
in vivo nature exposure, as psychological intervention 160–172

knowledge: declarative 48; scientific 128; sensory 216; of specific bird calls 117; translation of 253

lived body 85, 89–90
lived experience 84–85; of the natural world 85
lived other 85, 86–89
lived space 85, 90
lived time 85, 86, 91

mechanisms and green exercise 38–39
Merkevych et al.'s model *101*
Mission Himalaya 2018 240–241

mood disorders: and natural environment 14, 16; studies in populations with 14–16

natural environments: benefits on physiology 8–11; benefits on self-reported affect 8–11; and mood disorders 14–16
nature: and adventure 149–150; affective benefits of 7–17; and green exercise 35–42; and health 1–3; and humans 112; interventions and wellbeing 160–172; mood effects, theories for 11–14; and *parkrun* 214–218; *parkrun* as opportunity for physical activity in 209–211; phenomenology and human wellbeing in 83–93; and physical activity 1–3, 112; rich landscape of affordances in 116–117
nature and health models 96–100
nature-assisted therapies (NAT) 15
nature-based activities 3
nature-based APA: building brain resilience 70; building resilient, healthy, and happy youngsters 68–69; building resilient brains 75–76; promoting strength-based functioning in students 69, 71–73
nature-based therapeutic environments 255
nature intervention studies: Ballew & Omoto 167; current review of 161–169; Fuegen & Breitenbecher 167–168; Hamann & Ivtzan 167; Mayer et al. 161; Nisbet et al. 168; Nisbet & Zelenski 162–163; Passmore 168–169; Passmore et al. 168; Passmore & Holder 167; Passmore & Howell 163–167; review of 161–169; Ryan et al. 162
nature relatedness 152
Netherlands 3, 178, 179, *180, 181,* 251
NHS Mental Health Services 238
The Northern Care Coordination Partnership (NCCP) 238
Norway 130, 178, *181,* 223, 225, 251

Oculus 127
open skills 49
Outdoor and Adventurous Activities (OAA): Battle Back Centre Research 241–242; Canada 233–237;

Expedition Research and Mission Himalaya 2018 240–241; initiatives improving well-being of military personnel 233–239; research findings from Battle Back Recovery Courses 242–244; review of evidence of, for serving and ex-military personnel 239–240; supporting WIS-MP 233–244; UK 237–239; US 233–237
Outdoor Orientation Programmes (OOPs) 68
Outpost Charity 238

parkrun: and access to affective "green space" 215–216; affective and sensory experience 216–217; fostering affective communities 217–218; implications and conclusion 218–220; and nature 214–218; as opportunity for physical activity in nature 209–211; overview 208–209; research on 211–214
pathways to health and wellbeing 130–131
people with dementia 177–185
people with mental health problems 177, 182–183, 185–186
Perceived Competencies Scale (PCS) 72, *73*
perceptual fluency account (PFA) 12
perceptual-motor calibration 52
PERMA model 36–37
phenomenology 83–93, 84–85; corporeality or lived body 89–90; defined 83; eco-phenomenology, and lived experience 84–85; humans and rest-of-nature 83; integration and conclusions 90–93; in anthropocentric form 84; lived experience of the natural world 85; lived other 86–89; lived space 90; lived time 86
physical activity: and adventure 149–150; benefits of 130–135; and humans 112; and IVN 137–138; and nature 112; and type 2 diabetes 24–25; and virtual nature 127–142
physical activity in nature: affordances 113–116; contextualizing *parkrun* as opportunity for 209–211; ecological dynamics perspective 112–122; environmental constraints 118–119; humans, nature and physical activity 112; individual constraint 118;

interactive constraints 117–120; rich landscape of affordances in nature 116–117; suggestions for future research 120–122; task constraints 119–120
physiological benefits of virtual green exercise 132–133
pilot study 223–230
polyvagal theory (PVT) 196, 201
populations with mood disorders 14–16
Positive and Negative Affect Schedule (PANAS) 8, 10, 15, 161, 163, 167–169
Post-Traumatic Stress Disorder (PTSD) 3, 14–16, 191, 234, 239
Practice Guidelines for Treatment of Complex Trauma and Trauma Informed Care and Service Delivery 191
presence and virtual reality 138–139
Profile of Mood States (POMS) 8
Prospect-Refuge Theory 12, 13
pseudo-resilience 66
psychological benefits of virtual green exercise 131–132
psychological intervention: eudaimonic wellbeing 160–161; hedonic wellbeing 160–161; nature intervention studies 161–169; positive 160–172; *in vivo* nature exposure as 160–172
psychological resilience 64, 66; and APA programming in students 69–70
psychological wellbeing: in adventure 149–150; benefits of adventure 148–149
psychological wellbeing frameworks: adventure 150–154; for adventure recreation 147–155; basic psychological needs 150–154; for education 147–155; eudaimonia 150–154; hedonia 150–154; psychological wellbeing benefits of adventure 148–149; for tourism 147–155
psycho-physio-social benefits of virtual green exercise 131–133

relatedness, defined 75, 152
relational resilience 66
research: design IVN interventions for 135–141; on *parkrun* 211–214
resilience: APA intervention for young people 73–75; APA promoting

264   *Index*

strength-based functioning in students 71–73; characteristics of students' 70–71; concepts 66–67; nature-based APA building resilient, healthy, and happy youngsters 68–69; nature-based APA building resilient brains 75–76; origins 66–67; overview 63; positive youth development 67–68; psychological resilience in studentss 69–70; question of healthy adaptability 64–66; research endeavours 69–70; understanding 66–67

The Royal British Legion (TRBL) 238

Royal Yachting Association 238

Self-Determination Theory (SDT) 74–75, 152, 242

self-reported affect and physiology 8–11

Silkin, Lewis 237

situational taxonomy: for designing gait interventions 47–57; for evaluating gait interventions 47–57; guiding green exercise research and practice 50–52

Situational Taxonomy for Environment-Person Pairing In Natural Gait (STEPPING) 52–54, *54*

social return on investments, and epidemiology 253–254

solastalgia 89

"squirrel self" 87

Stress Reduction Theory (SRT) 3, 12–13, 95, 215–216

Stress-Refresh Scale 8

students: APA interactions promoting strength-based functioning in 69, 71–73; APA programming in 69–70; education outside classroom 223–230; psychological resilience in 69–70

students' resilience: characteristics of 70–71; as complex and unpredictable concept 70; descriptive characteristics 69; distinctive, amenable to change 70–71; inclusive 71; psychologically vulnerable, poor university readiness 70; and support for academic achievement 71

Subjective Vitality Scale 8

"Symbiocene" 35

Team Red, White and Blue (TRWB) 235

technological nature: and immersive virtual nature 128–129; and virtual reality 128–129

technology 253; defined 128; facial recognition 128; immersive-virtual environment 140–141; nonimmersive 131; use of 253; virtual nature 127; virtual reality 121, 127–129, 133–135

theories for nature's mood effects 11–14

tourism: adventure 147; and psychological wellbeing frameworks 147–155

treatment of complex trauma 193–194; integration phase 200–201; processing phase 197–200; safety/stabilization phase 195–197

treatments of type 2 diabetes 23–24

type 2 diabetes: comorbidities 23–24; green exercise for 27–29; green exercise, exercise adherence, and vitamin D for 26–27; green exercise and comorbidities of 27; green exercise as treatment strategy for 23–29; and physical activity 24–25; and risk factors 23–24; and treatments 23–24

United Kingdom (UK): NHS Mental Health Services 238; OAA 237–239; "Prevention Pays" policy 255; 25 Year Environment Plan 249

United Nations sustainability development Goals (goal 11) 250

United Nations sustainable development goals 2

United Nations Sustainable Development Goals (goal 3) 249, 251

United States (US): OAA 233–237; therapeutic recreation specialists in 234; wilderness therapy for youth at risk in 3

urban green infrastructure (UGI) 14

U.S. Forest Service 17

veterans: Canadian 234; OAA supporting 233–244

Veterans Affairs Health Care System 234

Veterans in Community 238

virtual green exercise 129–130; acute impacts on exercise behavior

133–134; duration of IVN exposure 140; future research on 140–141; green exercise concept 130–135; health and behavioral benefits of 127–142; immersive virtual nature 128–130; IVN interventions for research and health promotion 135–141; long-term impacts on exercise behavior 134–135; overview 127–128; physiological benefits 132–133; possible confounders 141; psychological benefits 131–132; psycho-physio-social benefits of 131–133; type of IVN technology 140–141

virtual nature and physical activity 127–142

virtual reality (VR) 127; cyber sickness 139; defined 128; immersion 138; and immersive virtual nature 128–129; issues for effective experiences in 138–139; presence 138–139; Sherman and Craig on 128–129

"voluntary attention" 38

"VR goggles" 129

"VR masks" 129

Walking With The Wounded 238

Warrior Hike Program (WHP) 234

The Warrior Programme 238

well-being: discussion 169–171; evidence for impact of care farms on 184–186; future research 171–172; hedonic and eudaimonic aspects of 160–161; impact of nature interventions on 160–172; nature intervention studies 161–169; RCTs of *in vivo* nature interventions **164–166**; two intertwining pathways to 130–131

Western empiricism 90

wilderness therapy: contextualizing complex-trauma 192–193; overview 191–192; phased treatment of complex trauma in 194–201; treatment of complex trauma 193–194

World Health Organization 23; *Health for the World's Adolescents* report 64

wounded, injured and sick military personnel (WIS-MP): adaptive well-being capacities of 233; inservice UK 242; OAA supporting 233–244

young people: APA as resiliencebuilding intervention for 70, 73–75; with behavioral and social problems 186; nature-based APA building resilient 68–69

Zuckerman Inventory of Personal Reactions (ZIPERS) 8

Printed and bound by CPI Group (UK) Ltd, Croydon, CR0 4YY
01/12/2024
01797780-0015